Love Entwined

Love Entwined

The Curious History of Hairwork in America

Helen Sheumaker

PENN

University of Pennsylvania Press
Philadelphia

Published by
University of Pennsylvania Press
Philadelphia, Pennsylvania 19104-4112

Printed in the United States of America on acid-free paper

10 9 8 7 6 5 4 3 2 1

A cataloging-in-publication record is available from the Library of Congress

ISBN-13: 978-0-8122-4014-6
ISBN-10: 0-8122-4014-6

Contents

Prologue

When I was sixteen I drove the family car to the Crossroads Mall in Omaha, Nebraska, to visit the antiques show being held there. I bought several old postcards, because they were cheap. I happily rifled through boxes of odds and ends, and remember bringing home an ornate brass doorknob, which at the time must have seemed a practical purchase for a teenager living in her parents' 1960s split-level ranch house. I also went through a shoe box of small, tattered objects at one stand. I came upon a button—a lightweight metal button fronted with some sort of woven brownish fabric. I held it carefully, trying to look experienced at evaluating antiques. "Is this hair?" I asked the vendor. "Nah," he muttered, "It's just dirty." I bought the button for twenty-five cents. At home I determined that it must be hair. I shivered with adolescent morbidity, voyeuristic and yet empathetic. Someone's hair had been woven and placed in this button frame; it must have been a woman; it must have adorned a dress; it must have been cut off the dress—when she died? When the dress was too frayed to wear? And then she died, and someone saved it; then they died, and someone who didn't know its story tossed it into the box of odds and ends. I shivered again, put the button in a small box, and forgot about it for years.

Revulsion, squeamishness, curiosity, and sometimes, a sentimental cooing: these have been the principal responses to hairwork that I have encountered in the years I have researched its history. Our own reactions raise the question: What has changed about American society that what was once acceptable is now unnerving and discomfiting?[1] The answer to this question resides in the complex history of consumerism and its aspects.

This book's title, *Love Entwined*, comes from a young woman's entry in her friend's album. When she attached a loop of her own hair to the page, Elisabeth Shrontz wrote to her friend Emma Miller,

Dear friend accept these lines
E'e[r] traced in friendship's hand

A token that love entwines,
Bound hearts with the mystic band.[2]

For eighteenth- and nineteenth-century white, usually middle-class Americans, hairwork was figuratively love entwined. What has been lost since then is the understanding that was self-evident to many Americans at the time: being made of human hair, hairwork was the person whose hair was used; it embodied the sincerity of those individuals; it demonstrated the emotions shared by the people involved. Hairwork existed in the contexts of changing ideals of gender, class identity, and the growing presence of the consumer market. But it also quietly asserts to us today that emotions played a role as well.

Changes in American culture since the nineteenth century have directly affected our views of decorative hairwork. Twentieth-century American ideas of cleanliness in particular contributed to its decline. Just the idea of working with hair seems unclean to many people today—if not because of religious prohibitions then because of sanitary standards. But wigs and hair pieces have remained popular in the United States throughout its history, and the most prized material for these accessories is today, as in the past, human hair. Nevertheless, germ theories, first introduced in the 1870s, and ideas about "dirty" bodily functions, have dominated American attitudes toward human bodily products. According to these arguments, human hair was one of many unclean materials that should be contained and disposed of, not made into decorative objects to be worn on one's person or displayed in the home.[3]

In addition, new fashions changed how most Americans dressed their bodies and furnished their residences. By the early twentieth century, clothing styles became looser and fabrics were lighter in color and weight, particularly for women. Hair jewelry had usually been dark, fussy, and ornamented, and it no longer appealed to consumers who embraced pastel colors, viscose fabrics, sheer blouses, and the uniform suit of men. Hair wreaths looked wonderful against the dark, richly patterned wall coverings of the nineteenth century, but the cleaner lines, lighter-colored walls, and less ornamented twentieth-century interiors made hair wreaths look awkward and weighty in contrast.

Above all, sentiments changed. Sentiment, or, in the broader sense, sentimentality, made hairwork alive to its audience in the eighteenth and nineteenth centuries. Today, we use sentiment to denote an intellectual position (such as being asked, "What are your sentiments on this?") or a narrative of emotional experience (such as selecting a greeting card which expresses the proper "sentiment"). For nineteenth-century middle-class Americans, sentimentality was a cultural perspective from which political and personal issues were framed. As cultural historians have demonstrated, debates over slavery, women's economic roles, and the rise of consumerism can be understood as outgrowths of, and contributors to, the sentimental understanding which permeated nineteenth-century white middle-class life.[4]

Sentimentality developed from the mindset of sensibility which dominated European and colonial American eighteenth-century thought. While today the terms are often conflated, "sensibility" and "sentimentality" once denoted quite different states of response. Sensibility was, in eighteenth- and nineteenth-century America, the ability to respond immediately and emotionally to an event, a thought, or a circumstance. Sentimentality, on the other hand, denoted a reliving of the emotional experience. In Jane Austen's *Sense and Sensibility* (1811), the younger sister, Marianne, is literally carried away by her emotion or sensibility. In this Romantic belief in emotional resonance, one's behavior directly mirrored one's emotional state. Of course, like all social stances, sensibility was a creation—a social way of acting that was adopted by individuals. Sensibility metamorphosed into sentimentality by the nineteenth century, and as we shall see, sentimentality was what gave hairwork its significance. While sensibility was embodied in an immediate reaction, sentimentality required a review of the past and then a narration of that experience. Swooning while hearing bad news was to be "sensible," that is, overwhelmed by one's senses; weeping while telling the story about hearing the bad news to others (for the fifteenth time) was to be sentimental.[5]

In both the eighteenth and nineteenth centuries, hairwork, being made of an individual's hair, was seen as an outward expression of that person's inner sentiments. Material objects such as hairwork were sentimental because they physically represented a past emotional state and they provoked the necessary reflection upon that experience. For example, the immediate grief a young husband felt upon the death of his wife was immaterial in that no matter how much psychic pain he had experienced, it wasn't "real" physical trauma. But his watch chain made of her hair upon her death physically manifested that grief and provided a constant reminder of the validity of the experience. The watch chain told the story of his grief to an audience of himself and anyone who observed his garb. Today, such display would appear mawkish; in the nineteenth century, open demonstration of sentimental grief was appropriate and validated a person's membership in the middle class.

Hairwork and its meanings reflected another transformation in American society in the 1800s. During the nineteenth century, white Americans were experiencing extraordinary economic change. Consumerism—the cultural rites of identifying the self through participation in the market of produced goods—took hold. Middle-class women were expected to stay at home, supposedly insulated from the vagaries of economic life, while men shouldered the financial responsibilities of the ever more demanding world of work. Of course, real lives of men and women differed tremendously from this scenario, but it remained an ideal.

The popularity of hairwork, which was at its peak from the 1850s to 1880s, was affected not by new technology (such as photography) or national traumas (the Civil War) but by issues of labor and production. When photography became increasingly available to everyday people by the 1860s, hairwork was not affected in the least. Hairwork, while it was created long before photographic images were possible, did not serve as a substitute for images but a complement to them. The Civil War, with its extraordinary cost in human life and the disruption for those who survived, did not lead to an intensification of the popularity of hairwork.

What the Civil War and its emotional toll, and the invention of mechanized portrait making, did do was make the question of how hairwork was created all the more important. Hairwork was supposed to be handmade, relatively inexpensive, and sentimental. If the manufacture of hairwork was depersonalized or mechanized, the meaning of hairwork was affected and it no longer served a purpose for middle-class Americans. In addition, hairwork was sentimental and its popularity stemmed from the validity of sentimentality itself. As middle-class Americans began to reject sentimental expressions as outmoded and hypocritical, which they did at the end of the nineteenth century, hairwork itself would become an anachronistic holdover. As Amelia Gere Mason wrote in 1901, sarcastically commenting on the newly unemotional approach, "there is no sentiment in business, and business is a controlling factor in the world today. In nothing does sentiment contribute to visible success."[6]

The late 1800s ushered in a new age in which middle-class culture valued "realism." While no more authentic than sensibility or sentimentality, and no more or less false than any other cultural expression, twentieth-century "realism" argued that open displays of emotion were shallow, hypocritical, and silly. In Henry James's *Washington Square* (1881), Mrs. Penniman's maudlin foolishness, and Catherine Sloper's lonely fate, presaged the decline of sentimental expression in the twentieth century.[7] James was not only ridiculing superficial people like Mrs. Penniman, but also warning the Catherine Slopers of the world to beware such overtly emotional fare. Hairwork was an obviously sentimental object. Once valued for its ability to provide evidence of one's sincerity, now hairwork represented a lack of honesty and integrity. It looked insincere.

Hairwork was also a product offered through the consumer market. The consumer market did not permeate the lives of nineteenth-century Americans as it does today, and there were large groups of people completely ignored by producers and sellers of market goods. Little attention was paid to African Americans, for example. But most Americans were facing a market that attempted to exert some degree of control in their personal lives. In this book, I argue that hairwork was one method of negotiating the demands of the market while asserting the primacy of the self. Hairwork was a fashionable market item and reflected styles that were socially acceptable at the time. But hairwork was made of a specific individual's hair. It was not only made of a person, it represented a person's emotions and sentiment. It was a unique kind of consumer product.

Historians have explored the relationships between sentimentality and consumerism. Sentimentality provided a way to consume goods in a way that expressed "one's 'higher' faculties and sentiments."[8] The nineteenth century was dominated by a "moral market culture," a consumer world driven by profits but which argued that sentimentality and religiosity could inhibit the naked greed otherwise rampant.[9] When one consumed in a proper sentimental fashion (whether the product purchased was sentimental, or the act of consumption was imbued with sentimentality), one demonstrated one's successful integration of the emotional attitude of sentiment through the action of selecting and purchasing a good on the market.

Hairwork was sentimental material culture which bound sentimental transcendence to the consuming body, thus inextricably linking the consuming individual to those characteristics so sought after. Not all hairwork was purchased "from the market," that is, created by professional hair workers. Amateur hair workers, women and only sometimes men, created their own hairwork. Through their fancywork, "women helped negotiate a new relationship with objects—one which blurred the boundaries between objects and the self."[10] Making one's own fancywork, including hairwork, formulated a relationship between the self and the market in which sentiment—an emotional stance considered innate and unaffected by market pressures (even while it was itself constructed through the market)—and one's own handwork created value and a product. This "sentimental enterprise" was one in which women, and sometimes men, created careers as fancywork experts, companies trafficked in fancywork supplies and ready-made objects, and women's periodicals and books produced copious instructions for crafters to follow. Fancywork offered its participants respite from the market yet was a haven created by the market to service sentimental customers.[11]

I argue, as other historians have, that consumption and production have a fluid relationship. Hairwork challenges notions of consumption, in part because hair and sentiments have been rendered into a commodity through a person's hand labor. And there is the question of what is actually produced when hairwork was created. Hairwork was a product, but was that which derived value in large part from the meaning invested in it by consumers. Without sentiment, hairwork stood for nothing; it was disembodied from its source of significance as a market product.[12]

Thus, hairwork resisted its own commodification even as it was marketed and sold. No matter how worked the hair was, how fancifully constructed, or however stylish it was rendered, hairwork was still made of the hair of a loved one. If fancywork negotiated the boundaries between the market and the self, hairwork took the self into the heart of the market. While we today may look upon this process as symptomatic of an era confronting new relationships with market goods, for most nineteenth-century white middle-class Americans who owned hairwork, the market had nothing to do with it. The hairwork was instead indicative of the ways individuals could, in the end, never become a part of the market.

We are the inheritors of the nineteenth century. Today, many Americans give hardly a second thought to the idea that they can express their "self" through the products they buy and use. American society, especially popular culture, has been dominated for several decades by an ironic stance that questions any attempt to be "sincere." Despite this, polls show that

Americans want politicians who are sincere, relationships that are honest, and corporations that act with integrity. But the dominant presence of the market, with its hyped-up appeals and constant claims of authenticity, suggests that those qualities of honesty are scarce. If we as individuals are reflected in the market, what does this mean about our selves?

Human hair does not hold the same meaning for different groups of people, and history can also influence what hair is intended to represent. Non-Europeans did participate in the long history of ornamental hairwork in the United States; African Americans, both before and after Emancipation, created and sold hairwork for white customers. But within the African American community of the nineteenth century, hair itself meant something very different in terms of memory and family. One powerful example from the nineteenth century is of free African Americans who, in an attempt to verify that their enslaved children were still alive, sometimes requested that the child's hair be sent to them as proof.[13]

Many non-European cultures shunned, and still avoid, the decorative use of human hair that has been detached from the head and is intended for a use other than augmenting one's remaining hair.[14] Most Native American groups, most African Americans, and Asian Americans had, and have, cultural and religious prohibitions against using human hair in the memorial fashion of Euro-American ornamental hairwork.[15] Yet all cultures share a fascination with the malleability of hair and contemporary society is rife with hair references. Phrases such as "let down your hair" suggest the dualistic nature of hair; it can be styled to society's rules or it can be "let down," that is, reveal the "true" self. Some societies cover the hair, particularly that of women, to avoid provocation of male passion. Others, including African, African American, Afro-Brazilian and other African diasporic cultures celebrate hair as a canvas of inexhaustible expression.

This fascination with human hair reflects the relationship between society and the self. Hair is grown from the human body. Hair (or the absence of it) is immediately visible to others. A hairstyle is the product of the individual self, howsoever a culture may view that "self." Individuals can do what they wish to the hair on their body. They can shave it off; they can cover it up; they can braid it, coil it, frizz it, or straighten it. They can dye it, cut it, cut shapes into it, or reveal the scalp in particular ways. Society also exerts pressure to imitate certain hairstyles or types. At times this pressure to conform can be politicized, even cruel.[16] In the 1950s, Malcolm X conked, or straightened, his hair until he realized that this struggle was misplaced. He was trying to be like whites, to imitate the very people that were oppressing him. And, as he states in his autobiography, upon that realization he let his hair go natural.[17]

Hair, then, reflects the position of the self in society. It is of the self, but can be modified to suit or to contradict society's dictums. The hairwork discussed in this book bears little relation to Malcolm X's struggle. Nineteenth-century hairwork was, though, a signal of acceptance in white middle-class culture. There were other markers of middle-class status, from income to education to dress to beliefs. But the sentimentality that hairwork visually and materially represented was a hallmark of being middle-class throughout the nineteenth century.

Hairwork asserted the importance of the individual in a physical and an emotional way. And it worked. Today, when we encounter hairwork in the odd bit of jewelry on display at a museum, or in a novel, or in a hair wreath at the local historical house, or in the loose bit of hair in an old letter, we confront a relic of the living, breathing reality of someone long deceased. Because these scraps of hair were saved to remember someone, we behold that person's self through a fragment of the body.

In the course of researching this book, I have looked upon countless pieces of hairwork, from the tiniest and most finely wrought hair feathers under glass, to hair blended with paints so that one can hardly tell human hair is part of the material, to enormous wreaths of bulbous flowers and leaves made of hair and rusting wire. As a woman born in the 1960s in an era and in a culture that frowned upon anything more sentimental than affixing a lock from baby's first haircut in a mass-produced baby book, I was in part discomfited by the texture of hairwork and its overweening (at least to me) sentimentality. And yet, . . . I was confronted over and over, with each different example of hairwork, with the tangible individuality of each worked piece. When you hold a brooch made of hair, you hold in your hand a memento of an individual, her life, and her emotions. There is no "code" to be broken in this regard: the hair came from a person's body, and the jewelry was made to represent someone's connection with that person. To add to the complexity of the object, the emotional connections and issues of self-identity were always filtered through the market. I was fascinated throughout the project by the intersection of emotion and economics each piece of hairwork represented.

The gift from the past—like the button I found in the Omaha antiques stall—asserts that, in the end, individual lives and selves are what matters and what persists through time. For this, I thank all those people of the past who saved those bits of hair, and those who treasured these memorials through the years.

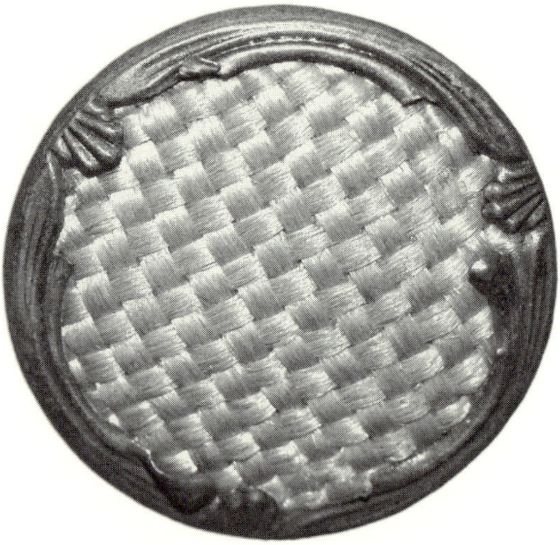

Figure 1. The material in the center of this metal button is woven hair. Hair workers used manufactured button frames, but the center was made "to order." The "fabric" that resulted complemented the colors and weight of fabrics popular for women's dresses in the 1870s and 1880s. The sentimental associations of the hair within the button provided its true value. Author's collection.

Chapter 1
That Curious Art

The practice of hairwork was a cultural import to the New World. European colonists in North America brought a tradition of making decorative objects made of human hair with them, but, more important, they carried a cultural outlook that legitimated sincere, emotional expression through material goods. Hairwork was always created by hand, whether those hands were professional artisans or skilled amateurs. As the nature of artisanship changed from an older apprentice-and-master relationship to that of independent entrepreneur, those who made hairwork changed, as well.

Eighteenth-century Americans who owned hairwork shared several things in common. First, they were white, free people. Africans brought to the colonies as slaves had neither the resources nor the cultural inclination to own worked human hair, while white lower-class people, including indentured servants, did not have the money for such a purchase. Second, owners of hairwork were people of wealth (even if of quite moderate means) who could afford to pay an artisan to craft such a good. Third, because hairwork was intended to represent a sincerity of self, those who possessed such goods placed a high priority on this idea. This was an ideal of personhood: one should be an individual of deeply felt, *sincere* emotions. One never flagrantly demonstrated these feelings; nevertheless, the heart of such a person was revealed through that person's taste in art, fiction, and possessions such as miniature portraits backed with hair. The desire to express sincerity led individuals to own objects that expressed sentiment. To our (twenty-first-century) eyes, these tokens of the heart appear overwrought, quaint, and even precious. But to their eighteenth-century owners, these miniatures with elaborately worked human hair were refined statements of the self.

Who Made Hairwork

In the eighteenth century, more hairwork was created by professionals than by amateurs.[1] Few examples of amateur hairwork from the eighteenth century have survived, and most artifacts in museum and private collections are of hair jewelry, which was professionally made. Instead, most amateur-made hairwork was hair embroidery, that is, needlework that used human hair as the thread or floss for stitching elaborate designs. These sentimental and commemorative pieces usually combined two individuals' hair and memorialized an event such as a death. One example, a pincushion made of silk, has a design chain-stitched on its front in two colors of human hair. Hair embroidery often depicted these popular mourning scenes of the day, such as a Grecian-robed woman standing next to an urn-topped cenotaph, with cherubs hovering above her.[2]

Hair embroidery examples are the only "amateur" hairwork evident in collections today.[3] Far more common was hairwork professionally created by artisans: certain jewelers, silversmiths, or goldsmiths as well as miniature artists also offered hairwork. One reason for the lack of amateur creations may be that the popular styles of hairwork were too difficult for an amateur to execute well. Unworked and unadorned hair was often included in a locket, and for this no expertise was required. But other kinds of popular hairwork, including elaborately worked hair placed on the back of miniatures, put into brooches, or slid under glass in a ring, required the experienced and patient hand of a hair worker. Most of these pieces required special tools and techniques of the artisan. It was not until the nineteenth century that styles of hairwork encouraged amateur productions.

Hairwork, and the miniatures it backed, was widely advertised in the 1770s through the 1800s. The development of advertising for personal consumer goods marked not only a change in how goods were exchanged but also what goods could mean. Late eighteenth-century American advertisements reveal that shops began to be used for the creation of new identities as well as for simply restocking households with material goods.[4] Miniature-portrait artists and hair workers were not immune to these changes. Most hair workers saw themselves as workers in a craft that was sometimes understood to be an "art" but not to be of artistic stature. Thus, the small businessmen and businesswomen offering hairwork presented their craft as a combination of business and art, as befitted an occupation understood as an artisanal trade.[5] In 1782, Hamilton Stevenson announced that "he will follow his business of Painting in Miniature, and executing designs in Hair." In 1785, James Askew expressed gratitude for "the great encouragement he had been favoured with in his business in general, particularly in his much improved art of railed Hair work." Customers were often referred to in genteel terms, so Francis Rabineau's clientele were "encouragers of this elegant art"; but even he did not overlook the business side. While Rabineau characterized his past sales as "the many favors he has received from the Ladies and Gentlemen" of the community, he also assured his customers that "he continues to execute all kinds of Drawings . . . [and] Hairwork for Lockets, Rings and Bracelets, in natural or dissolved hair . . . in the neatest manner."[6]

Some hair workers were primarily jewelers, and hair ornaments were a minor part of a varied inventory of stock. In a typical advertisement, the jeweler listed his entire inventory, and hairwork appeared among a multitude of other items. Jeremiah Andrews, a jeweler in Baltimore, "informs the Public, that he has a neat assortment of Jewellery, of his own manufacture, equal to any imported. Ladies paste shoe buckles, garnet hoop rings, with every other kind of rings, lockets, and broaches, plain or with stone, hair work'd, in the neatest manner, mourning rings, made on the shortest notice, with every other kind of Jewellery, by their humble servant."[7] Jewelers such as Andrews were small shopkeepers who offered hairwork as part of a varied line of purchased and self-produced wares. Other hair workers concentrated on hairwork alone. M. Sauvage advertised her craft in 1799: "Those Persons who are desirous of having Hair Work plaited for Rings, Bracelets, Lockets, will please apply to M. Sauvage, at the house she resides in, in Meeting street, between George and Boundary Street."[8]

Working from lodgings was a common practice for many jewelers, goldsmiths and silversmiths, miniature-portrait artists, and hair workers. Some hair workers simply conducted business from their residence, but other hair workers and miniature-portrait artists were itinerant workers who traveled from city to city. In 1796, Edward Malbone announced to the city of Boston that "Edward G. Malbone, from Newport, takes this method to inform the Public, that he intends to practice the above art [of miniature painting and hairwork] during his stay in this town. As he has hitherto been uniformly successful in his Likenesses, he flatters himself he shall be able to give satisfaction to his employers."[9] Five years later, much of Malbone's business was still conducted by traveling a circuit between Providence, Newport, Boston, New York, Philadelphia, Charleston, and Savannah.[10] Hamilton Stevenson outlined his own travels in his advertisement that informed the public that "having returned to this place, and intending to remain some time in it, [he] begs leave to acquaint the publick, that during his stay," he will be available for employment.[11]

The stock required of a hair worker and miniaturist was minimal. Paints, brushes, and prepared ivory or glass discs were the necessary tools, and, once he or she took up temporary residence, an advertisement was published to attract customers. Many hairworkers provided examples of their expertise, such as those seen in one tray of a sample case (Figure 2). Jewelers, however, often established shops.[12] William Coleman, a goldsmith and jeweler in Baltimore, had a shop at Fell's Point, "adjoining Mr. Lindsay's Exchange Coffee House." Coleman explained in his advertisement that "he plats hair and forms it into cyphers, sprigs, figures, or any other devise for rings, lockets, &c. patterns of which may be seen at his shop." In 1784, the jewelers Cooke and Company boasted of their "new wholesale and retail manufactory and commission store" in Baltimore. Ten years later, Daniel Carrell likewise characterized his place of business as a "manufactory and sale shop," where he offered "a number of articles [that] are of his own manufactory." In 1800, John B. Dumoutet referred to his own shop as a "Hair-work & Jewellery Manufactory."[13]

Whether one was a jeweler, miniature-portrait artist, or hair worker was determined by the breadth of one's training, abilities, inclinations, and monetary resources. Most hair workers were also miniaturists and could provide a complete "token of self" in the form of a miniature portrait or mourning scene that was mounted in a gold frame with elaborately worked hair on the back. Jewelers commonly offered hairwork and the mounting of the miniature as a service alongside a variety of other personal adornments.

It is difficult to know how much hairwork usually cost. While it was advertised relatively widely from the 1770s to 1800, prices are rarely given in the advertisements. Instead, vague phrases alluded to the cost. In 1784, John Walters boasted of the quality of his work, "joined to his (really) moderate charges." M. Sauvage likewise assured her customers of "the moderate prices she asks for her work." In 1795, Joseph Cooke reassuringly guaranteed the "most equitable terms."[14]

It can be estimated, however, that most complete miniatures, which included the sitting for the portrait, the completed portrait on an ivory or glass disk, the hairwork plaiting for the back of the miniature, the glass overlay for the front and back, and the gold finished frame, cost around twenty-five dollars. (Again, most hair workers were also trained in jewelry work, and probably offered the complete package.) In 1800, Raphaelle Peale notified the Philadelphia community that he offered "Likenesses, For a short time, Fashionably set in Gold, with platts and cyphers complete, for twenty-five dollars; the miniature alone, ten dollars."[15] The "likeness" was, of course, the miniature. "Platts" were the plaited hair on the back, and probably refers to the basket-weave pattern and not the also common

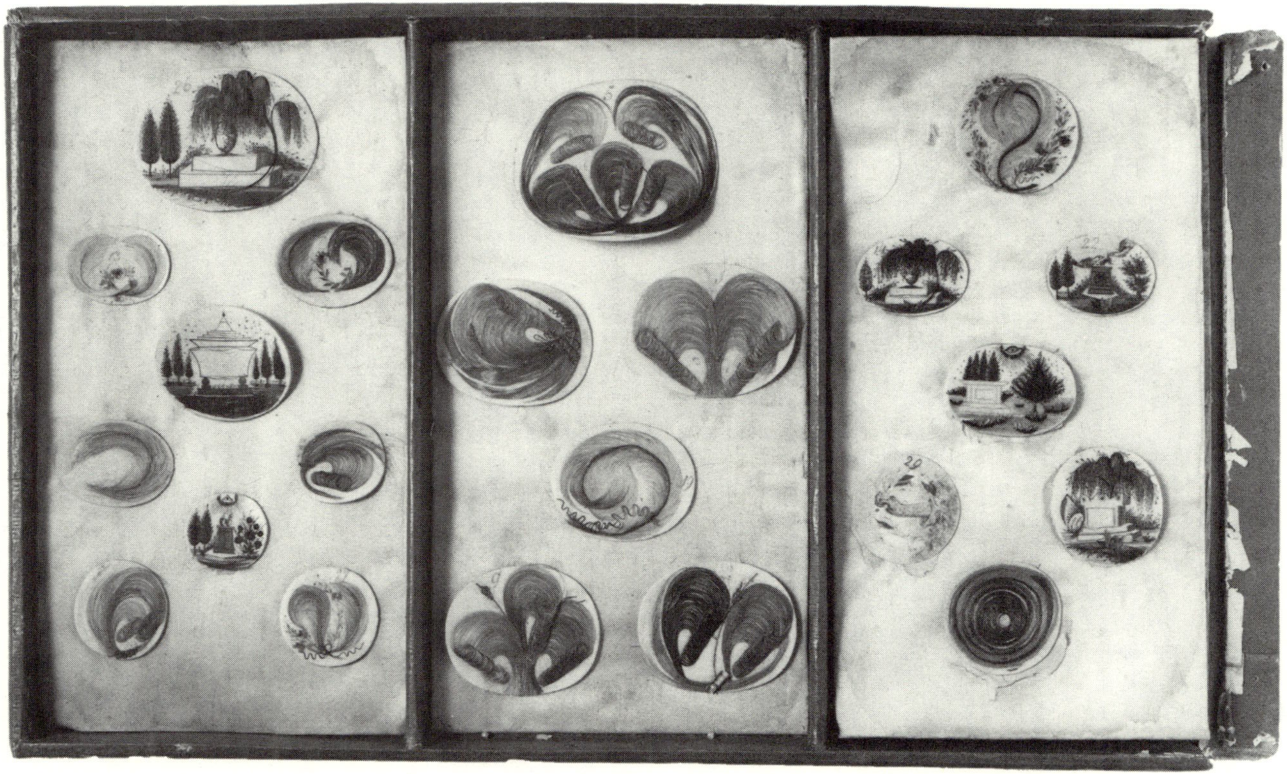

Figure 2. This tray of hairwork samples is one of five trays that fitted into a wooden box. A hair worker, jeweler, or, more likely, a miniature portraitist, would have used the box to advertise his or her expertise. The medallions are examples of palette work, with the hair glued flat onto the discs of ivory. In the case of the mourning images, the hair is chopped finely and affixed as a kind of "paint." Courtesy Winterthur Museum and Country Estate.

feather style. "Cyphers" refers to the fine gold work adorning the worked hair.

Another successful miniature-portrait artist and hair worker, Edward Malbone, charged prices similar to Peale's. Traveling his traditional circuit, Malbone recorded in 1801 that he received fifty dollars for two "miniature sittings," and twenty-two-fifty for "one sitting." These may have been for the miniature portraits alone, for which the customer had a "sitting." Malbone received sixteen dollars for "two framings," and seventeen dollars for "a miniature setting," both of which probably included the hairwork as well as the gold frame.[16] Peale's and Malbone's price structures suggest that at the end of the eighteenth century, even when hairwork was an integral part of the miniature it was not a costly addition to the piece. Most miniature-portrait artists were also hair artists, and apparently saw no need to provide pricing for the hairwork alone. A craftswoman like M. Sauvage, who advertised only her skills as a hair worker, would have struggled with a far lower income than would a prominent portraitist such as Peale or Malbone.

Although hairwork was subordinate to the portrait, it was nonetheless integral to the piece. Most miniatures were sold with worked hair on the back. There were other kinds of hairwork available to customers. For example, Daniel Carrell advertised in 1794 that he could offer "a great assortment of lockets, miniature frames and rings, devices and hair put in them at the shortest notice and most reasonable terms."[17]

Carrell's term "devices" was a general term to denote the worked quality of the hair, that is, that the hair had been worked into some kind of design, and was mounted into a piece of jewelry. For example, in 1787, Peter Leret offered "Mourning Rings and Lockets engraved and enammelled in the neatest manner, at the shortest notice. Likewise hair worked in any device, and set in gold on the most reasonable terms. Also, Miniature pictures elegantly set."[18] Samuel Folwell offered "Mourning Lockets, Bracelets, Breast-Pins, Rings, &c. furnished with Devices in Hair, or Likenesses in Miniature, at a short notice," and elsewhere spoke of his talents at "that curious Art of working Devices in human Hair." "Devices" evoked the artisanal nature of hairwork, and perhaps as important, the assurance that hairwork would be done to the customer's satisfaction. Thus, the jewelers Cooke and Company promised "hair worked in any devise to the greatest perfection."[19]

Hairwork was a "fancy device." It was an object of fashion as well as a product of an artisan's craft.[20] In 1762, the jewelers Rivington & Brown prescribed "Lockets set in gold to preserve Lover's hair." In 1772, Philip

Tidyman reminded Charlestonians that he "continues . . . [to] plait and make Hair in all Fancies." John Miot also offered "hair worked in all Fancies," while a year later G. Smithson elaborated on the forms of those fancies, for he "works Hair in Platts, or other curious Forms, such as Landscapes, Flowers, Figures of all kinds, Mottos, Posies, or emblematical Devices, without any Assistance from Coulers." Fancy and fashion could inflect even mourning, as when James Askew offered "Mourning Rings, Lockets, &c. made and worked . . . in any device that fancy can suggest, in the most modern taste with dispatch" (Figure 3).[21]

Because hairwork was a commodity of fashion as well as of craftsmanship, artisans employed an elaborate protocol in their advertisements. Customers were, as Hamilton Stevenson characterized his clientele, "Such Ladies and Gentlemen as may wish to employ him," while Francis Rabineau "Respectfully acknowledges the many favors he has received from the Ladies and Gentlemen" who patronized him. Desaignes expressed gratitude for "those who will honor him with their custom," while Josiah Flagg appreciated those who "may please to honour him with their commands," and Joseph Cooke's potential customers were those "who chuse to embrace the opportunity" to have their likenesses taken. Others were more blunt in their acknowledgment that they were seeking employment. M. Sauvage thanked in advance those who "may please to employ her," and John Walters was pleased to note "the attention the subscriber has always paid to his employers."[22]

While such language had been used in previous decades, by the 1790s these flattering encomiums were common in advertisements for hairwork. As shopping itself began to represent the shopper's identity, shopkeepers and artisans became more adept at obscuring the base, monetary relationships they held toward the customer. Hairwork, as a personal commodity, was especially likely to be advertised in intimate terms. Brooks and Warrock were particularly effusive and wrote that being "impressed with a grateful sense of the encouragement they have experienced since their commencement on business; [they] desire to return their sincerest thanks to their numerous friends and customers, and hope their future exertions to please will shew their gratitude for past favors. From the decided preference and flattering approbation their work has everywhere met with, they feel a confidence that their labours in future will have the same success."[23] Brooks and Warrock presented a curious if effective blend of a recognition that their craft was a form of work and yet encompassed a personal relationship. Theirs was a "business" of "the future exertions" of "their labours." At the

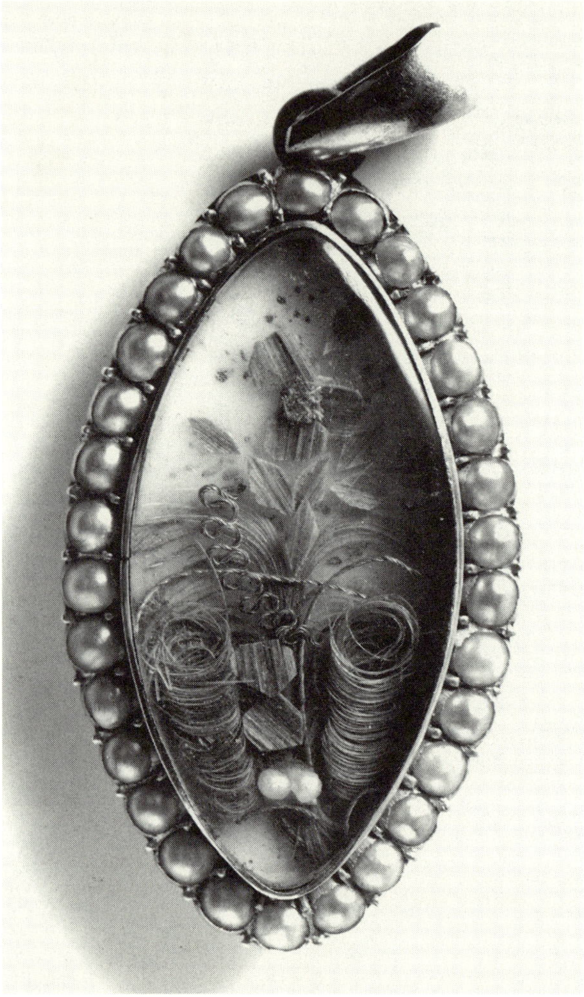

Figure 3. A good example of what "fancy can suggest, in the most modern taste": a hairwork "device" from 1800 to 1820, which is also a locket. The hair was looped, glued, cut into petal shapes, and also twined around wires. It was then fixed onto an ivory base, placed under glass, and framed in seed pearls. Courtesy Winterthur Museum and Country Estate.

same time, Brooks and Warrock framed their customer's patronage—and their goods—in terms removed from a commercial relationship.

The "Real" Hair Worker

Hairwork's appeal lay in its position as a craftsman's product and as a personal good nominally distant from the world of commodities. Yet in the

1780s, hairwork was as likely to be produced in manufactories by apprentices as by the lone artisan. Samuel Folwell, a young hair worker breaking from his apprenticeship past, used authenticity as a mark of value of his work and products. This idea of authentic production nicely dovetailed with the post-Revolutionary American emphasis on sincerity. To be sincere was to be honest and virtuous, qualities highly valued in the new republic. Hairwork of the eighteenth century, made by Folwell and others, was understood in its time to represent this honesty and the authenticity of the maker and the consumer.

In 1786, at age twenty-two, Samuel Folwell placed his first advertisement in the *Pennsylvania Packet*, a Philadelphia newspaper. He announced that he could conduct "Miniature painting, and Hair Work, Executed in the neatest Manner, and as much as possible imitating Nature." He could also provide engraving—a hint of his training as a jeweler.[24] Two years later, in 1788, Folwell still conducted business at Laetitia Court in Philadelphia, where he had been two years prior. Having been briefly absent from town, Folwell announced to Philadelphians that he "wishes those Ladies and Gentlemen to be informed, who have enquired for him during his absence, that he is now arrived in this city and ready to execute their Commands. As he is the only real Hair-Worker here, and his residence will be but six weeks, they may be disappointed without applying soon."[25] The response to his advertisement was swift, though perhaps a bit unexpected. Four days later, three jewelers, Jeremiah Boone, J. Anthony, and Joseph Cooke, in their own advertisement, "Present their compliments to the Public, and beg leave to inform them, that Mr. Folwell is not the only real Hair-Worker in this city, as the Master who taught him, and afterwards employed him at 7s.6 per day, is now here, with several others who are capital Workmen in that Branch, and far superior to Mr. Folwell."[26] There were several points of difference between these three and the upstart Folwell. At question was the central assertion of Folwell's that he was the "only real Hair Worker." Another source of the jewelers' anger, though, was that one of them, Joseph Cooke, had been Folwell's master, and had even deigned to employ his former apprentice. Finally, echoing their conservative outrage at Folwell's entrepreneurial activity, the three asserted the primacy of their workmanship.

As expected, Folwell returned with his own prompt volley. Folwell noted that the advertisement of the three jewelers was, to say the least, "injurious to my character and profession as a Hair-Worker."[27] Folwell then turned to what was the most volatile issue: the assertion of, as Folwell phrased it, "my being instructed by a master [Mr. Cooke it is supposed is meant]." Mr. Cooke's claim that Folwell's knowledge of hairwork was the result of Cooke's tutelage was, according to Folwell, pure "fable and will." Folwell continues, "Mr. Cooke understands just so much of the business of hairworker, as the ass therein represented did of the lyre."[28] Folwell explained the arrangements between himself and his former master, Cooke. Folwell had agreed to work for Mr. Cooke for—as Cooke stated in his advertisement—7s.6 per day. However, Folwell sarcastically instructed his readers to consider "how vastly profitable a business [such as Cooke's] must be, and how generous the master who, whilst he taught, would employ his pupil at that rate, in an occupation which was to be his support through life."

Joseph Cooke responded with furious condemnation. Folwell, wrote Cooke, was (among other things) "malevolent," "false," "ungracious," and "pusillanimous."[29] Folwell was the "Viper of the fable" who "excites only detestation, because it manifests the disposition without the power to injure." Folwell came to his former master, according to Cooke, "ignorant of the first and simplest principles, of the art which he alludes." It may be that Folwell now demonstrated some "ingenuity and talents," but those were the result of Cooke's careful training. And, yes, Cooke had been "willing to contribute something to his support; but it cannot be a proof of his proficiency." Folwell's "attempt to depreciate my abilities in my profession," wrote Cooke, "indirectly denies the services which I have hitherto rendered him."

Cooke and Folwell, unhappily conjoined through an apprenticeship system inherited from Europe, demonstrated the ways this tradition was changing by the late 1780s.[30] Hair workers, who were often also jewelers, silversmiths, and goldsmiths, relied on apprentices as did other artisanal craftspeople. Jewelers and hair workers sometimes advertised for apprentices. In 1794, Daniel Carrell, whose advertisement welcomed "orders from the country," also stated his need for "two or three journeyman." Claudius Chat, a silversmith, jeweller, and hair worker, stated in 1794 that "two or three apprentices of honest parents, are wanted." A year later, Chat was again advertising for a "Lad of 16 or 17 years old, of honest connexions, wanted as an apprentice."[31]

A boy apprenticed to a jeweler to learn the trade usually worked with a written contract and ideally received training from his master, as the apprentice supplied labor for him. At the end of the contract, apprentices were released. They could become journeymen—not quite a master, lacking capital resources, but free to choose their employment. Journeymen often became masters themselves, once they saved enough money to set up their own "manufactory."

Traditionally, the relationship between a master and an apprentice was one of mutual obligations and responsibilities. By the 1780s in America, however, that system was eroding. The dispute between Folwell and Cooke was rooted in shifts in the apprenticeship system that were themselves linked to changes in how goods were produced in post-Revolutionary America.

By the 1780s, some masters had begun to define their role as providing only food and shelter, and no longer seeing themselves responsible for the moral and intellectual development of their apprentices.[32] Masters evaded their traditional duties in part because in changing economic and labor conditions it no longer served them well to provide intensive, years-long training to those who would inevitably become their future competition. The end of the Revolutionary War saw a surge in demand for consumer goods, including specialty items such as jewelry.[33] The increase in demand encouraged more young men to enter the trades as apprentices. At the same time, changes in shop structures led many masters to hire only apprentices and half-trained journeymen. Apprentices and journeymen were now cheap labor rather than inheritors of a traditional artisan craft.

Masters were also changing their traditional shops into enterprises based more in retail trade than in direct production. In 1784, the jewelers Cooke and Company (the same Cooke who jousted with Folwell) boasted of their "new wholesale and retail manufactory and commission store" in Baltimore.[34] Their new business of wholesale business and retail store, combined with the more traditional direct fulfillment of customer orders, encompassed the changes experienced throughout American industry. Such businesses demanded larger reserves of capital and also required larger labor forces to complete the orders.[35] Cooke's own advertisement attested to this. Dismissing the recalcitrant Folwell, Cooke had employed "several others who are capital Workmen in that Branch [of hair working] and far superior to Mr. Folwell."[36] This was in part the central dispute between Cooke and his ex-apprentice. In Folwell's eyes, Cooke, by offering him an inadequate wage, had broken a traditional faith. This was occurring in other industries as well. In 1805, for example, Philadelphian shoemaking journeymen accused their masters of being "capitalists, not producers."[37] From Folwell's perspective, Cooke, a mere retailer and wholesaler, was intent on employing skilled labor cheaply, and could not be considered a "real" hair worker. As Folwell stated in his rebuttal, "Jewelers and Silversmiths, whose occupations do not enable them to execute this branch themselves, take order from their friends, and employ those who are in the particular line, while they receive a greater price than the person who execute their commission."[38] Cooke had moved from being the master of master craftsmen to the master who was the mover of goods. Although this shift did not come into effect fully until later in the nineteenth century, Cooke demonstrated that immediately after the Revolutionary War, such changes had begun to affect individual lives.

The differences between the two men lay in their different ideological approaches rather than in their practices. The traditional inequity among apprentices, journeymen, and masters colored their view of the others' actions. By the 1780s, these economic differences within the working class made for sometimes volatile relations.[39] Both men were, they believed, on the side of tradition. Folwell was faulted for his rejection of the traditional subservient position of a trained apprentice, while Cooke was a nonproducer, a mere distributor of goods who profited from others' labors.

Both men represented the emerging consumer economy. While Cooke focused on building capital reserves, expanding his trade, and employing inexpensive labor, Folwell developed a multifaceted business whose appeal rested on Folwell's self-inscription as an "artist."[40] In March 1791, working in Charleston, Folwell effused in an advertisement that he continued to offer "the most correct likenesses in Miniature and Profile Painting and in Shades, by a method entirely new. . . . He also executes in a very elegant stile, mourning devices, fancy pieces, etc. in hair." In addition, Folwell guaranteed impatient customers he could take a portrait in less than five minutes, for four dollars to three guineas.[41]

In addition to his hair working and portrait painting, Folwell, described by one historian as a "methodical artist of moderate ability but relentless energy," worked in his wife Elizabeth's fancy embroidery school.[42] Five years after his advertising skirmish with Cooke, Folwell announced that a "Drawing School for Young Ladies, By Desire of many Parents, Is intended to be Opened in Philadelphia, under the Tuition of Samuel Folwell, Limner." Folwell promised tutelage in pencil work; painting on satin, ivory, and paper; and "that Curious Art of working devices in human Hair, in which he has long had professional Practice in this City." Folwell promised that for "those who discover a natural *propensity* to this polite Art, no Attention shall be wanting, to enable them to delineate Nature in every striking Form."[43]

Between the two of them, Samuel and Elizabeth Folwell created a relatively successful empire of fancywork crafts. Samuel Folwell's own career was a forerunner of the following century. Folwell's position as an "artist" was important because of the legitimacy that designation lent to his instructional enterprises. Folwell did not teach "grand art"; rather, he taught the art of decoration. And he pursued his career in a variety of ways, from traveling a portraiture circuit between Philadelphia and Charleston to creating his own school for ladies. Folwell did not advertise or train apprentices in a "shop"; he trained young ladies whose social and economic position suggested that they would never be in the situation of M. Sauvage, a woman earning her livelihood through hairwork.

A fancywork school was usually a woman's enterprise. While Mr. and Mrs. Folwell's school was successful, most such efforts were made in desperation by women motivated by a lack of any other ways to make money. Jane Chancellor Payne, living in Parkersburg, Virginia, and saddled with an alcoholic husband, had first retreated into fervent prayer and temperance activities. However, with two children and after nearly ten years of her husband's self-inflicted decline, she had little choice but to find employment for herself. In 1843, the family moved to Clarksburg, Virginia, where she noted in her diary, "Last Monday I commenced teaching Fancy work in this place I find the scholars easily instructed affable and agreeable."[44] The students and their parents were well satisfied with their instruction, but Jane found teaching an empty practice. Two months later, the family returned to Parkersburg, Virginia, after settling their debts in Clarksburg. Jane wrote in her diary on June 4, 1843, "Last Monday I commenced my school I commenced with the hope of deriving benefit for my family for all our earnings has passed off from us and we are again almost penny less my husband for a while listened to reason and promised to relinquish the fatal evil which has been the cause of both loss and sorrow . . . if there is a hell on earth it is that experienced by the wife of a drunkard." By July of that same year, the family had moved yet again, to Zanesville, Ohio, where Jane vowed to "make an effort to form a class of fancy scholars." In October, with the family still in Zanesville, Jane wrote of her effort to start yet another class of fancy scholars. She told of walking from house to house, showing her work and asking if the parents would consider sending their children to her. "I turned out among strangers to try and make a school and after walking in the hot sunshine 2 days I suceeded in geting 5 scholars. . . . The next day I commenced my little school one of the scholars and never shall I forget her for it seemed to look in pity our situation at once and advanced money from which together with what flowers I was fortunate to sell and 2 quilts mr. P. sold kept us in provisions and necessaries during my first class." When she returned to the boardinghouse where the family lived, "I was tole by the Landlord that he wanted the room we occupied that evening I afterwards learned that it was because we were out of funds."

Jane's efforts to raise money—giving fancywork lessons and selling flowers (these were paper flowers made by Jane and her husband) and quilts—were vital to the family's subsistence. In one month, with a class of ten fancywork students Jane earned $68. The paper flowers brought in $26. In addition, Jane sold fourteen quilts. After bills for the boardinghouse, food, and clothing were paid, the family had about $20 left.

Jane's family did survive. The final pages of her diary are devoted to locks of hair from herself and her children. Ironically, the last entry of hair is Jane's. Two ribbons are glued onto the page, and written next to the ribbons is the caption, "Jane Chancellor Payne (d. 1863)." Her lock of hair is missing.

Jane's skills in fancywork, most likely learned in a school similar to Samuel Folwell's, were not used to ornament her household domain; instead, they kept the family alive. Her struggle to engage students was constant, and her dislike for the public nature of her new life never abated. Moving from town to town, in part because each town could supply only so many students for her "schools," Jane lived a highly visible life. At each town, she went door to door seeking students and then, after the month-long course ended, she held a public exhibition of the students' work in an effort to gain new students.

Although Jane Chancellor Payne's fancywork school was little more than a small group of students meeting in a boardinghouse room, the Folwells' school represented a more organized and commercial effort. For a hair worker and miniature-portrait artist like Folwell, a man's livelihood as an artisan was not found in the subordinate position of journeyman nor was it in creating a "manufactory" with many workers, as his master Cooke did. Rather, it was in offering innovative products, creating less capital-intensive opportunities such as a Ladies' School, and traveling to promising markets.

A similar consumer-driven stance is evident in an advertisement by Raphaelle Peale. Peale, working in Philadelphia in 1800, set his advertising copy within a fanciful locket-shaped frame. He announced that "Raphaelle Peale, Portrait Painter, in Miniature and Large, Will deliver Likenesses, For a short time, Fashionably set in Gold, with platts and cyphers complete."[45] His advertisement is something new in the world of hair working and miniatures, for the eye-catching visual device emphasized the decorative aspect of his consumer good. And, on the cusp of the nineteenth century, it was hair workers such as Peale and Folwell, and their customer-oriented production and advertisement of consumer goods, that characterized the coming decades of the hairwork trade.

Hairwork and Portrait Miniatures

Folwell, Peale, and many others were offering painted miniatures backed by worked hair. These were tokens of the self, intimate yet intended for public display. The pairing of hair and a personal image was meant to represent the sincerity of the individual depicted and the individual owner. Popular from the 1760s to the 1820s, portrait miniatures were small oval portraits, usually slightly over two inches high. The portrait was placed under a convex piece of glass on the front and often was backed by a braided or flat woven hair ornament. The resulting small oval piece could be kept in a leather case similar to later daguerreotype cases, displayed on a small stand, or mounted as the center of a choker, bracelet, or ring and worn.[46] Portrait miniatures were intimate in scale and in what they represented—the personal bonds between individuals.[47]

Portrait miniatures often asserted a relationship between individuals and, indeed, sometimes played a central role in the construction of a new relationship. In the 1820s, Mary Todd Lincoln's father, Robert Todd, wrote his fiancé Elizabeth Humphreys to encourage her to marry him. He sent a miniature portrait of himself to Elizabeth, writing "this remembrance is a small testimonial of my sincere regard for you."[48] Miniature portraits were not only to be accurate depictions of the physical appearance of the sitter but also were character studies revelatory of the individual's inner nature and true self. Portrait miniatures were satisfying because of their ability to reach beyond mere representation. In fact, later forms of depiction, such as daguerreotypes in the 1840s, often were faulted for their verisimilitude and their lack of insight into the human character.[49] Thus, to be both artistically and commercially successful, miniature-portrait artists had to produce a "likeness" that also reflected larger, cultural contexts.[50]

While the pictorial representation of the individual was the prominent feature of a miniature, the artistic quality of the human hair on the back of the image was also important. The worked hair (which typically was glued into feather plumes or woven into a basket pattern) was another way an individual was depicted. Painted images could be like a person, but they could never capture the person's true character. Hairwork was absolutely like; not only was it of the person's body but it expressed, through its fanci-

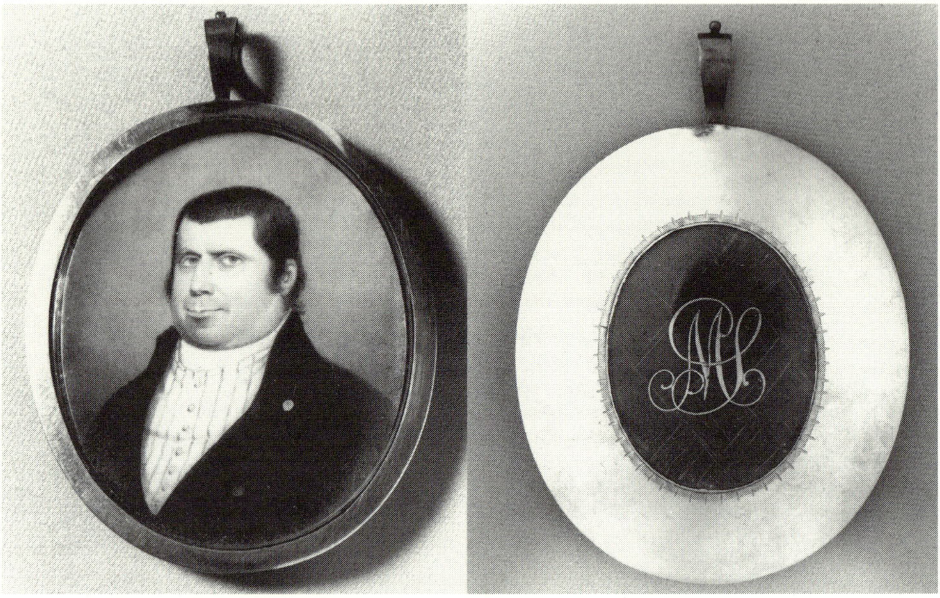

Figure 4. Hairwork could convey facets of character not well represented through the physical characteristics of a person. Here is a man whose appearance suggests an unemotional approach to life, yet the hair and fanciful initials on the reverse suggest someone closely connected and beloved by others. 1824–1840. Courtesy National Museum of American History, Kenneth E. Behring Center, Smithsonian Institution.

ful working, some otherwise fleeting attributes of character—the lightness and ease that came with familiarity, for instance. For this reason, the artistry of hair working was a selling point for painters (Figure 4).

So, miniature-portrait artists often boasted in their advertisements of their equally important talents in working hair. Cooke and Company assured customers in 1784 that it could provide "hair worked in any devise to the greatest perfection," while in the same year Josiah Flagg countered that "he purposes Miniature Painting and working Hair Devices, for Lockets, Brasslets, Rings, &C. in a neat and elegant manner." Likewise, James Askew, in his advertisement of 1785, assured readers that he provided articles "worked with the real hair given, in any device that fancy can suggest, in the most modern taste with dispatch."[51]

Portrait miniatures backed with hair were a vital tool in the construction of a middle-class identity in eighteenth-century America.[52] Successfully combining sentimental expression with a doubled form of representation, portrait miniatures were emblematic of the sincerity and assertion of authenticity so important to the white, eighteenth-century consumer. James Askew, quoted earlier, asserted that his products were worked with "the real hair given" *and* he promised that which "fancy can suggest" stamped with the "most modern taste."[53] Hair guaranteed both a true likeness and a like interpretation, because it was the literal body reworked.[54] The hair itself and the expressiveness of the portrait imparted sincerity. Fancy was simultaneously conveyed in the intricate working of the hair and in the miniaturization of the depiction. Modernity was evident in the fashionableness of the display and the wearing of the portrait miniatures. Thus, miniatures were popular among those middle-class individuals who prized sentiment, fancy, and modernity as status markers.

Hair's natural property of flexibility was exploited in hairwork. Hair could represent mourning, romantic love, kinship, or even a yen for fashion, and it could be manipulated into a variety of forms to adorn miniatures. Many jewelers simply stated, as did Peter Leret of Baltimore in 1787, that they could offer "hair worked in any device." The variations were endless. For example, the jewelers Oliphant and Henderson, working in South Carolina, offered "hair framed into squares, ovals, sprigs, flowers, cyphers, hearts, &c. for rings or lockets."[55]

Such elaborately worked hair, no matter how finely done, usually did not appear on the front of the miniature but was placed on the back of the case. As with portraits, mourning scenes were painted on small ivory discs and mounted in jewelry-like settings.[56] However somber in tone, mourning scenes combined the sentiments of love, sorrow, and fashion. For instance, a typical miniature was adorned with a common, late eighteenth-century mourning scene, complete with disconsolate mourners and a tomb under weeping willows.[57] The William Dunklin miniature (Figure 5) typifies these images. It simultaneously evokes the arcadian fantasy of the garden of Eden, the death of George Washington (whose demise provoked a fad of depicting an imposing tomb surrounded by sad, attractive young women), and the redemptive nature of mourning itself.[58]

Such generic images were individualized by the inclusion of human hair. For instance, the Dunklin mourning miniature is backed with ornate Prince-of-Wales feathers made of hair. Curving around Dunklin's thick curl of dark brown hair is a carefully arranged twine of blonde hair (Figure 6). The female mourner on the front of the miniature is reiterated on the back, and the gently protective arrangement is extraordinarily evocative of the

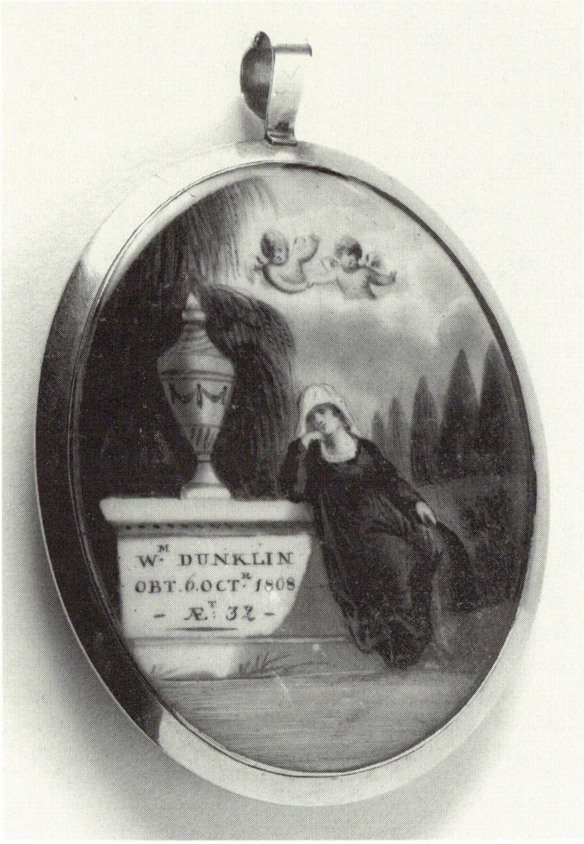

Figure 5. This image was generic in the early 1800s; what distinguishes William Dunklin's memorial is the reverse side with its worked hair. Mourning pendant dated 1808. Courtesy Winterthur Museum and Country Estate. Gift of Ms. Jeannine Mannebach.

lives of those left behind. The often repeated image was rendered intensely personal. Despite its prosaic appearance, then, the Dunklin brooch acted as a potent avenue between the living owner and the deceased William.

The popularity of hairwork did not lessen as miniatures were less favored. By the 1830s, hair jewelry was linked to what is termed sentimental fashion. Eighteenth-century hairwork styles were modified to provide even more open displays of the hair and the affections it represented, and new styles developed that did not simply include hair but were wholly composed of hair. While portrait miniatures and miniature mourning scenes never completely disappeared, they were replaced in the mid-nineteenth century by more "modern" styles that were far easier to wear and display.

One feature of miniatures that increasingly became a drawback was

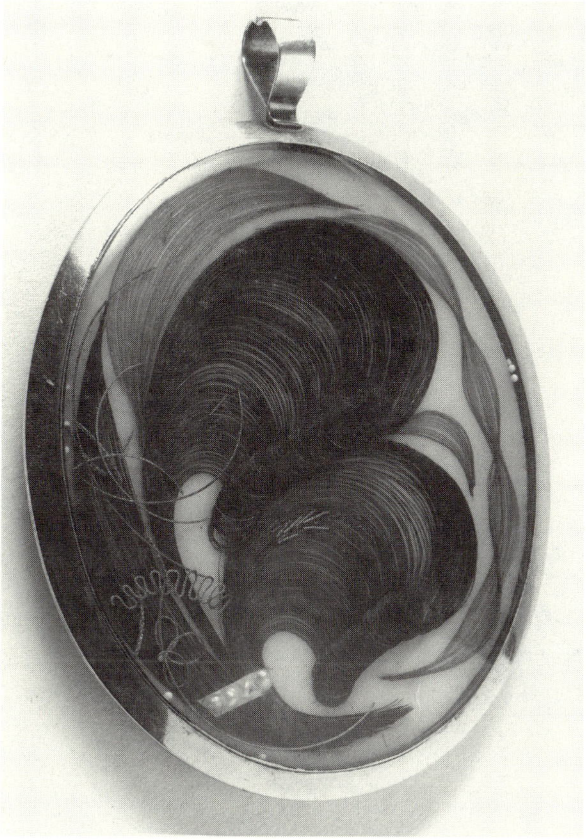

Figure 6. The reverse side of the Dunklin mourning pendant has artfully worked hair. The individuals—at least, their hair—embrace. 1808. Courtesy Winterthur Museum and Country Estate. Gift of Ms. Jeannine Mannebach.

that they were difficult to display openly. Early miniatures were sometimes made with a loop attached to the top of their oval frame. The loop provided a way to slide the miniature onto a neck chain, or later, to hook it onto a watch chain. Miniatures could then be displayed with either the image or the hair facing the viewer. For instance, in her portrait of 1808, Sarah Bell prominently displayed a finely worked miniature case with the letter "C" in hairwork.[59] Sarah Bell could reverse the chain to hide the hairwork and display the miniature that surely lay on the other side of the pendant (Figure 7).[60] By the 1830s, mourning and portrait miniatures were no longer made to be worn. Miniatures were being made larger and into bulkier rectangular shapes; they were increasingly displayed as parlor decorations rather than jewelry worn on the person.[61]

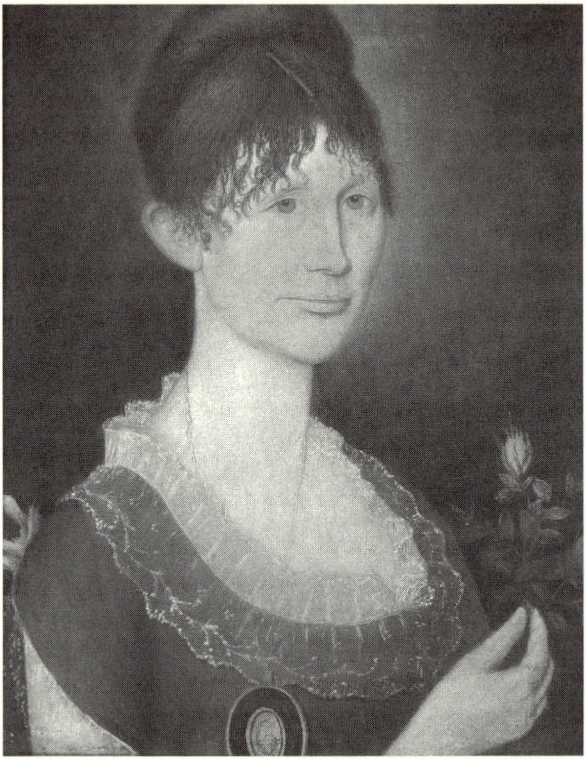

Figure 7. In this portrait, Sarah Bell has adorned her body with a pendant mourning miniature, hairside out. Her dress, curls, and single flower tell us she is young, romantic, and yet has experienced loss in her life. Aldridge (or Oldridge), *Sarah Bell*, circa 1808, The Colonial Williamsburg Foundation, Williamsburg, Virginia.

Hairwork and Sentimentality

When new forms of hairwork appeared in the 1830s, the meanings of the jewelry shifted from an explicit relationship to mourning practices to a broader idea of fashionable sentimentality. From the 1830s to the 1880s, hairwork was a fashion, albeit a highly sentimentalized one. In 1844, a women's magazine noted that "sentimental bracelets, composed of hair . . . are now considered indispensable."[62] One did not need mourning and melancholia to legitimate the expression of sentimentality because by the 1830s sentimentality had been accepted as fashionable.[63]

In the eighteenth century, the sentimental associations of hair were obliquely displayed; by the nineteenth century, hairwork and the sentimentality it conveyed was worn for others to observe. This practice revealed a paradox about sentimentality. While display of one's sentimentality was essential to being regarded as sentimental, that same exhibition could easily be construed as ostentatious, vulgar, and insincere.[64] Fashion was constantly in flux, it was superficial, and it was self-aggrandizing. It opposed the sincerity that women in particular were supposed to possess. Fashion was expressed with goods, and therefore was opposed to the domestic sphere. Thus, those constant fluctuations in styles threatened to undermine the premise of sentimentality itself.

Even as hairwork revealed the dissonance between genuine emotion and frivolous fashionableness, it attempted a remedy. Hair's undeniable relationship to an individual asserted a sincerity of character that transcended the hypocrisy that fashionableness implied. The mid-nineteenth century was the height of the popularity of hairwork perhaps because as fashion was criticized as being particularly hypocritical, hairwork's genuineness was being asserted.[65] On the one hand, hair jewelry was very much a commodity, buttressed as it was by marketing and salesmanship; on the other hand, it was exactly that which could not be completely commodified. Hair jewelry provided a way to forestall the apparent effects of fashion in the market and in the social world.

The shift from eighteenth-century sincerity to the far more elaborate sentimental expressions of the nineteenth century is evident in several short stories from the 1840s that feature hair and hairwork. Associated with the power to evoke distant or deceased individuals, to provoke emotions, and to represent the individual in the marketplace, hair and hairwork provided authors with a convenient plot mechanism. Hairwork was made of human hair and, because of this, it had the power to reveal a fictional character's true nature. In a short story of 1843, a young woman has lost her dying grandmother's dearest possession, a ring made with hair from the grandmother's first husband and that of the father of our heroine's father. The young woman's grandmother accused her granddaughter of pawning the ring, saying "I've faith to believe, Mary Richardson, that you've sold that ring. It cost ten dollars when it was new." The father, long lost, found himself in an "intelligence office," an employment agency in the same city as his daughter and mother (both of whom, he was unaware, lived in that city). The father came across a young woman wearing a stolen hair ring, and immediately recognized her guilt. Asking her, "Where did you get that?" he pointed to her ring. "That ring I mean, and you know it, for you never came by it honestly."[66] The father had, of course, recognized his father's hair mounted in a ring he had himself given to his mother years before. This was hair jewelry's gift—it could forever preserve an individual, protecting the person from the vicissitudes of fortune and time, and connecting individuals thrown apart through those same changes in time. The hair in the ring was, literally, the man's father, and thus recognizable even when stolen from its rightful owner. This was the sincerity and authenticity of hair at work.

It was also believed that hair could, through its ability to represent the individual, evoke emotions just as the person might. D. Ellen Goodman, in her short story "The Two Shreds of Hair," of 1848, embroidered an intricate tale around "a simple lock of hair—glossy and black as night—coiled into a delicate curl, and nestled down in . . . folds of . . . snowy paper." The narrator wondered at the evocative power of that "simple lock of hair": "A single tress of jetty hair, soft and silken—strange that it should thus touch the chain of memory link by link till it vibrates almost painfully—strange that it should awaken such emotions, and cause my heart to beat thus heavily."[67]

Here, then, is an array of metaphors of the transcendental characteristics of hair. The "simple lock" was sinuously "coiled" and "nestled" in its "snowy" bed; the hair's physicality sounded the first chord of the narrator's psyche. Then memory, compared with a chain, was mirrored not only in the intricate links of hairwork but also in the ephemeral emotional ties that acted as a vinculum of time. Indeed, the force of these emotions in turn provoked a physical reaction ("and cause my heart to beat thus heavily"), returning the narrator and reader to the tangible reality of the hair itself. In this way, hair's physicality triggered the emotional and ephemeral and was then returned to its own genesis point in the lock of hair. Hair told a story or, at least, sparked a narrative. Men and women who owned hairwork relied on these assumptions about the meanings of hair to tell their own elaborately woven stories.

Although the rhetoric applied to hairwork was its authenticity—Samuel Folwell's "real hair worker" creating devices from the hair of the individual is echoed here—there was a problem. Hairwork was popular because it *was* a product of the commercial market. By the 1800s, hairwork was very much a commodity and, as such, it stood in contradiction to the values of sincerity it purported to represent. The dilemma of the good can be seen in a short story, "The Hair Neck-Lace," that appeared in the *Ladies' Companion* of 1843. This story sounded a warning about the risks of participation in the consumer market while it affirmed the process of production and consumption. Lucy, the central character, does not escape her venture into the market of commodity goods unscathed. In the end, Lucy's shorn head was emblematic of the treacheries of the market of sentimental, personal goods.[68]

"The Hair Neck-Lace" is a literary fantasy of ownership and the body. First, the story asserts that the self is not enough. One's identity must be created through and for the market in order to be worth something and to be of value. Lucy remarked to her own image in her mirror, "'Ah! . . . would these ringlets were strung with diamonds, then might I have something to offer to my poor suffering country. But can I not turn them to some advantage,' continued the girl thoughtfully, and after a short pause, she exclaimed joyfully, 'yes, yes, I will weave necklaces out of them, and offer them for sale—hair neck-laces will be very pretty, if handsomely woven.'"

Hairwork was "very pretty, if handsomely woven"; that is, braided into intricately worked jewelry, laboriously wrapped around wire, tediously coiled into flowers. One's body, one's self, as represented by the bit of hair, functioned as a raw material that must be worked. Hair and, consequently, the self, then, had to be transformed through handwork in order to have value and function as a market good. But all the work of braiding, twisting, and twining could be undone if the sentimentality coating the object wore thin. Thankfully, hairwork such as that created by Lucy enjoyed a "tripled insurance" against being taken for a mere commodity. First, hairwork was of human hair and thus recognized as inherently individualized; second, it was made by hand, not machine; and, third, it represented a "true" sentimentality—an expression of emotion resistant to either machine or market.

These three elements of hairwork are evident in the story of Lucy's production of hair necklaces for the market. Having "a want of wealth" and wishing to make money to donate to the (American revolutionary) war effort, Lucy mused over a variety of plans. "But all her schemes prove impracticable" until she came up with the idea of cutting and working her own hair, for *that work* "will bring me something—and I can well spare a few locks." Lucy took her highly wrought hairwork to a jeweler. "The man [was] attracted by her luxurious tresses, as they waved in the gentle breeze, and [was] surprized at the novelty of her offer, for, at a glance, he discovered that the neck-laces were composed of her own hair." He assured the young girl, "I will soon dispose of the neck-laces, my noble girl. . . . Every lady will purchase, when they learn of whose hair they are made, and for what purpose they are sold." Lucy cut her own hair, worked that hair, and, in so doing, produced a commodity, but that hair, even in its worked state, was not to be wholly divorced from Lucy herself. Indeed, it was the persistent connection between the hair and her self through its sincere desire for a noble, selfless cause, that established the market value of her hair necklaces.

Lucy's own hair, her own handwork, and her most sincere sentiment provided the "triple insurance" of authenticity. Despite this, her necklaces were vulnerable to depreciation in market value because of their popularity. "All the inhabitants of Philadelphia, both male and female, flocked to [the jeweler's] store to admire and purchase, and very soon hair neck-laces, marked with the single word Lucy, became all the rage among the fashionables." Authenticity was firmly affixed by the device of the name tag that was attached to the necklace by the jeweler, not by Lucy. With Lucy's act of selfless sacrifice, the authentic presence of Lucy in the hair fancywork was confirmed. In addition, the base material was of Lucy, the handwork was of Lucy, and, finally, the necklaces were labeled as "Lucy." While this increased the commodity status of her product, that same integrity ramified the cost to her self. Lucy was well aware "of the sum which might be raised, should she consent to part with all her hair, on the one hand, the sacrifice by which that sum was to be purchased, presented itself on the other, and all her sensibilities were aroused."

That risk was real. Lucy's fiancé Edwin had told Lucy (one hopes with all due sincerity), "I love you for yourself . . . but I certainly do idolize these rich, bright ringlets." Lucy refused to give Edwin even one curl of her hair, saying "Were you once in possession of your idol, then I would be forgotten, or perhaps forsaken! No, no, I will not give you one hair, but prove yourself worthy, then I promise to give you the whole of it, into the bargain." Lucy understood that her hair may have represented her self but did not wholly constitute it. However, Lucy relied on Edwin's attraction to her hair to "win" him in marriage. Although she had refused to bestow the locks on the loving Edwin, Lucy, in his absence, conceded to selling those curls. In doing so, she risked losing his love, for Edwin identified Lucy's very self with her "rich, bright ringlets." Lucy's gamble was a risky one. While her hair brought a high price on the market as a worked piece of fancy, the loss of that hair, and its subsequent commodified status, threatened to lessen Lucy's literal self-worth as measured by Edwin's love.[69]

This story is an illustration of the constitutive process of production and consumption. For Lucy, her self—her hair—garnered a financial reward but at a high psychic cost. "As curl after curl disappeared beneath the operation of the scissors" Lucy cried, "they are my all—and Edwin will love me no more—but I give them for America." The scene closes: "All the beautiful hair of the patriotic girl was manufactured into neck-laces, and sold, bringing very high prices, thereby yielding a very considerable sum."

Poor Lucy suffered in two ways. First, Edwin had clearly stated that his love of her hair was second only to his love for her self; second, Lucy had sent her hair out to parts unknown. Luckily, her motivations were pure and worthy, at least in nineteenth-century eyes. She had selflessly sacrificed for a virtuous cause and, thus, could not be scorned. The severing of the hair represented the threatened loss of self to the demands of the market. But within the safe confines of sentimentality, the possibility of misuse was ameliorated. Lucy's hair, while worked into a commodity and sold on the market of "fashionables," nevertheless could not, in the rhetorical parameters of sentimental culture, be misused. She had given of herself through the cutting of her locks and the work of her hands, and all for the cause of freedom. Her actions guaranteed her safety.

There was the possibility that others would not recognize this, though, and its resolution depended not on Lucy but on Edwin. How will he react to her now nearly bald head and her great sacrifice? Edwin returned from the war and, finding his shorn love, was asked, "Can you not love me as well without it?" Edwin assured Lucy he could, for two reasons, neither of which directly answered her question. First, he reiterated the redemptive promise of sentimentality that her sacrifice "twas a noble, a glorious act!" and therefore, could be forgiven. Second, he has himself purchased a "Lucy" necklace—to give to Lucy! Reunited, the lovers marry, and "Lucy, in a simple dress, of white, with no ornament save the hair neck-lace which Edwin has clasped around her neck, gave her hand to him."

When Edwin clasped around Lucy's neck her own hair necklace, made of her own hair, worked by her own hands, priced as a commodity, sold on the market, and bought by Edwin himself, Lucy was reunited with her very self—the person Edwin loved. This short story was a fantasy of reconciliation and unification. In it, the dilemmas and tensions that the growing consumer market posed for middle-class Americans were neatly, satisfactorily, and artificially resolved. The story's plot outlined how, through sentimental consumerism, nineteenth-century middle-class Americans could retain a sense of self in the face of a depersonalized "stranger" world of industrial urban life. Hair fancywork offered this tantalizing promise to middle-class Americans in the nineteenth century. As an object of sentimental consumerism, hair fancywork provided a material representation of authenticity and naturalized value in a context of dangerously unstable values.

Hairwork and the Friendship Album

A similar effort at personalization can be found in albums that coupled verse and hair. Albums of different sorts—autograph, hair, and, later in the nineteenth century, scrap—were popular among middle-class women throughout the nineteenth century. Autograph albums are part of a larger genre of albums called *album amicorum*, or friendship albums.[70] Intimate and personal, albums were also a means of displaying affiliations of heart and soul. In the nineteenth century, hair began to accompany the verses. Sometimes the hair is a simple lock, glued or sewn onto the page; other times, women wove the hair into lace patterns. Hair albums were a tripled form of display: inscription, the individual, and the relationships represented. The album's owner, in turn, through her selection of those included, was the center of a network of individuals.

This open display of self could prove troubling, especially because it was women who were the main participants in autograph album making.[71] In 1827, an author bluntly appraised the self-referentiality of autograph-album collecting and giving as "the tribute, too, of remembrance which we delight to pay to others, [that] we desire for ourselves." Nevertheless, this "wish for applause; the thirst for fame; the desire that our names should shine down to future posterity . . . [is remedied] with the unambitious desire to retain, even beyond the span of life, the affections of the warm hearted few who shared our joys and sorrows in the world."[72] Thus, the act of memorializing was not a grab for fame and recognition, but rather a selfless "entombment" of "the only lasting bond of affection; which alone can secure our affectionate remembrances." Through memorializing others, one negated the hypocritical urge for egotistical self-display. Women were wonderfully positioned to do just that as they were supposed to be a self constituted of others. Thus, the feminine form of the album provided women with an avenue of self-expression that paradoxically functioned as an effacement of their own selves for the beneficial display of others around them.

Verses accompanying locks of hair echoed similar ideas about the relationship between hair and the individuals that we saw in the portrait miniatures and jewelry. While many of the verses were hackneyed, for recipients, some of the handwritten verses were deeply meaningful. In an 1834 memoir, a woman noted that "I have always loved albums, much as they have been ridiculed . . . and it interests me to see the ardour of a young lady, when, opening the gilt leaves, she finds there sentiments dedicated to her alone."

The verses, in this woman's eyes, were not redundant but rather were "contributions from native poets."[73] This effect was intensified when the verses were paired with the hair of the author.

Hair, detached from its original owner, could nevertheless stand in for that individual. Emotional repercussions that would otherwise be the result of the interaction between individuals could be triggered by the hair itself. In 1827, an anonymous author asked, "Have you an ancient Album—the repository of the mementos of early affection?—Turn over its leaves, stained by the finger of time—sit down and ponder upon the names enrolled upon them; each says *remember me*. . . . There are not two other words in the language that call back a more fruitful train of past remembrances of friendship, than these."[74] These remembrances were intensified by the inclusion of hair with the friend's handwritten verse.

In Mary Edes's album of 1828, a friend wrote

One short *line*, and then we *sever*, *Alas* perhaps forever;
Though far distant *you* may *be*
Sometimes *deign* to think of me.
Affectionately yours M. . . .
M. Holt Greenfield [emphasis in original][75]

Hair accompanied the emphatic verse. Hair, severed from the body but still always of that body, acted as a physical marker not only of an individual but of the memories and thoughts of that individual. Thus, Greenfield hoped to reach over distances, past the shortcomings of "one short *line*," and move his young lady friend to at least "sometimes *deign* to think of me."

That severed piece of self, when tied together with an evocative verse, was a token of an individual's relationships and emotions. Many verses commented on the physical reality of the hair that is a part of the self being memorialized within the pages of the album. For instance, elsewhere in Mary Edes's album:

Please to accept this as a momento of affection
from your friend R. Holt Greenfield N[ew] H[ampshire] 1828

Please to accept this as a token of friendship
from Sally Fletcher, January 29 1828

These verses pointed to the tangible quality of hair—the token of friendship was not simply the handwritten verse but was in the jointure of emotion and sentiment, the self through handwriting, and the self through the hair. "This from your friend Anna L. Duncan," wrote Anna herself. Such presence of self on the pages of an album added impetus to an ongoing life for the album itself. Owners of albums browsed through their books, adding, amending, and never simply allowing the memories of friends and family to remain ignored and static. In this album, Sally Fletcher's verse was later emended by Mary Edes, when Mary noted sadly, "now is slumbering with the dead 1833" under Sally's inscription.[76]

Many verses referred to the public dimension of the album, although most often "display" was veiled by the metaphor of memory. That is, memory was to be triggered by the review of the verse, signature, and hair, and the stimulation of memory in others was the means of display of self and affiliation. In another album, this of 1839, one correspondent wrote evocatively,

How dear to my heart are the scenes of my
childhood. The friends of my youth
O I neer shall forget. Angels fly [illegible]
Mary when memory recalls the scenes
of bye gone days. Think with some
dear recollection your *warm friend*
Julia, whose best wishes you ever have.
Those cranberries are not to be forgotten. [emphasis in original][77]

Accompanied by a lock of braided hair, the verse was to maintain the memories of "scenes of bye gone days" that "are not to be forgotten." In part, hair accomplished this fixation of fleeting memory through its physicality. Having been an actual part of the human body, hair represented one's "warm friends" through their living presence.

Sentimentality, like this verse, looked backward as it attempted to fix memories in the present. One of the hallmarks of sentimentality was its practitioners' efforts to construct the present as both the past and the future. This was one reason its emphasis was on immediate emotional reaction. When you are leafing through the pages of a scrapbook on which individuals' locks of hair are affixed, and their thoughts penned, it is difficult not to react. Sentimentality pulls reactions from its onlookers by confronting viewers with locks of human hair and with fervent expressions of human emotion. Hair albums, like the miniature portraits that preceded them, were intended to be deeply personal, intimate, and yet testimony to the emotional connections that made the individual exist in her or his social setting.

Hairwork signified the fixed quality of those relationships, but the meaning and uses of hairwork did change from the eighteenth to the nineteenth centuries. In the eighteenth century, hairwork indicated class status and an individual's sincerity. The wrought hair in a miniature portrait accompanied the honest, straightforward image of the person. But nineteenth-century Americans were practicing two seemingly contradictory forms of display. Sentimentality was an outwardly directed mode of emotional expression, whereas sincerity depended on a reserve that miniature portraits neatly personified. An eighteenth-century miniature portrait fronted the more grandiose lines of the wrought hair and in effect hid that emotional flurry behind a somber image of the person, but nineteenth-century sentimentality demanded visibility. So hairwork became the object itself. Samuel Folwell's new career direction in the earliest years of the 1800s suggests this. Once specializing in portraits and hairwork, he, along with his wife, began generalizing in an array of sentimental goods for young ladies. The proud artisan who had fought with Cooke became the teacher of the soft arts of sentimental appeal.

As we shall see in the following chapters, the burgeoning market of consumer goods and the practice of consumerism, that is, the purchase and use of manufactured goods, increasingly informed the meanings of hairwork. Consumerism linked the individual self to the goods the individual selected from the market; a person was, in part, what they bought. Hairwork demonstrated a self-evident relationship between individuals and objects for those women and men who wore miniature portraits, created albums, and contributed verses and locks of hair. The self lived on or perhaps even gained life through its material representation in hair and its metaphorical representation in image or verse. These forces intensified well into the latter third of the nineteenth century. As individuals increasingly demonstrated their character through consumer goods, hairwork's value as a piece of the self that was also fashionable and sentimental increased as well.

Chapter 2

An Article of Commerce

In the 1850s and 1860s hairwork jewelry and hairwork parlor decorations were very popular among white, middle-class Americans. The sincerity of the eighteenth-century consumer, which was so convincingly expressed through the ownership and display of another's hair, had by the 1850s and 1860s been modified into a public statement of sentimentality. This measured display of emotion was offered as a remedy for the ills of the market, but that anodyne was suggested and created by the market itself.

Sentimentality validated emotions when they were reflected on and then expressed. Thus, sentimentality required the narration of experience and had broader applications than sensibility. For example, when a child died it was understood that for the parents that experience was harrowing, agonizing, and often crippling. Nineteenth-century middle-class culture often memorialized the death of children through innumerable poems, essays, memoirs, and novels based on the event. These artistic representations of grief were not necessarily produced by grieving parents. Instead, the *idea* of the death of a child was the impetus behind producing these works. (I am not suggesting that children did not die in the nineteenth century, or that parents did not grieve, but, rather, that childhood death itself was an artistic motif.) Why did a culture that frowned on hypocrisy iterate such an intimate experience? Because sentimentality legitimated the constant retelling. Sentimentality provided specific and consistent narrative frameworks and a language of emotion that allowed for the public expression of private suffering. Middle-class culture emphasized control over one's emotions, bodily movement, and self, but sentimentality allowed for the structured loss of control.[1]

The public display of emotions that sentimentality provided for also explains why sentimental expression and market goods worked so well together. Gift books; scrap and, later, photograph albums; diaries; novels; jewelry; and lithographic images are just some of the products created by the market to aid consumers in the proper display of sentimental character. The market posed a threat to sentimental claims of intimacy and sincerity, but it was the market that offered visible, instantly recognizable emblems of sentiment.

At the same time, sentimentalism seemingly contradicted the emergent forces of the market. For most Americans of the 1850s and 1860s, economic changes such as larger-scaled commercial enterprises and the ever-increasing importance of the market to individual fortunes, reputations, and lives, seemed to endanger the basis of society, the family. (Keep in mind that African Americans, whether enslaved or not, were purposefully banned from full participation in these larger economic shifts, and enslaved African Americans were precluded from the legal right to family.) The presence of the market, with its tendency to convert all relationships into monetary transactions, contradicted the concept of the family as the institution exempt from such "cold" relations. Hairwork, a product of that market, affirmed the continuing importance of the family even in the face of market arguments against the central role of the domestic circle.

Hairwork was especially useful in providing middle-class individuals a way to signal their own sentimental character to others. In eighteenth-century elite culture, one demonstrated one's "true" response through sensible (that is, emotional) and sincere reactions. One's mind and body reacted in accordance with one another, and thus the integrity of character was revealed through the coherence of emotional response. But nineteenth-century sentimentalism demanded a reiteration of response: the immediate reaction was to be relived and reenacted. Hairwork, whether jewelry or parlor decorations, was wonderfully suited to aid a performance of emotion, especially if the hair was presented more openly. For example, eighteenth-century portrait miniatures were backed with hair and displayed on small stands placed on parlor tables. A visitor would have to pick up the miniature, or be handed it, and turn the object around. By the 1850s, these small pictures were replaced with jewelry that was made entirely, or almost entirely, of hair, or large parlor decorations that were made entirely of worked hair. A parlor visitor was directly confronted with hair (often a large quantity of it) and thus the owner's emotions were delineated in the hairwork. There was no chance of escape for an onlooker, nor was circumspection desired.

Hairwork made tangible the narrative of experience demanded by sentimentality (as laid out in countless sentimental fictional tales) because it physically embodied the emotional relationships between individuals. When a young man wore a watch chain made of his wife's hair, he testified to a relationship of love, physical closeness, and all the other experiences that sharing one's life with another entails. As one advertisement argued, "these gems of *Hair Jewelry*, interwoven with a starry way of brilliants, or the pearl, that gem which is interwoven with the pure image of our little eternity of time—they call into being thoughts and emotions of affections—remembrances of husband or wife, lover or child, parents and children."[2] Hairwork would "call into being thoughts and emotions of affections." And that was not only for the owner but for anyone who could see the jewelry on the wearer. This was necessary for sentimental expression because the "thoughts and emotions" were reiterated.

As in the eighteenth and early nineteenth centuries, hairwork remained a fashionable item. In 1853, a fashion writer of a popular women's magazine reported that "many novel and elegant designs for brooches, bracelets, &c., have been introduced. Among the most remarkable productions in the beautiful art of hairworking, is a set wrought with small globes, resembling beads of various sizes. These globes are transparent, and are wrought in a style of such exquisite delicacy that they seem to be made of the finest lace."[3]

Another issue of that magazine noted in the same year that "hair ornaments of jewelry were never more in favor than at the present time."[4] Hair's aesthetic and plastic attributes were exploited by skilled artisans. For example, the texture and colors of woven hair were used to create pleasing patterns and even to complement more common jewels. For example, in 1858 one writer effused that "hair jewelry may be said to have arrived at perfection. We have just seen a bracelet, the band of which is formed of a plait of light, silky hair, and the clasp, which is of blue enamel, is set with fine pearls in a most tasteful and elaborate design. Another clasp, destined for a bracelet of dark hair, is of ruby enamel set with small diamonds."[5] Some of these new forms could be quite elaborate and expensive. In 1859, for example, there were "NEW STYLES OF JEWELRY.—Many novelties are *bijouterie*, in which hair forms a part, have recently appeared. Bracelets composed of hair are studded with jewels. Brooches are encircled in a framework of richly wrought gold, ornamented with pearls. Some very elegant ear-rings have been formed of hair and turquoise."[6]

How Hairwork Was Made

Even when paired with the most expensive jewels, hairwork still denoted sentimentality. It took a highly trained and skilled professional to create these elaborate pieces and the increasing popularity of a sentimental market goods heightened the demand for commercially produced hairwork. Hairwork was not made by machine, it was made by hand, and by skilled hands at that. In fact, hairwork's value as an object of sentiment came in part from the fact that it *was* hand-produced. From the 1850s to at least the 1880s, hairworkers thrived in large urban areas such as Philadelphia, New York City, and Chicago, as well as in small towns throughout the country.

In 1862, Mark Campbell, a prominent hairwork dealer and author, noted proudly that "it is only a few years since the first introduction of Hair Jewelry as an article of commerce."[7] He had his chronology wrong, of course. And while the hairworkers of the 1850s and 1860s introduced several innovations such as mail-order services, most hairwork jewelry in the country was still made by hand, by craftswomen and craftsmen in small independent shops and manufactories similar to those of the eighteenth century. (Most hairwork parlor decorations, however, were made at home by amateurs.) In fact, until the 1870s, almost all jewelry, not just hairwork, was made by hand in the United States. The technology for machine-based production of jewelry simply did not exist until then, and even after machine dies and cutters were introduced, jewelry manufacturers continued to use small-batch production techniques.[8] For the hairworkers, then, the threat was not machine production; their greatest challenge was something beyond their control—their customers' perception of whether hairwork was stylish (that is, closely aligned with the market), and yet intimate enough to be sentimental. As long as hairwork was seen as both fashionable and sincere, hair workers would find an audience for their trade.

Both professional and amateur (that is, women making hairwork not for wages but as a hobby or home craft) hairworkers depended on the same published instructions to create hairwork. Most professional hairworkers apprenticed or trained under an artisan, as in the eighteenth century, but, by the 1850s and 1860s, even professionals could rely on books and magazines to help guide them. Mark Campbell of Chicago; the National Artistic Hair Work Company, also of Chicago; and others published instructions for the trade and for home crafters. Women's magazines, such as *Godey's Lady's Book and Magazine*, also provided serial instructions for their audiences. Thus, both popular magazines and craft books were sources of techniques and styles for professional hair workers.

For a professional hairworker, the trade was in hair jewelry, not parlor decorations. Hair jewelry was not particularly difficult to create, but its production was tedious, time-consuming, and required specialized training in order to be efficient. The procedure for making hair jewelry was the same for amateurs and professionals. First, most hair-jewelry instructions suggested that the hair be cleaned before being worked. *Cassell's Household Guide* earnestly recommended that "all hair in its natural state will be found to be more or less greasy and dirty, and should therefore undergo a thorough purifying before being made use of."[9] This ritualistic purification probably related more to the eventual use of the jewelry than any necessary step in its manufacture, for most hair-wreath directions skipped this step. Indeed, *Godey's Lady's Book and Magazine* noted that "hair, as it is cut from a person's head, provided it be not very greasy, is in a fit state to work with at once."[10]

But *Godey's* immediately followed this with detailed instructions for cleaning the hair. Most recipes for doing this involved water, washing soda, and borax. After soaking the hair in this mixture, the hair was well rinsed and dried. More complicated instructions involved "drawing" the hair by laying it flat and pressing the dirt and grease off of it. Both palette-worked and table-worked hair was to be cleaned before being worked. While cleaning the hair may have made it easier to work with, the ritual was also related to the future intimate contact between the jewelry and the wearer's body.

The two specific techniques for making hair jewelry were palette-working and table-working. Palette-worked hair resulted in pictures composed of hair glued on a flat surface, while table-worked hair resulted in braids that were either tightly woven into elaborate patterns (similar to hemp bracelets and necklaces popular today) or into more open tubes of woven hair. Both kinds of hairwork were then mounted into jewelry casings. Palette-worked jewelry and table-worked jewelry could be made by amateurs or professionals, but the complexity of jewelry meant that there was a demand for professionally made pieces until the end of the nineteenth century.

Palette-worked hair required several tools that could "be bought at some shops . . . but the articles are so simple that such an outlay is by no means necessary."[11] Tools included a "palette," a flat hard working surface made of china or glass. This could form the base of the actual jewelry, and

Mrs. C. S. Jones recommended to her amateur hair workers that "it is well to procure one of the tablets used by the regular hair-workers, or opaque glass, upon which to affix the device." In addition to the palette or ground, an aspiring palette worker would need scissors, curling irons (metal sticks resembling knitting needles), a knife, pliers, a "spatula" or flat razor blade, and camel's hair brushes. Gum glue and gold-beaters' skin would also be required. Finally, for adding decorative touches, a hairworker might need fine annealed wire, artificial pearl beads, India ink, watercolor tints, and metal beads.[12]

The hair was smoothed flat and laid on top of a piece of gold-beaters' skin that had been moistened with gum arabic.[13] Once these squares of glued hair dried, they could be cut into geometric shapes that could then be arranged to form patterns of stars, plaits, or far more elaborate designs, such as crosses, flowers, and leaves. In the 1880s, the National Artistic Hair Work Company even offered dies to aid hairworkers. These were metal shapes that could cut the glued hair into the desired shapes (much like a cookie cutter) of leaves, flowers, and symbols. The patterns did not have to be flat because the hairpieces could be affixed on edge to achieve a three-dimensional effect. To create an even more elaborate appearance, Jones suggested that "the hair of several persons, and of different colors, may be beautifully arranged, so that the contrasting colors will produce an artistic effect." Combining hair was also a useful sentimental technique. As *Cassell's Household Guide* stated, the "pretty effect" that resulted when several colors of hair were used "will sometimes increase the sentimental interest of the ornament." *Cassell's* suggested that the greatest sentimental impact came "when the hair of a husband and wife, mother and child, or that of the different brothers and sisters of a family, is used together."[14] Thus the manufacturing technique had a role in the affective purpose of sentimental hairwork.

Another palette-worked technique was hair painting. Hair painting was literally painting with hair. The hair was ground up, mixed with glue, and painted into designs. Hair painting had been popular in the eighteenth century and had been used to back miniature paintings.[15] The National Artistic Hair Work Company called for "gum of tushmer," which one researcher has suggested was "gum water" that was produced by companies around the country.[16] Most examples of hair painting used hair as a pigment, and even finer details such as fences, the sides of tombstones, and the like, were delineated using straight, single hairs. Often, glue was simply spread in the desired shape and finely chopped hair sprinkled on top to create a "whiskery" look.

A third palette-worked technique was hair feathers, or what was known as Prince-of-Wales feathers. The hair was smoothed flat and then wrapped around the curling iron. The body of the iron was heated until the curl was set. Then the curl was fixed with glue and weighted flat for several hours. This produced a flat, flaring curl. Three of these curls arranged together constituted the Prince-of-Wales style. Usually these feathers were mounted in a small, oval jewelry frame to create a brooch.

All three palette-worked techniques produced relatively small-scale hairwork, although large "pictures" of hair were possible. The completed project was affixed to a glass or an ivory base and mounted in brooches, pins, and rings. Alexanna Speight recommended in 1872 that instead of the typical black-bordered brooch frame, hairworkers try "plain or burnished gold" and even consider "at all events in their earlier efforts . . . our artist [should] dispense with any mounting in jewelry at all, but place the work in an ordinary frame."[17]

Table-worked hair required a very different technique than palette-worked hair, and its steps echoed the artisanal roots of the craft. Table-worked hair was hair braided into flat or cylindrical lengths that were then used for everything from rings, necklaces, and earrings to fobs, watch chains, brooches, and stickpins. *Godey's Lady's Book and Magazine* suggested that an "ingenious hair-worker will think of many little domestic articles which could be either made of hair or ornamented with it." For example, *Godey's* helpfully continued, one could make hair "bracelets, brooches, ear-rings, rings, chains, necklaces, shawl-pins, cravat-pins, purses, bags, book-markers, pencil-cases, guards, studs, stud-chains, scent-bottles, walking-sticks, and riding-whips."[18]

Whatever might be produced, the tools required were not, at least according to *Godey's*, expensive. "To do the finest, most delicate, and most beautiful descriptions of hair-work, nothing is wanted which is not already in every one's possession."[19] First, a braiding table was needed. Thrifty *Godey's* recommended a bandbox, but most writers suggested an actual, albeit small, table. The round top of either needed to have a hole cut in its center. In addition to the table, a hairworker would need thread, scissors, knitting needles, weights (Campbell required wood and lead bobbins, but *Godey's* made do with pennies), and hair.

The hair was separated into sections of equal numbers of strands, and then into subsections whose number depended on the complexity of the pattern. For example, to braid a standard "snake chain," one of the most common braids, Campbell instructed readers to "take thirty-two strands, or any number that can be divided by four, twelve hairs in a strand, and sixty strands for usual size [of finished braid]."[20] Although hair could be spliced to make it an adequate length, this was a challenge for inexperienced hairworkers. Each of these strands was weighted on one end with the bobbins and arranged with the bobbin ends hanging off the outer edge of the table. The opposite ends of all the strands were tied together, weighted with a bobbin, and hung through the table's center hole. Each strand was numbered and placed along a circular chart that rested on top of the braiding table, and the hairworker simply moved the strands over other strands, repeating all steps of movement precisely, and a regular braid emerged in the center of the table.

Cotton or elastic cord often was used as the center of the braid and, sometimes, although not always, removed after the braiding was completed. Once the braid had reached its desired length, *Peterson's Magazine* and other directions instructed that it "must now be immersed in scalding water, and suffered to remain there for ten minutes" or so.[21] The hair was then dried either in open air or in front of a warm stove.

Hair could be braided over wood forms that were inserted into the emerging braid and, again, when the braid was finished (and pregnant with its encased forms), it was boiled and dried and the forms were squeezed out. This produced a braid shaped as the mold was, and usually the braid was an "open-work" net. Molds in the shapes of acorns, drops, crosses, and the like were usually made of wood. Cylindrical molds (to form the open, tubular shapes that were mounted, for instance, on the sides of a brooch frame) could be made, as *Godey's* recommended, with plain metal knitting needles or lengths of brass wire. Iron and steel, readers were warned, would rust in the boil bath. An openwork piece, however, did not always need to have a mold, since the hair could simply be braided to take on the desired shape.[22] A popular molded style was a "bead" necklace where the hair looked like a joined length of separate beads. Actually, this style was made by braiding the hair around a series of consecutive round wood beads. The necklace, with the beads still inside, was boiled and dried, and then the forms were carefully squeezed out. A small gold band was clipped around the connecting "link" of narrower hair between each round shape, and the entire necklace was mounted on jewelry clasps. The necklace now looked like a string of hair beads.

How Hairwork Was Purchased

Most hairwork businesses were small-scale enterprises that made standard pieces of hair jewelry, albeit by custom orders, such as breastpins and, later, watch chains. In 1859, C. Linherr of New York City wrote a receipt for a Miss Colgate, who had purchased a hair breastpin for six dollars. T. A. Linherr, his brother, could provide "Every description of Ornaments made in Hair," including "Hair Designs for Albums."[23] In 1866 in Philadelphia, Madame K. Schmitt advertised her hairwork manufactory. Her business was a one-woman effort at this point (she was in business in Philadelphia until 1900, and in later years employed several young women and family members), as she notified the public "that I have REMOVED my Hair Jewelry Manufactory to my old stand" that was located in a glove store.[24] Robert Link and his brother were "Artists in Hair and Jewelers" in New York City. "Being desirous of obtaining the good will of the public, it shall be their aim," they promised in an advertisement, "to make not only a superior in style [*sic*], but a durable article, at reasonable prices."[25]

These hair workers advertised in local newspapers, and even local entrepreneurs exploited the combination of fashion and sentiment that made hairwork so popular in the 1850s and 1860s. Vincent Brandly, an "artist in Hair and Jewelry," advertised in New York City's *Le Bon Ton*: "Citizens:—Would you have Hair Setting and Hair Braiding executed in the most chaste and skillful designs? Would you, friends, preserve the hair of living or deceased relatives as mementos of your affection? . . . You answer "Yes," to all these questions. Then call at once on VINCENT BRANDLY."[26]

Brandly excelled at selling the *idea* of hairwork. He promised affection in a material form. He understood that hairwork appealed to customers because it was unique, fashionable, and sentimental.

While some customers, especially those in urban areas, may have visited a hair jeweler in person, most people probably ordered their jewelry from their local jeweler, who then sent the order (including the hair provided by the customer) on to an actual hairworker. Most customers had no idea that their hairwork order was subcontracted out by their jeweler. In fact, retail jewelers often used other workers to complete miscellaneous tasks in addition to hairwork. For example, Samuel Parrott, keeping a small jewelry store in Philadelphia in the 1860s, used both a "jobber" to do repairs, and a hairworker for his hair-jewelry orders. On July 28, 1863, Parrott paid three dollars to William E. McCale for "repairing jewelry," and in February 1864, Parrott made another payment to McCale of $13.80 "in full for jobbing jewelry" for, among other items, the repair of several watchcases. The next month, Parrott paid F.T. Dressler four dollars "for hair jewelry."[27] Parrott recorded payments in April and March of 1864 to F. T. Dressler, and on April 4, 1867, Dressler received $11.37 from Parrot "in full for hair jewelry." On August 6, 1867, it was ten dollars to Dressler from Parrott, again for "hair jewelry."[27] Parrott, then, used separate contract workers for different kinds of business. McCale, a jobber, completed repairwork for Parrott, while Dressler provided Parrott with the hair jewelry Parrott had sold from his own shop. Did Parrott's customers know about these arrangements? It is unlikely. The customers would have brought the hair to be used to Parrott's shop, selected a style from a design book, and left the hair to be worked. The fact that Parrott himself did not actually create the hair jewelry probably went unnoticed.

Independent hairworkers (even those bereft of a store) did not have their livelihoods threatened when mail-order hairwork appeared in the 1850s. If anything, mail-order services increased the demand for the products. Whether ordered from the hairworker him- or herself, subcontracted by a retail jeweler, or subcontracted by a mail-order house, the jewelry still needed to be hand worked by a trained worker. The intricate styles of hair jewelry popular in these decades ensured that.

The first mass marketer and large mail-order dealer of hair jewelry was the women's magazine, *Godey's Lady's Book and Magazine*.[28] As *Godey's* remarked, hairwork, "hitherto almost exclusively confined to professed manufacturers of hair trinkets," was now available (through *Godey's* publication of instructions and through its mail order service) to everyone.[29] Mail order was a popular way for women in smaller towns and rural areas to attain fashionable items and to avoid the high prices at local retailers. Many years later, in 1887, Marion Edmonds Roe, in a column titled "How to Dress Well on a Small Allowance," criticized the high prices at local retail establishments. "In buying at country stores, you get about forty cents' worth of goods for each dollar expended, while in buying of large dealers, you get your money's worth." She informed her readers that "shopping by mail is one of the blessings of the age to women who wish to dress tastefully."[30] And it was seen this way by women in the 1850s as well as in the 1880s.

Godey's trafficked in mail-order items from 1852 on. In November 1854, the magazine began offering hair jewelry made to order. That *Godey's* began to offer such a service was not inconsequential for the continuing popularity of hairwork. By the Civil War period, *Godey's* boasted over

150,000 subscribers, and estimates of actual readership are much higher because of the prevalence of "buying clubs" and shared copies of issues.[31]

Godey's did not simply suggest hairwork as one possible good to be ordered. *Godey's* actively promoted hairwork by publishing fiction that relied on hairwork as a motif, and by featuring hairwork as a fashionable accessory. For example, in July 1854 *Godey's* presented a fashion-plate illustration of two young women in off-shoulder evening dresses. As was *Godey's* method, the plate was accompanied with a careful description of every visible component of the outfits. The first figure wore a blue taffeta evening dress with a heart-shaped bodice and a "light hair necklace and gold cross about the throat."[32] Of course, in this issue, as in every issue, the magazine also promoted its mail-order business of selling jewelry, hair jewelry, patterns, cloth, and assorted goods. And such marketing strategies worked. Following on the heels of *Godey's* fashion plate in July, in November 1854 the "Philadelphia Agency" listed for the first time two hairwork orders. "A.V.R.—Sent hair necklace by mail 29th," and "N.P.S.—Sent hair bracelets by mail 23rd."[33]

Godey's provided images of the kinds of hairwork it could supply, complete with prices. In January 1857, they published illustrations of a hair breastpin and a rotund hair bracelet, priced at seven dollars and four dollars, respectively. The following month *Godey's* provided a complete price list that offered seven different styles, ranging in price from $1.50 to $15.00. By 1857, *Godey's* was conducting a brisk business in hairwork and, in April 1857, the magazine listed twenty-nine orders that were filled.[34]

Godey's apparently received the hair loose in an envelope, with a precise description or drawing of the style desired. One careless customer left the magazine at a loss. In October 1857, the author of the "Philadelphia Agency" list exasperatedly wrote, "Will the person who sent us a draft for thirty-two dollars in one letter, and some hair in another, please write us as soon as they see this?"[35]

As noted earlier, *Godey's* also specialized in providing instructions for fancywork such as hairwork. These how-to directions did not undermine the magazine's mail-order business; in fact, they probably encouraged it. For example, many of the books that promoted hairwork were offered by *Godey's* at the same time that it was providing hairwork by mail order. In February 1862, *Godey's* notified its readers that "messrs. J. E. Tilton and Co., Boston, . . . are publishers of that valuable illustrated guide to drawing of all varieties, called "Art Recreations," which they will also send, post-paid, on receipt of price, $1.50."[36] This was Levina Urbino's book, and it presented instructions for crafts ranging from taxidermy to hairworking. In October 1862, *Godey's* offered for $1.25 copies of "Martha Pullen's" (Matilda Pullan's) *The Ladies' Manual of Fancy Work*, a book of instructions for palette-worked hair. Making one's hairwork one's self ensured a sentimental value, even if the final product wasn't as pretty or refined as those professionally made.

The Market of Human Hair

The presence of the human hair market directly interfered with the business of hair workers. In February 1858, *Godey's*, the major national retailer of hairwork in that decade, informed readers that "we don't purchase hair to make hair-ornaments. This answer will do for about a dozen inquiries."[37] What were customers asking about? There were two possibilities: either customers were concerned that the company would substitute ready-made hairwork for that requested, or customers assumed that the company would supply market hair with which to create the hairwork. The presupposition that Godey's trafficked in human hair bought on the market undermined the sentimental premise of *Godey's* hairwork business: that it was not like the rest of the market of goods.

The popularity of hairwork rested on an uneasy balance between its role as a commercial product (and, hence, one of fashion) and as a sentimental good (and, thus, immune to the vagaries of fashion). There was also the problem, and it was a problem, that hair itself was a market commodity, bought and sold like other raw materials. Human hair was sold in bales or lots, as hemp or cotton might be. And then there was the wig and artificial-hair market, for which much of that "raw" hair was sold, which was an even greater threat to the market of sentimental hairwork because artificial-hair accroutements were personal items made of other people's hair. Finally, the wig trade's affiliation with theatrical products challenged the sentimental connotations of hair jewelry because the pretense of the theater was a metaphor for the superficiality of fashionable life itself.

In 1860, the *English Cyclopaedia* outlined the market of human hair. It described the "young women in England, who have beautiful tresses, [who] are sometimes urged by poverty to part with them for money to the hair-workers." The *Cyclopaedia* distinguished between the wig-making industry that relied on bought hair and the "minor manufactures of human hair." For hair jewelry and the like, "no hair-harvest is necessary for a supply of materials; the ordinary clippings are sufficient."[38] That did not really answer the question, though, since it was suggested that it was still sold hair that was used to make hair jewelry.

Selling their hair was a tempting option to make at least a bit of money for some American women. In 1863, Virginia Penny listed "growers" [of hair] as one occupation open to women in her review of women's work. She suggested that women might, as some young European women do, line up, sell their hair to the highest bidder, and the "hair then, after being cut as closely as possible to the head, is weighed and paid for, and the girl goes home to let another suit grow out for shearing time."[39] Louisa May Alcott famously depicted a more traumatic, albeit fictional, moment of selling one's hair in her novel, *Little Women*. As the March family's fortunes dwindled in the face of the father being absent at war, Jo sold her hair for money to contribute twenty-five dollars—a sizable sum in the mid-1860s. Asked where she could have possibly earned so much money, "Jo took off her bonnet, and a general outcry arose, for all her abundant hair was cut short." Jo vividly described the scene of her hair sale to her horror-struck family. "In a barber's window I saw tails of hair with the prices marked; and one black tail, not so thick as mine, was forty dollars. It came over me all of a sudden that I had one thing to make money out of, and without stopping to think, I walked in, asked if they bought hair, and what they would give for mine." Drawn in by the display of hair and a calculus of value, Jo bargained the sale of a part of her. Asking the barber if he would buy her hair, the barber "rather stared. . . . He said he didn't care for mine, it wasn't the fashionable colour, and he never paid much for it in the first place; the work put into it made it dear."[40] Jo learned where the "true" value of hair lies: the hair itself was relatively worthless. The object of value was the worked hair, in this case, hair worked into artificial hairpieces such as wigs or the switch Jo had seen in the window. Artificial hairwork was a commodity, and like other manufactured goods, it could be marked down in price. In 1872, Mrs. S. W. Holbrook advertised that "I propose to sell the best human hair goods, of all kinds, for 60 Days! without regard to cost! . . . Now is your time to purchase hair goods! At half the Regular price!"[41] Thus was the potential fate of Jo's hair.

Alcott dramatized what must have been the experience of at least a few women in America. Most discussions about hair selling, and where hair for wigs came from, argued that it was Europeans who sold their hair for the market. For example, Virginia Penny advised that "most of the hair made up in [America] is bought in France and Italy."[42] However, in the United

States, some wig makers advertised their willingness to buy hair. For instance, Francis Bailey informed customers that "raw hair [was] purchased at the Highest Cash Prices."[43]

Once the hair was bought, it was transported to large cities, such as London, Paris, New York, or Chicago. The hair was warehoused and sold to individual wig makers. In an 1869 article that ran in various English publications, the author described a hair warehouse. "The place, in fact, was redolent of hair. There was hair in all the drawers, hair in cardboard boxes, hair hanging from the ceiling and clinging to the walls, hair upon the counters, upon the chairs, and in the very inkstand; there was even hair in the air itself, moving about as it were in clouds, which when you agitated them disagreeably caressed you."[44]

The hair warehouse was the site of the bizarre contrast of the commodity of hair, stored in piles, bags, and drawers for resale, and the inescapably intimate character of hair itself. Hair used for such a purpose seemed both distressingly "dead," hung from the ceiling like recently butchered animals, and yet animated as it "disagreeably caressed" our narrator, the walls, chairs, and the inkstand. This was a nightmare vision for nineteenth-century sentimentalists, for here hair was cruelly dissociated from its owner and from any possible sentimental meaning. The hair was merely the leavings of the uncaring market.

Thomas Gardner, a hair-goods dealer, represented the ways in which the boundaries between sentimental hairwork and artificial hairwork could be blurred. In an advertisement, Gardner boasted that his business was "the oldest established hair goods manufactory in the state, established in 1837." He sold wigs, various kinds of artificial hairpieces, and "hair jewelry in the most fashionable styles."[45] In addition to these goods, Gardner offered disguises of several kinds, such as "theatrical wigs, beards, moustaches and imperials [both] on hand and made to order." And customers found "costumes to rent for balls and private parties . . . [and] masks in great variety, clown sticks, grease paints and burnt cork."[46] Gardner's advertisement conflated three different areas of ornamentation: wigs, sentimental hair jewelry, and theatrical costumes (Figure 8).

Gardner's offerings also indicate a shift in middle-class culture's relationship to sentimentality. In the 1850s and 1860s, private parlor theatricals were very popular. In contradiction to the emphasis on sincerity and sentimentality of the 1840s and 1850s, these parlor-room plays dramatically represented the "new worldliness" of middle-class culture. Private theatricals focused on elaborate special effects and melodramatic actions, such as ex-

112 HOUSEHOLD GUIDE.

GEORGETOWN (D. C.) Pop., 12,598; Dist. from N. Y., 230 m.; Take Penn. R. R., then B. & O.

The Oldest Established

HAIR GOODS MANUFACTORY

IN THE STATE.

ESTABLISHED IN 1837.

Ladies' Wigs, Half Wigs, Bandeaux, Back Hair Waves, Saratoga Waves, Newport Waves, Langtry Frizzes and Switches

In Great Variety. Also

HAIR JEWELRY IN THE MOST FASHIONABLE STYLES

Gents' Wigs, Toupees, Theatrical Wigs, Beards, Moustaches and Imperials on hand and made to order.

COSTUMES

To Rent for Balls and Private Parties. Costume Trimmings, Gilt and Silver Bullion Fringe, Tassels, Stars, Laces, Cords, Braids, Spangles, &c.

MASKS IN GREAT VARIETY,

Clown Sticks, Grease Paints and Burnt Cork.

THOMAS GARDNER,

104 Orange Street, - NEW HAVEN, CONN.

GREENWICH (Conn.) Pop., 7,965; Dist. from N. Y., 28 m.; Time 1 h Fare, $0.71; Adams Ex. Take N. Y., N. H. & H. R. R.

Figure 8. Sentimental hairwork and artificial hairwork (that is, wigs) coexisted but not happily. Thomas Gardner's undated advertisement for wigs and costumes reveals just why nineteenth-century Americans associated wigs and hairpieces with hypocrisy and insincerity. Sentimental hairwork asserted the "true" self, but artificial hairwork attempted to disguise who one really was (thin hair and all). Advertisement, courtesy Warshaw Collection of Business Americana, Archives Center, National Museum of American History, Smithsonian Institution.

pressing love by "kissing a miniature or embracing a lock of hair," and suggested that all behavior was, at its roots, artificial.[47]

At the same time, theatricals and costuming recalled the constant threat of fakery and deception. Sentimental hairwork, because it provided for so many layers of apparently authentic sentimental expression, experienced sustained popularity because of its supposed antagonism to the vagaries of fashion. So Gardner's advertisement was a contradiction in terms in many ways. By implicitly suggesting that hair jewelry was similar to masks and greasepaints, Gardner raised a troubling issue. Was hairwork equivalent to the blatant insincerity of costuming?

Hairwork as a Gift

In the 1850s and 1860s, hair jewelry was a common gift. In the nineteenth century, the meaning of gift giving shifted as goods were increasingly manufactured and as participation in the market intensified. In the face of a growing consumerism, gift giving offered the possibility of a more intimate level of attaining and possessing objects, because a gift was what another had personally prepared or selected, purchased, and endowed on the recipient. Hairwork, and especially hair jewelry, traditionally was a gift to others, and that practice continued throughout the nineteenth century. But just as hairwork was an unlikely commodity, so it was also an uneasy gift—in part, because gifts were transformed commodities. When objects were given as gifts, the transaction attempted to mutate a common good into a personal possession. With the rise of mass-produced, market goods, gift giving provided a way to personalize commodities through the acts of selection and endowment.[48] Commodities derived their value in part from their abstract existence. Their alienation from the human labor required for their production meant that a stable, unchanging value could be attached to them. But such anonymity required some sort of personalization to become a truly valuable, personal possession. To be given something and to accept that gift as an offering of a person's feeling for you was to fully appropriate the object. Thus, gift giving transformed objects into possessions through the process of giving and thus provided an effective remedial check on the impersonal nature of commodities themselves. But whenever the meaning of an object shifted, as it did through the transaction between individuals (as an object becomes a *gift*), the danger existed that the object might be rendered meaningless and, hence, emptied of value as an object able to transcend the market's distant and abstract designations.

In addition, some kinds of things simply made "bad commodities." Objects with personal histories and identities resisted fixed values and pricing and made for uncertain transactions. Part of the difficulty was that "bad commodities" were those things whose immaterial values rested tenuously in the material itself.[49]

Ironically, such "bad commodities" made wonderful gifts. But like other "bad commodities," hairwork as a gift posed as many difficulties as it did remedies. Hair jewelry and other hairwork were of unstable value because the sentimental and emotional characteristics of hairwork were not inherent in the material used despite the concerted effort on the part of middle-class culture (in the form of periodicals, poems, short stories, and advertisements) to argue that they were. Sentimentality's role in stabilizing the values of certain kinds of commodities (such as hairwork, photographs, and other "gift-like" objects) was to link the self with the object. Sentimentality provided an emotional mechanism that associated goods with individuals in a seemingly indelible and lasting fashion. Hairwork was a principal device of sentimental consumerism, for its meaning stemmed from the association of the individual (through the hair) and the emotions that hair represented (which were sentimental). Despite these attempts to affix meaning to the object, hairwork, as with other forms of sentimental goods, could lose its close affiliation with the self and the emotions it was supposed to embody. Even as a gift, hairwork proved fluid in its representation of relationships between individuals.

Gifts represented the identities of both the giver and the receiver, and this intimate relationship between object and human suggested that *how* an object was produced was indeed important.[50] If handmade, and thus directly a product of human action, a gift could be supposed to be more closely related to the individuals involved. But by the end of the nineteenth century, handmade gifts were less common than before, and most gifts were more likely to be manufactured and purchased. This shift from handmade to manufactured gifts occurred gradually throughout the nineteenth century. In the face of a preponderance of manufactured gifts beginning around 1880 to 1900, "the symbolic messages conveyed by handmade gift items were intrinsically superior to those conveyed by manufactured ones."[51]

Handmade gifts were considered more expressive of the self because they were simultaneously a gift of the time it took to make the object and of the actual self that "had a hand" in its production. Handmade gifts were also distanced from the detached values of the market.[52] At the same time, gift giving was meant to erase the presence of the market and allow the "true characters" of the giver and the recipient to be revealed through the transaction and through the gift. For this reason, historians have argued that gift giving became a more integral practice among the middle class as the reach of the market expanded.[53]

Hairwork, of course, was an ideal gift, for while it was handmade and of the bodily self, its role as a sentimental good meant that the market recognized the value of hairwork as a commodity. The affiliations of hairwork with the market needed to be balanced by the overt sentimental meaning of hairwork. In the short story, "Gift-Making," from *Godey's* in 1857, Mrs. Cooper wished to buy the perfect Christmas gift for her husband. She used a variety of methods to overcome the impersonal market, but she failed spectacularly.[54] She and her husband had read a story about a faithful man who died wearing his beloved's hair as a band on his arm. Mrs. Cooper, inspired by the romance of the tale, planned on having a similar band made of her own hair for her husband. Being thrifty, she had already made a fancy braid herself, and this should, if all goes well, ensure the personal significance of the gift. She took her braided hair to the local jeweler. Explaining in detail the kind of armband she desired, the "principal of the large Broadway establishment which she turned to" argued it would be very expensive. Besides, he pointed out, her braid "will wear very easily in this style" as he "produced several specimens of fanciful hair-work from a drawer close by."

Mrs. Cooper was increasingly worried that the jeweler did not understand the style she desired, and he wouldn't answer her plea for a promise that he "be very sure [the hair braid] not be touched." Pressed for time, she finally acceded to his demand that she "leave it to his taste and judgment." She did and, to her ultimate dismay, the final gift, wrapped securely and presented to her husband and unseen by his harried wife, was not greeted with joy. Rather, Mr. Cooper exclaimed as he opened the box, "Hallo, Matty! what's this? a dog-collar?!" And indeed, the gold encrusted monstrosity "would have encircled the brawny arm of "the village blacksmith"; and, as for all sentimental associations, the "dog-collar" had nipped them in the bud."[55] As a final insult, the "dog-collar" was accompanied with a bill of $37.75—far out of the reach of the moderate Mrs. Cooper.

Mrs. Cooper eventually sold the gold back to the jeweler and had to forfeit her hair as well. In the end, "Mr. and Mrs. Cooper exchanged only a very fond kiss, and the promise that even in gift-making they would hereafter let appropriateness and thoughtful consideration stand in the place of lavish expenditure."

For the knowledgeable audience of *Godey's*, Mrs. Cooper made several errors that doomed the success of her gift-giving attempt. While she had done well to braid the hair herself, she allowed the market to interfere too much in the remaining portion of the manufacture of the gift. Hairwork, even when made by the hand of the giver, could still be marred by the market, here in the form of an uncaring, avaricious jeweler whose eye and heart were not focused on the fine sentiment of the gift but on profit and monetary value. Mrs. Cooper's efforts were complicated by the fact that the jeweler was male, because his insistence relied in part on the prerogative of masculinity over Mrs. Cooper's more accommodating femininity. Interestingly, the moral of the tale suggests that women, as nascent consumers, must be more assertive for their own—and their families'—interests.[56]

Even when made into a highly unique form ("what's this? a dog-collar?"), hairwork still required the distance from the market that commodities—and especially the self commodified, as Mrs. Cooper's hair literally was (at the cost of $37.75)—could sometimes simply not reach. Because of Mrs. Cooper's inability to keep the market at bay, her gift of herself is a failure. Although she received a piece of hairwork that was certainly unique and undeniably a part of herself, it nonetheless fell short in its lack of sentiment, its taint of the market, and its shortcomings as a true expression of her love and consideration for her husband.

Mrs. Cooper's attempts to create the perfect gift failed, but perhaps her effort was inevitably doomed. Perhaps, the story suggests, one can never really give of oneself, truly, through an object. Even when a gift is a part of oneself, it is vulnerable to mishap and distortion. In the end, Mrs. Cooper and her husband satisfied themselves with "only a very fond kiss." The qualifier "only" is fitting, for, as the last lines conclude, Mrs. and Mr. Cooper did not intend to never participate in the market of goods. Rather, they vowed to be more careful, and to value "appropriateness and thoughtful consideration . . . in the place of lavish expenditure." While cautionary, their dilemma could be resolved by a more self-conscious participation in the act of selecting, buying, and consuming commodities.

Hair jewelry was commonly used as a gift because hairwork and, in particular, hair jewelry, was a fluid good whose meaning could shift from being a "product" to a "present" to a "possession." One reason for this was that hairwork was seen as a commercial product of fashion and as a sentimental token. It was a valued gift because the market valued it, and the market valued it because it was manufactured by hand and heart.

Hairwork and the Photographic Image

Hairwork was a way for individuals to represent themselves to others in the form of a gift. Nineteenth-century middle-class Americans found an ever-increasing variety of ways to represent the self to others, through photography, for example, which was invented in 1839. Commodified likenesses of the physical self were an effective means of negotiating between the demands of the market and the need to retain a sense of integrity of the self. Hairwork and photography were two of the more common methods of presenting another person with a likeness of one's self. They served quite different purposes of self-representation, however.

One of the attractions of having a photographic image taken was that photographs were the self unadorned. Photographic likenesses simply presented an image of one's true appearance, and thus marked a return to the eighteenth-century ideal of the sincere self. But that image was often more harshly revealing than was comfortable for the depicted individual or the onlookers. It is important to note that the popularity of hairwork did not wane as photographic images became more readily available. Indeed, all evidence suggests that hairwork gained market presence as photographic likenesses were introduced. Why? The popular understanding of photography may have been a factor. As one writer observed, "Photographs are not, in the highest sense, art. . . . They are at best mechanical products."[57] Hairwork was a product of hands *and* emotions, and it was therefore understood as a truer representation of one's self.

Two examples of how nineteenth-century Americans thought about hairwork and photography as a gift are instructive. Sarah Heywood resorted to hair jewelry when her photographic likenesses repeatedly disappointed her. Rachel Cormany, however, was well satisfied with her fiancé Samuel's gift of a daguerreotype. How each of these women discussed her role in the gift exchange illustrates how photography could satisfy and disappoint its participants.

In a series of letters to her fiancé, William Folwell, Sarah Heywood detailed the pitfalls photography's consumers encountered. Her solution was to present William with both a photographic image and a watch chain made of her hair. Her reactions to the many attempts at securing a decent photographic image of herself reveal how photography challenged her desire to convey not only "reality" but her emotions.

Sarah Heywood was engaged to William Watts Folwell in 1860. They had met in 1859, and Folwell noted in his diary that "there was something about her looks and manner that affected me, and I got leave to call."[58] Soon after they became engaged, William's parents offered him a two-year tour of Europe, which he joyfully, if a bit callously, accepted.

Sarah Heywood was enamored of her "dear Will," as she addressed him in her many letters. After an unhappy childhood, she glowed in her letters to William, basked in the knowledge of someone else caring for her, and referred to herself often as "your own dear child." With William soon leaving for his long absence, Sarah searched for a way to physically substantiate the emotional attachment they shared.

Sarah had an ambrotype made for William to take on his journey, but she was discontented with the image. "You're are [sic] very foolish," she chastised Will, "to show that ugly picture of me, I do not think your relatives will ever accuse you of marrying for beauty, but, I flatter myself. I am not quite so ugly as that ambrotype."[59] Three days later, Sarah wrote Will that she has "had a colored ambrotype taken for you, which I would like to send you, also . . . I had three pictures taken but everyone thinks, this, the best likeness they ever saw of me—I hope it will please you."[60] While the image may or may not have pleased William, it certainly failed to fulfill Sarah's own needs at self-representation. She wrote William a few weeks after having sent the picture, which had at the time satisfied, but now, having shown her ambrotype around, "Miss Mary agrees with Auntie, but her sisters, and Mrs. Langdon, say, there is a determined haughty expression about the mouth—which is not natural. My poor unfortunate mouth! which is *naturally* so ugly, it will not take well in a picture. Will, pet, I am afraid you will have to be responsible for some of its *newly acquired* ugliness, for you kissed it's slight beauty all away."[61]

It is on receiving others' reactions that Sarah reevaluated her own perception of the ambrotype. This is, of course, an element of the social function of a photographic image. While nominally a "true" likeness, photography presented a literal image of the self that was metaphorically understood. "There is," reported Sarah, "a determined haughty expression about the mouth—which is not natural." This "flaw" was noticed and remarked on by others, and Sarah conflated the technological interference of the photographic process with a conception of a true likeness—an image natural in its honesty. Somehow, the camera had lied. Yes, Sarah acknowledged, her mouth was "*naturally* ugly," but then again, the camera revealed this so emphatically as to be unnatural.

It's an uncertain venture, then, how a photographic likeness would appear to others. As "natural" as the mouth may appear—and we must assume that, being a photograph, Sarah's mouth was depicted much as it looked on her face—it nonetheless can, and does, look "unnatural." The process of having a photograph taken has been likened to gambling, in that both acts are, in the end, speculative ventures.[62] Sarah, in being photographed, risked being revealed as something more, perhaps, than she is. To be photographed was to risk a too-telling likeness whose claim for truth telling was substantiated by the technological processes that, for Sarah at least, distorted her self.

William's watch fob, as his daughter noted, was "worn all his days." Sarah reached a happy compromise: she gave William a likeness of herself that could be publically displayed, yet protected her from the "all-too-like" qualities of a photograph. She is able to reify the "looks and manners" of her self that first attracted William, while avoiding the "all-too-like" appearance of a photographic likeness. Sarah neatly resolved the problematic venture of commodified likenesses, in that she was able to represent herself without revealing too much of her own character (Figure 9).

In contrast to Sarah's trying experience, Samuel Cormany's gift to his fiancé Rachel Bowman of a daguerreotype was a great success. In her diary, Rachel recorded her enthusiatic response to his gift. "I[t] does me good to look at his miniature [the daguerreotype] only, and infinitely more to look on himself in reality. That miniature is the dearest little thing I ever saw . . . and in my estimation not another man in the world could grace it to better advantage than he. He is good, pretty and smart."[63] Rachel's favorable appraisal certainly satisfied Samuel's goal of maintaining their ties over long distances. Only a few days before Rachel received Samuel's gift, he noted in his diary that he found his leave taking of Rachel after a short visit difficult. Samuel "went over to give the dear one the parting hand—It seems hard to part. . . . and I tarry at Allentown to sit for a Daguerreotype and send back to honey."[64]

Samuel's gift fulfilled another of Rachel's positive evaluations of him. Just after Samuel had left her, she briefly noted in her diary that "I love him so, to me he seems the dearest object on earth. It is so sweet to love and be loved."[65] This sentimental characterization also aptly described Samuel's image. A few days after receiving the daguerreotype, Rachel showed "her Darlings likeness" to a friend. And Samuel's effort to create a living conduit

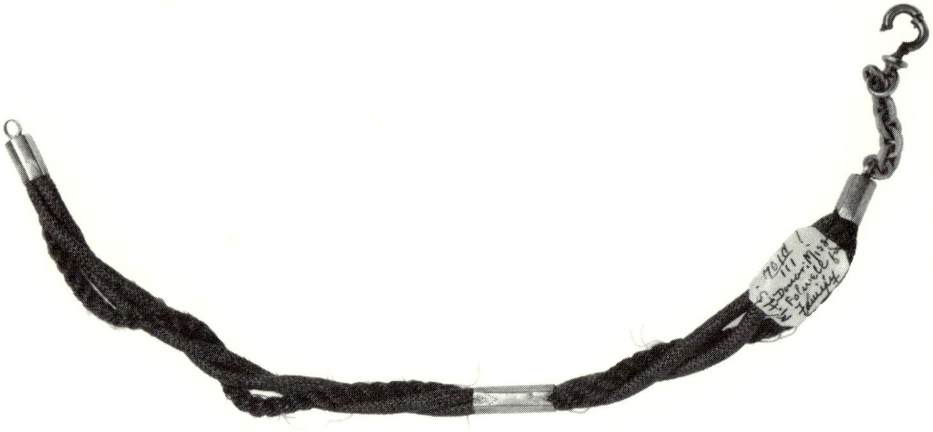

Figure 9. The watch chain that Sarah Heywood made for her fiancé William Folwell is unprepossessing and rather frayed. But that wear was the result of William's use of the watch chain his entire adult life. That, in itself, is testimony that Sarah was able to give William an "image" of herself, embodied both in the hair and in her work creating the chain. Courtesy Minnesota Historical Society.

between himself and his fiancée was also successful, for less than a month later, Rachel had her own "miniature" taken and sent to Samuel.

The concept of a true likeness involved the ability to represent the true authentic interior self. For Samuel, his image evoked his own supposed goodness—as Rachel commented, it "is in such a pretty case. He is good, pretty and smart." The affect of goodness and prettiness was shared, at least in Rachel's eyes, by the daguerreotype and by Samuel himself. In contrast, Sarah Folwell struggled with the supposed haughtiness of her expression. Portrait photographs "serve[d] as a vehicle for expressing the subjectivity of the self to others."[66] For Samuel, this served his purposes and even increased the intensity of his relationship with Rachel. For Sarah, though, the withering comments by Miss Mary, "Auntie," "her sisters," and Mrs. Langdon contributed to her insecurity. Sarah feared that she could not measure up to such disinterested viewing. In a manner, Sarah rendered herself into a portable object so that William can "show that ugly photograph" of her to his relatives. While William himself said that it was "something in her look and manner" that attracted him, Sarah feared that her gamble—her attempt to give William something of herself—could not and would not relay anything other than herself as an object, and in that capacity she would lose the value William had earlier recognized.

Unlike Samuel and Rachel, Sarah was caught in the classic and clichéd horns of a dilemma. Newly engaged and facing a long separation, Sarah wanted William to have an image of her beyond the mental, yet the ambrotypes were simply not suitable. They were too similar to one another. As an alternative self-representation, Sarah Heywood had "an engagement gift made of her own hair" made for William for his journey.[67] The watch chain is an example of the sort of hairwork sold through mass marketers such as Sears and Wards, with pinchbeck findings in a common, unexceptional design. Nothing distinguishes William Folwell's watch fob from the thousands of others made in the latter half of the nineteenth century, except, of course, for its exceptional, individual material—Sarah's hair. In giving William this fob made of herself, Sarah accomplished what the photographic image failed to do. She presented Will with her true self undistorted by any unnatural process.

Mourning and Hairwork in the 1850s and 1860s

The gift of hairwork was intended to be a living conduit between individuals. The hair's filaments would transmit one's self to another, and as the recipient took possession of the gift, he or she accepted the giver's self. Death alone, it would seem, could break the relationship. Hairwork was used to transcend the effects of death as well. Just as gift giving could provide a method of exchange that rose above the rational transactional concerns of the market, mourning offered middle-class Americans during the 1850s and 1860s a way to participate in the market of goods while standing apart from that world.

By the 1850s and 1860s and then throughout the rest of the century, mourning was increasingly expressed through market goods. What were considered to be appropriate, genuine, and sincere expressions of grief were those items that were *marketed* as such. Mourning products that incorporated hair of the deceased and, sometimes the living, had the same advantages that other forms of hairwork enjoyed. Hair was a material of the body, requiring bodily exertion to transform it into a sentimental object. By working the hair into a decorative form, the labor of mourning was rendered explicit and visible. And, finally, by incorporating hair, commercial products were no longer of the market but were creations of the heart.

Nineteenth-century middle-class mourning was a public act replete with commercial goods, specialized dress, and elaborate etiquette. These traditions of mourning were criticized in the 1970s by historian Ann Douglas as "a curious exhibitionism [that] seems to be doing the work formerly expected of self-scrutiny."[68]

Grief was measured by its visible enactment, and its success depended on its public appearance. Mourning, in fact, amplified the expressive power of nineteenth-century hairwork as well as highlighting its ambiguous commercial status.

Hair, unlike the bodies of the deceased and perhaps even the sentiments of the living, promised to remain forever "alive" and active. In Lydia Sigourney's 1860 poem, "The Lock of Hair" (1860), the unfortunate heroine died all too young. But her brief life is relived "at thy talismanic touch" of a lock of hair. "How full thou art of memories, severed tress!" the narrator exclaimed as various scenes of the departed's life are recalled. The narrator's daughter is seen first as a small child with "clustered ringlets," then as a school-girl, a bride, a widow, and finally a dead young woman. All these images of her life are arranged around an image of a lock of hair in a mourning brooch (Figure 10).[69]

In a social world that valued work and the visible results of labor and expressed these through the body, mourning encompassed both the demand of continual labor and that of demonstrative effort. In "The Lock of Hair" and "The Last Good Night," sorrow was an active, physical enterprise. In "The Last Good Night," a young girl dies. "Close her eyelids, press them gently / O'er the dead and leaden eyes," its parents (and the reader) are instructed. Then,

wipe the death drops from her forehead,
Sever one dear golden tress,
Fold her icy hands all meekly,
Smooth the little snowy dress;
Scatter flowers o'er her pillow,— . . .
Lay the bud upon her bosom;
There,—now—softly say Good night.[70]

"Sever one dear golden tress," and then begin the exercise of mourning the departed, who, of course, having left the hair, would never really be gone.

As it had been in life, hair was so persistently drawn into relationship

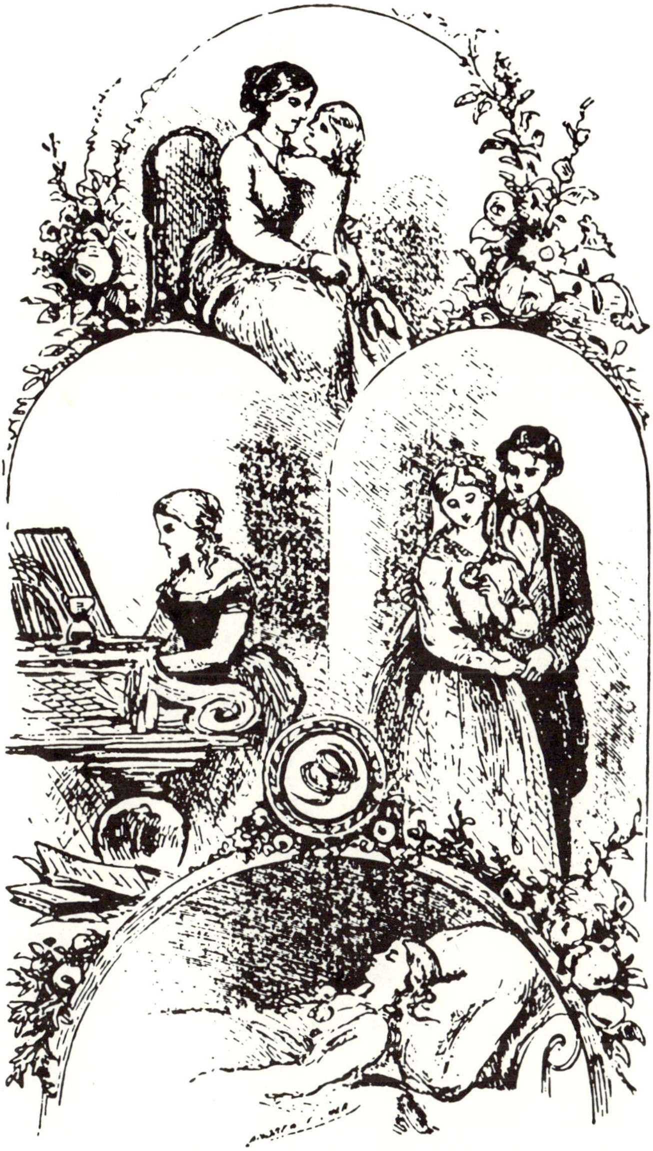

Figure 10. "Back at thy talismanic touch return . . ." Through "The Lock of Hair" (the title of her poem), Lydia Sigourney led her readers in 1860 through the life of her heroine. Memories of the deceased's childhood, marriage, motherhood, and death reside within the treasured brooch, itself encircling a lock of hair. Illustration from *The Lady's Almanac for 1860*.

with the individual that it could indeed stand in for the deceased. In a short story of 1862, a mother's last act reinforced this connection. "I smoothed back the bright golden ringlets that had won for him the pet name of 'Sunshine . . .' I folded up the golden curl in the tissue envelop."[71] Another author cautioned readers to be good to their mothers for "Too early, death, led on by care, / May snatch save one dear lock away. / Oh, revere her raven hair!"[72] Another bereaved parent, again, years after the death of his child, says to his wife, "'I need not ask what this is,' says the husband, as he unfolds a little packet [containing his deceased child's hair]."[73]

Hair could provide impetus for two stages of mourning: first, tears; then, memory. Memorial hair—that is, hair saved on the event of a person's death—triggered tears and thus began the necessary process of mourning. In one story, as the father opened the packet of his child's hair, "tears come into his eyes, as he looks at a silky curl cut from the head of their dead child."[74] Such tears, especially from men, were encouraged. "There is something peculiarly touching in manly grief. The eye of woman overflows as readily as her heart; but, when waters gush from the rock, we feel that they are extorted by no gentle blow," observed one writer.[75]

After this initial stage, hair could move the mourner along the path of grief to a more transcendent stage of remembering. A commercially produced epitaph poem adorned with a lock of real hair suggested that once this storm of grief had passed, recollection and transcendence of the experience could begin for the living.

I've received a lock of hair,
Once worn on thy gentle brow;
. . . .
Tender, pure, and much lov'd brother,
Though thy form no more I'll see;
Still, beloved, too, with mother,
With this lock I'll think of thee.[76]

In the calm that followed tears, recollection could begin. "It is the divine nature of their qualities to conquer pain and death itself: to turn the memory of them into pleasure."[77] "With this lock I'll think of thee," an epitaph card promised to the departed individual (and instructed the owner of the card).

In "My Treasures," several individuals were recalled through their respective hair. The departed were equated with riches, and the ironic difference between the lowly objects in the narrator's treasure box (locks of hair, broken rings) and the rich "jewels" of her memory highlighted the act of recollection. First, a young child was recalled:

This is a curl, a tiny thing
  Cut from a wreath of golden hair.
Dear little head! it's buried now,
  And the curls have withered upon its brow!

Then, a young woman, for "here is a lock from a long-loved head, / Look, how soft the raven hair!" And yet another young woman was called forth, "Here's a glossy auburn tress, / I cut it off when Fanny died." The poem concluded,

Curls, and rings, and tresses of hair,
  Notes and flowers, books they have read;
Gems and things I have seen them wear . . .
'Tis a sacred place to me,
Where my guarded treasures be![78]

Memories were objects—both literally (hair, rings) and figuratively—to be hoarded and fondled, just as a miser might caress her piles of gold. The hair was not valuable so much for being *of* the person but for being an objectified version of the departed. Hence, hair was a talisman for Sigourney, or it was a jewel in a treasure box.

Hair and hairwork acted to metaphorically entwine the past and present, the deceased and the living, by either braiding the hair of the departed or combining the hair of the departed with that of the living. For example, a commercially printed mourning card of a poem had one lock of hair sewn onto it. The verses on the card expressed the deepest sorrow and "personal" recollections of a childhood together. "Brother—brother, I remember / All our little playful days," began the poem. "We were knit, *us* twain, as one," mourned the narrator. Mourning and grief were understood as deeply personal and idiosyncratic experiences. The poem directly addressed the deceased ("Brother—brother") and the narrator of the poem posed as the grieving individual ("I remember"). In addition, the title of the poem, "Lines; on the reception of the lock of hair from my only—my departed brother" provides instructions for the owner. And, yes, someone did in fact carefully sew onto the commercially printed card (Figure 11).[79]

There were other kinds of mourning products made of hair that were not jewelry. E. C. Shriner offered to create "mementoes of the dead," in-

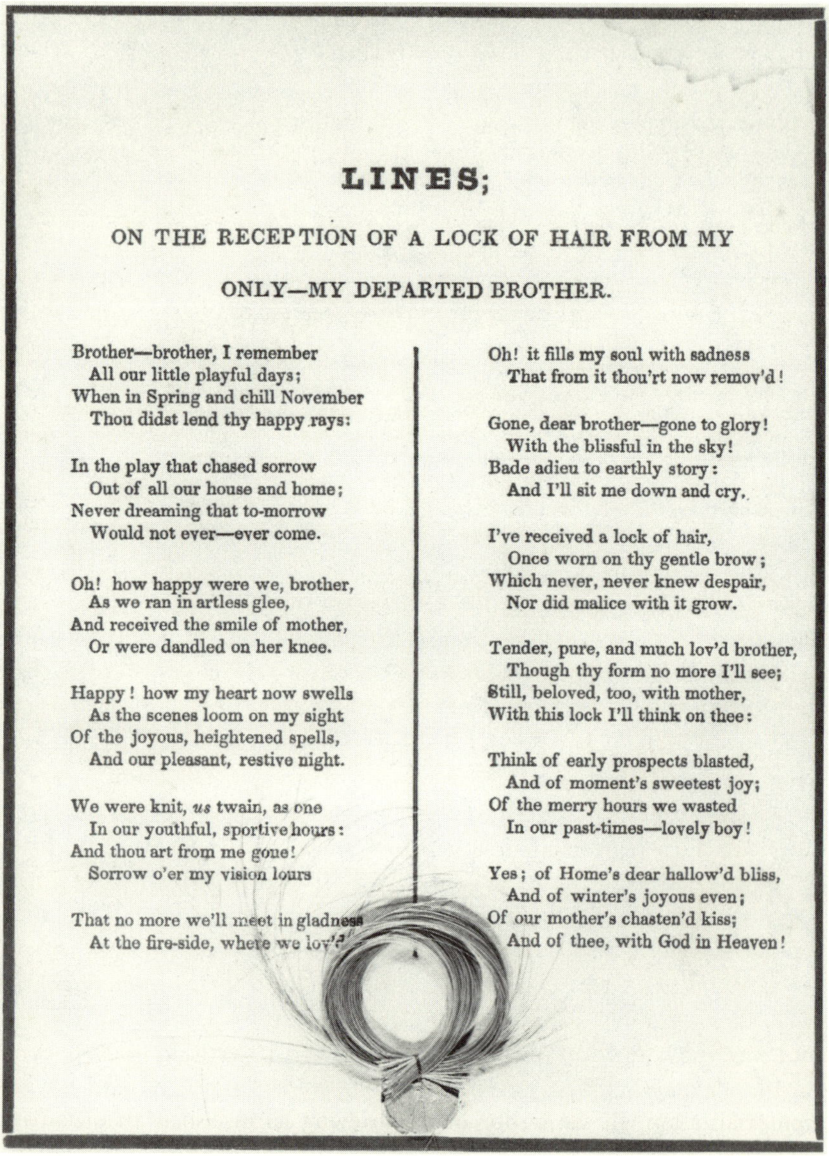

LINES;

ON THE RECEPTION OF A LOCK OF HAIR FROM MY ONLY—MY DEPARTED BROTHER.

Brother—brother, I remember
  All our little playful days;
When in Spring and chill November
  Thou didst lend thy happy rays:

In the play that chased sorrow
  Out of all our house and home;
Never dreaming that to-morrow
  Would not ever—ever come.

Oh! how happy were we, brother,
  As we ran in artless glee,
And received the smile of mother,
  Or were dandled on her knee.

Happy! how my heart now swells
  As the scenes loom on my sight
Of the joyous, heightened spells,
  And our pleasant, restive night.

We were knit, *us* twain, as one
  In our youthful, sportive hours:
And thou art from me gone!
  Sorrow o'er my vision lours

That no more we'll meet in gladness
  At the fire-side, where we lov'd

Oh! it fills my soul with sadness
  That from it thou'rt now remov'd!

Gone, dear brother—gone to glory!
  With the blissful in the sky!
Bade adieu to earthly story:
  And I'll sit me down and cry.

I've received a lock of hair,
  Once worn on thy gentle brow;
Which never, never knew despair,
  Nor did malice with it grow.

Tender, pure, and much lov'd brother,
  Though thy form no more I'll see;
Still, beloved, too, with mother,
  With this lock I'll think on thee:

Think of early prospects blasted,
  And of moment's sweetest joy;
Of the merry hours we wasted
  In our past-times—lovely boy!

Yes; of Home's dear hallow'd bliss,
  And of winter's joyous even;
Of our mother's chasten'd kiss;
  And of thee, with God in Heaven!

Figure 11. A lock of hair is given a home and sentimental meaning. The hair represents the brotherly relationship and the untouched purity of a child who has died young. Courtesy The Winterthur Library: Joseph Downs Collection of Manuscripts and Printed Ephemera.

cluding "wreaths made from Relics of Deceased Friends." Shriner could use almost any material to do this, from hair to "pieces of their Clothing, Shrouds, Coffins, Old Shoes, Stockings, or articles found among their effects," all to "be wrought into Wreaths or Boquets." "How pleasant to preserve in so beautiful of form the Relics of our loved ones," urged Shriner's advertisement. In addition to wreaths, "single Locks of Hair [could be] made into Flowers as low as fifty cents" could be used.[80]

Later in the century, W. R. Seymour and Company specialized in mourning products, and one of their premier offerings was wax flower memorials.[81] "These are really the finest and richest memorials that can be made," assured an advertisement. Composed of an elaborate frame, gathered silk border, and numerous wax flowers, customers provided personal touches that, when incorporated into the memorial, would convey the most sincere of emotions. Customers were asked to "send name, age and date of death; the number of the verse or prayer you desire. State whether you desire walnut, bronze or gold frame. Send hair and photography." The verses were supplied by the company, which also sold memorial cards. Customers had a choice of forty-four verses in either English or German, and if the customer had a "verse of your own (different from ours and not exceeding eight lines) they can be placed on any number of copies free of charge."

Number 8 of the W. R. Seymour and Company line noted,

'Tis hard to break the tender cord,
  When love has bound the heart,
'Tis hard, so hard to speak the words,
  We must forever part.
Dearest loved one, we must lay thee
  In the peaceful grave's embrace,
But thy memory will be cherished,
  'Till we see thy heavenly face.

And the W. R. Seymour and Company memorial wax flower and hair wreath would, the company suggested, augment this process of grieving and memorialization. In the parlor of the grieving family, such an ornament openly demonstrated the family's ability to both reconcile themselves to their loss and maintain the memory of the deceased, and all in a "unique," decorative form.

All these objects, from the simplest locks of saved hair to the most expensive commercial goods, wedded the living with the deceased in a socially visible manner. Given the emphasis in the nineteenth century on the relationship between an individual and his or her hair, and given the often transcendent properties assigned to hair, it is understandable why hair was used in this way. But the elaborate array of mourning objects made from hair is not so readily explicable. Why use hair in such repetitious, ornate, and fanciful ways? Why continue to harbor the bodies of the family's dead ones long after their departure?

We have already seen the answer to this question in the other cultural work hair performed. Mourning practices were not enacted for the dead but for the living. The need to personify the dead and to engage them in the continuance of life was not a relevant activity for the departed but a necessary action of the living. In her examination of contemporary nostalgia, Donna Bassin labels such activity as "mourning play." "Through memory," she argues, "the self is provided with a sense of history and the potential for renewal." With the deceased rendered into an object, mourning becomes, as nostalgia does, "an attempt to reenact reunion with the lost object."[82]

Thus, the nineteenth-century, middle-class use of hair to create such objects of affection was an active response to the experience of death. By working the hair of their departed loved one, nineteenth-century Americans reconstructed and renewed their own living self. And, at the same time, the mourners enacted the set strategies of sorrow by constructing self-possession of their own. Creating mourning hairwork, then, was not so much a moribund practice as a self-transformation. Hairwork itself represented transformation: Bits of hair became fashionable jewelry in the hands of professional artisans, and then that market good was transformed into an intimate possession by virtue of its material of hair and through its emotional significance. When hairwork was given as a gift or created to mourn a loss, middle-class Americans in the 1850s and to the end of the century were able to position themselves as fashionable and sentimental.

Chapter 3
The Gem That Binds

Market-produced hairwork was increasingly criticized for its relationship to the market at the same time it was becoming more popular and more readily accessible to a growing middle class in the 1850s and 1860s. Hairwork made at home by a woman's own hands for the pleasure of herself and her family was encouraged as an alternative. Promoted by a mini-industry of instructional manuals and guides published in popular women's magazines, hairwork became a popular fancywork craft for middle-class American women. While market-produced hairwork was valued in its own right, amateur-made hairwork claimed a more comprehensive expression of women's domestic role and of the integrity of the physical and emotional labor invested in it by its maker. Hairwork crafting was marketed, however, like other kinds of fancywork—as a pleasant activity for middle-class women. Fancywork itself was seen as an ideal women's activity, requiring discipline, a regulated sort of self-expression, and, above all, a willingness to give of one's self. Hairwork made at home was understood to be not only of a woman's hand but of her heart. For this reason, amateur-made hairwork was considered superior in its emotional integrity to the increasingly popular market-produced hairwork.

If one were to evaluate nineteenth-century women's lives by what is found in today's museums, the conclusion would be that women were consumed with the making of things. The parade of seemingly useless and overworked objects, from needlework to featherwork, shellwork, seed wreaths, quilts, and the like, give us a very narrow image of women's lives during the 1800s. But museums collect objects and, in the case of middle-class white women, fancywork is often what we have left of their lives. Why did fancywork crafts, including hairwork, become so popular in the mid-nineteenth century? The answer stems from the role of women and the family in the time period. Fancywork was a woman's activity. Women's ideal roles were circumscribed by home, husband, and children. To be a mother was to embody the highest honor accorded women. Making fancywork replicated what a mother was supposed to do. Just as she was to knit together the members of her family, she was to knit together materials to create ornamental objects for the home.

Fancywork and Middle-Class Women in the 1850s and 1860s

Fancywork added value to a home. The result of making fancywork was, as a book for ladies in 1851 asserted, the "difference in the furnishing of a bachelor's house, and one where a lady presides; the thousand little elegancies of [a lady], though nothing in themselves, adding, like ciphers, prodigiously to the value of the solid articles they are appended to."[1] These improvements in home capital came from how fancywork was actually made. First, fancywork was supposed to use otherwise wasted materials (for example, a lobster claw used to create toothpick holders, penwipers made of "spare" felt), which, skillfully combined, make an object of value from nothing.[2] Second, fancywork both *looked* and *was* very time-consuming. That was in part its worth. While women's domestic work was sight unseen (the "within" part of the home), fancywork made that work "without" and thus visible and knowable. Objects of fancywork, replete with visible traces of production, testified to a woman's ingenuity and resourcefulness and stood as a statement of her taste and refinement.

Although representative of a woman's obedience to the dicta of true womanhood and to her non-economic but valuable role in the home, the material character of fancywork also allowed women an avenue of self-expression. Women created fancywork—in particular, hairwork—which illustrated their ties to children, family, friends, and husbands. Creating objects offered some individuals an opportunity to counter the assumptions of domestic ideology. It also legitimated creative activity that was defined by assumptions of what was valuable in a woman's life.[3]

That women's intellectual and mechanical talents were especially well-suited for the labors of fancywork was obvious to many prescriptive authors. The groundwork for such associations was laid much earlier in American culture. In 1777, Mrs. Hannah Robertson noted that fancywork was a wonderful teaching tool for young girls, for "even those whose genius seemed so bad as to appear void of any inclination to learn any thing, yet [even they] would have learned to make flowers as soon and well, as those of the brightest parts."[4] Even dullard girls with no other talents (for Mrs. Hannah Robertson, despair was found in a girl's reluctance to learn "plain-work, embroidery, [and] sattin work"), could find interest in the "lighter" fancywork efforts of making hair and wool flowers and other fancies. Exactly a century later, Mrs. Robertson's wisdom still held true. "There is," assured Annie Frost in *The Ladies' Guide to Needlework, Embroidery, etc.*, "no occupation so essentially feminine, at the same time so truly lady-like, as needlework."[5] George Blakelee agreed, noting that "there is a certain class of ornamental or fancy work that seems to belong especially to girls. Their tastes and deft fingers appear to be particularly fitted to the performance of the same."[6] The characteristics of creating fancywork—its numbingly infinite articulation of tasks and its finely, minutely wrought character—was really just an expression of woman's very nature.

But even guidebooks acknowledged that girls and women might need some persuasion on this point. Fancywork was discussed as a way for women to balance the rigors of self-discipline and the freedom of self-expression. In a short story of 1851, "Duty. A Tale.," a mother used fancywork to teach her daughters their duties as women. The mother instructed her two daughters that "duty, [is] not cold and stern, as it exists in your imagination, but tender and gentle amid its high and firm resolves." Yet her daughter Lucy debated her mother on this point, and argued that such formalized constructions of emotion were cold-hearted and disinterested. She observed that "it is so much easier and happier to obey you and papa because *I love you*, than because it is my *duty* to do so." But her mother cautioned that "affection is never so pure or steadfast as when it is guided and controlled by duty." Her daughter apologized for her disagreement and then, "resuming her embroidery, seated herself once more at her mother's side."[7]

The mother repeated her lesson on duty through fancywork. With her worktable to her right, she watched worriedly as her daughters obediently completed their fancywork and sketching even as they simultaneously rejected the tenets of domesticity. After their mother's death, each of the sisters married. However, each depended on the "easier" response of heartfelt, although undisciplined, love, and each sister ultimately was alone again and filled with regrets for having squandered her respective chances at love and fulfillment. They were now those "whose most ardent affections are swayed by the firm yet gentle hand of duty." They had, unknowingly, finally learned this lesson of their mother's through their edifying, lifelong practice of fancywork. Fancywork was a fitting metaphor for the successful maturation of the daughters into true women of the home.[8]

Fancywork was an ideal tool of instruction with its demands to follow carefully detailed instructions, for repetitious hand motions, unswerving attention, and daily practice. As noted earlier, this was why fancywork was often a part of a young girl's formal education.[9] It encouraged the development of the proper, feminine self through its integration of sentiment and beauty with discipline and structure. Through fancywork, a woman demonstrated a character that was deeply emotional and affectionate and whose egoistic desires were successfully subsumed in the care for her family. For instance, rhetoric and practice carefully regulated fancywork's imaginative aspects through step-by-step instructions.[10] When the daughter Lucy and thousands of her real-life counterparts sat down to do their two or three hours of Berlin work, tatting, embroidery, or hairwork, they immersed their bodies and selves in an act of instructional discipline.[11] They worked to create a self that could more readily accept the duties of womanhood. Fancywork was an act of creation not only of the actual physical object but also of the intangible self.

This womanly self succeeded when domestic ideology was not simply enacted but was truly a part of one's character. Yet for nineteenth-century middle-class Americans it was the visibility of discipline that counted, for it provided evidence of an individual's attainment of a proper character. Women's work from the eighteenth to nineteenth centuries became less and less recognized as labor. Middle-class women were no longer seen as the "Good Wife," the eighteenth-century partner of the household, but as the "Good Mother" whose refining influence wafted throughout the home. Of course, while the measures of women's work were altered, women's work did not cease.[12] Women's domestic work was just as gritty, difficult, and arduous in the nineteenth century as in any preceding time. The larger culture, however, especially by the mid-nineteenth century, no longer acknowledged that labor. Instead, a woman's influence (not work) was ephemeral and seen, if at all, in the "touches" of luxury and refinement of the home.

Above all, a nineteenth-century woman was defined as "Mother." A mother's duties, according to one adviser, were best fulfilled when "she weaves her child's *habits* through conduct; and does it, too, as clothes are made, stitch by stitch."[13] To methodically mold a child's nature through countless acts of guidance was a mother's gravest responsibility and her greatest honor. Influenced by the Enlightenment concept of childhood as a malleable and therefore dangerous period of an individual's life, nineteenth-century ideals of motherhood placed much of the burden of nurturance on women.[14] The ideal of motherhood argued that the home was a woman's true domain and the family was her craft. Sentimental domesticity rested on highly idealized images of the mother and her children. Those images prominently featured the mother and her children (*white* mothers and children), who were considered to be outside of the world, of the market, and of competition.

To live out the ideals of sentimental domesticity was, as Mary J. Muckle wrote in 1882, to transcendently wend together "Mother, Home, and Heaven."

There are three words that sweetly blend,
That on the heart are graven;
A precious soothing balm they lend—
They're Mother, Home, and Heaven!

They twine a wreath of beauteous flowers,
Which placed on memory's urn,
Will e'en the longest, gloomiest hours
To golden sunlight turn!

They form a chain whose every link
Is free from base alloy;
A stream where whosoever drinks
Will find refreshing joy!

They build an altar where each day
Love's offering is renewed;
And peace illumes with genial ray
Life's darkened solitude![15]

Performing such actions as to "twine," to "form," and to "build" produced the physical evidence of a mother's labor: "a wreath of beauteous flowers," "memory's urn," "a chain whose every link / Is free from base alloy." In these sites of containment (an encircling wreath, an urn, a chain), women produced children who would never forget the mothers who performed such self-sacrifices. In that remembrance and through their children's everyday actions, a mother's work found its legacy.[16] Her work was, quite literally, never done. A mother's influence accompanied her adult children as they confronted the harsher realities of competitive life. In addition, mother love was understood as an Edenic refuge: an earthly paradise of acceptance and nurturance before mother and child were separated—before markets and money intruded in an individual's life.[17] In addition, maternal love could, theoretically, knit back together home and market.

Hair jewelry physically and actually entwined individuals together, and its characteristic of incorruptibility powerfully embodied the ideals of motherhood's affect. Through the creation, wearing, and ownership of hair jewelry, women provided irrefutable evidence of their own success at accomplishing this boundless existence. In addition, hair jewelry was intended to evoke memory and sentiment. A mother's influence transcended earth and heaven because her love lasted in the memories of her children. Because children were born of their mother, not only did they retain the effects of her guiding love, they were themselves a corporeal talisman of their mother's life.[18]

Making Hairwork at Home

Many women were persuaded that making hairwork at home, with their own hands, was a far better way to meet these demands "to effect evaluating influence." The earliest example of handwritten instructions for hairwork is an 1812 receipt book that included directions for table-worked hair.[19] Throughout the eighteenth, and nineteenth centuries, women (and men) were able to make hairwork themselves. But it was not until the mid-nineteenth century that doing so was desirable. As the market for consumer goods was increasingly becoming a part of American life, the handcrafted nature of human hairwork offered a respite from the market. But professionally made hairwork was created by those who did not necessarily share the customer's sentiment. Making one's own hairwork could guarantee that. In addition, women's roles were defined as a counterpoise to the market. In the 1850s and 1860s, "Woman" was that which the market could apparently never be: She was where sentiment could be found; where people cared for one another; where profit and competition had no place. Ironically, making one's own hairwork was appropriate because the market deemed it so.

Those in the business of promoting the amateur craft of hairwork were quick to suggest how the market posed a threat to the sanctity of sentimental hairwork. Hair jewelry, no matter the sentiment behind the purchase, was a product of the market, and in nineteenth-century eyes, the market denigrated the more intimate realms of life. Writers of hairwork guides assumed that this concern, properly inculcated, would increase the appeal of their own product.[20]

For Mark Campbell, hair jewelry "inspired a love for personal embellishment, which has made it popular and sought for, far more than the flashy jewelry, which have no souvenirs of affection entwined as remembrances of the loved and the lost."[21] Hairwork contradicted the changes in American culture so vividly represented by "flashy jewelry." Owners of hairwork treasured their pieces for the material used to make their watch fob, their earrings, and their necklace. It was the hair of a loved one "encased in cunningly devised objects of gold, to remain 'a joy forever,' as [to be] treasure[d] as a souvenir in the remembrance of the loved."[22] The base material was even more valuable than its hand production. Hair jewelry's sincere representation of affections was a reprieve from the influx of increasingly available goods that threatened to overwhelm individual and class distinctions. Hairwork was handmade, it was of the heart, and it came from one's sincere affections, and thus seemed very different than the other kinds of commodities easily available in the market of consumer goods.

One way to guarantee the authenticity of the hair in the jewelry was to make it one's self. Again, how-to marketers argued that making hairwork by one's own hand was preferable to having hair jewelry professionally made, because, as *Cassell's Household Guide* argued in the 1870s, "in all hair jewelry or ornament the chief value is a sentimental one, and when any doubt exists of the hair itself being genuine all real interest attaching to the article is lost."[23] As *Cassell's* helpfully pointed out, "any person would prize a device of this kind when worked by his or her own hand—and of the genuineness of which no doubt could consequently exist." Therefore, making hair jewelry was a kind of insurance policy against possible sentimental fraud. "In a word," as the National Artistic Hair Work Company concluded in 1886, "to become his or her own artist in hair-working" was the only way to gain certainty.[24]

Godey's Lady's Book explained in 1850, "By acquiring a knowledge of this art, ladies will be themselves enabled to manufacture the hair of beloved friends and relatives into bracelets, chains, rings, ear-rings, and devices, and thus insure that they do actually wear the memento they prize, and not a fabric substituted for it, as we fear has sometimes been the case."[25] *Godey's* laid out a logical sequence of argumentation that remained consistent throughout the century. By making one's own hairwork, the maker could effect the transformation of "friends and relatives into bracelets, chains." The control of this process would ensure that the sentimentality represented by the memento was sincere. Its authenticity was guaranteed because the "fabric" was a known quantity.

An additional reason for a woman to choose to make hair jewelry herself was because many hair workers did not seem honest. In 1869, Levina

Urbino began her instructions in making hairwork with the arresting claim, "To make hair flowers we need live hair, that is, hair from a living person."[26] In 1885, a domestic encyclopedia issued the same caution, warning that, in making hairwork, "The hair used must be obtained from a living person."[27] Hairwork was intended to represent the private affiliations and affections of individuals. What Urbino and others were concerned with was the use of human hair—that is, dead hair—for wigs and artificial hairpieces. This use of hair was wholly commercial and seemed far from the cozy world of hair fancywork. For Urbino and others, the hair of the living person was hair animated by affection, affiliation, and love. Hair used for any other purpose, for making money, was dead.

And that was dead hair. In an advertisement for her mail-order business, Matilda Pullan assured her potential customers that she would "carry out with the utmost exactitude; and to guarantee that the hair sent shall be that actually used—a point of much importance to the wearer, though often and very cruelly overlooked by the worker."[28] Even more frightening, the National Artistic Hair Work Company (which, like Pullan, offered directions for making hair jewelry and provided a retail mail-order service for purchasing pieces) mournfully explained, "Now, to the everlasting disgrace of those who practice it, there are persons whose greed to gain leaves them no regard for the finer feelings of the living, no respect for the dead. The hair of a departed friend is taken to a tradesman to be worked up into some little device, and what is frequently done is this— . . . they throw the hair away and supply other in place of it, which is already made up."[29]

Instead of seeing the process of transformation worked by one's own hands, customers who relied on professional hair workers sent off a loose hank of hair, and received in return the hair now utterly transformed into a commodity of a necklace, a pair of earrings, a watch chain that they then paid for. This "invisible" step of transformation was useful in establishing the value of hairwork as a marketable commodity. But because hairwork's marketability was related to its ability to convey sincere emotions in an undistorted fashion, professional hair workers had to address the issues of fashion and sentimentality simultaneously. For many customers, the issue was avoided by home manufacture.

To embark on a hairwork project was not easy, and many instruction writers granted this. As Mrs. Jones conceded, the "ability to so arrange and secure each strand of the sacred treasure, becomes an accomplishment truly valuable, and worthy all the patience and skill required in its performance." A decade earlier, in 1869, Madame Urbino warned that "practice in this art is of more value than precept. The artist will find the difficulties gradually disappear as the work is persevered in, and to study specimens of hairwork, now so common, will assist the learner in many points."[30]

Instruction writers also positioned amateur hairwork as an explicit move against the monopolistic control of professional hair workers. Not only were professionals suspected of dishonesty and heedless treatment of hair, but they were the jealous conservators of an old tradition. In 1850, *Godey's* remarked that hairwork, "hitherto almost exclusively confined to professed manufacturers of hair trinkets," was now available (through *Godey's* publication of instructions) to everyone.[31] Mark Campbell touted the fact that his *Self-Instructor* broke these bonds. "Heretofore the Art of making these goods has been jealously guarded by a few dealers, who have accumulated fortunes, and would still retain it a profound secret but for the publication of this book" (Figure 12).[32]

Women who chose to delve into these "profound secrets" used the same tools and techniques, and created styles similar to those of the professional hair worker. As noted earlier, both amateurs and professionals had access to the same books of instructions. Of course, guides aimed at amateurs alone, such as instructions published in women's magazines, framed the activity as most suitable for women. For example, *Godey's Lady's Book* recommended hairwork because it was "as free from all the annoyances and objections of litter, dirt, or unpleasant smells, as the much-practiced knitting, netting, and crochet can be."[33] For women's magazines, making one's own hairwork was not only a way to circumvent the market, to ensure the authenticity of the piece, and to insulate the hair of loved one's from uncaring hands, it was also a way to enact the discipline required of women themselves.

The hairwork that women made themselves varied dramatically from the simplest locks of hair held in a locket or sewn onto a page of a letter, to unique brooches and bracelets, to very large hair wreaths that were hung on parlor walls. Amateur-made hair jewelry is often accompanied with notes describing the piece's home manufacture, or the frayed, awkward appearance of the piece suggests an amateur hand. Some amateur-made jewelry looks much like professionally made, as professionals and amateurs used similar braid patterns and jewelry mountings.

Most hair-jewelry instruction writers assumed that amateur hair workers would take their finished projects to professional jewelers to be mounted into their intended jewelry frame. In 1859, *Godey's* ended its directions by announcing to at-home workers, "the work is finished, and ready

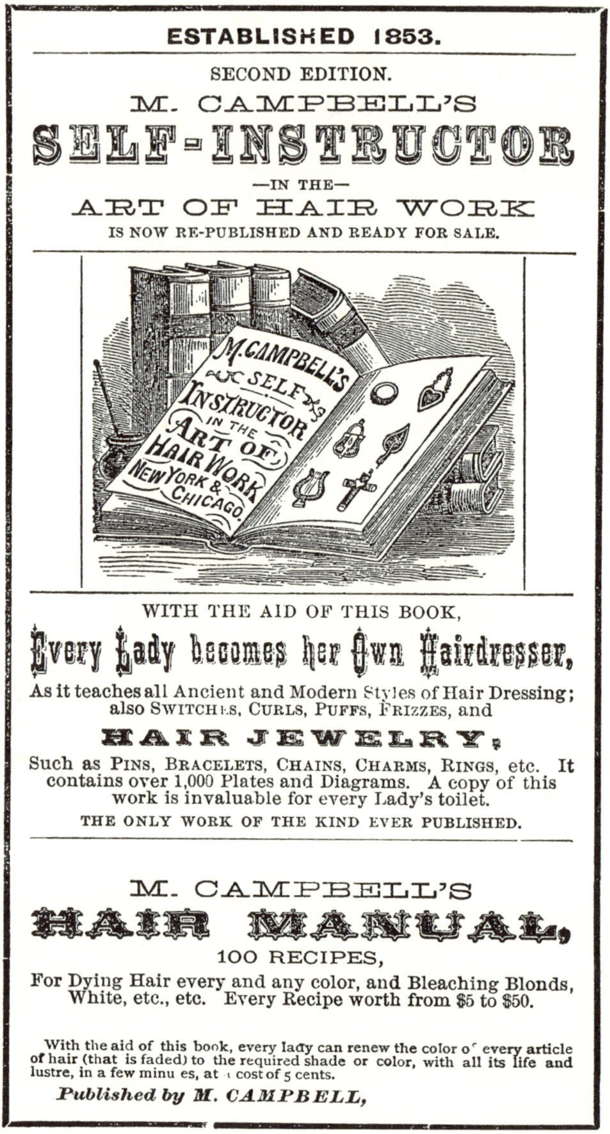

Figure 12. Another of Mark Campbell's efforts to become the leader of both sentimental and artificial hairwork, his *Self-Instructor* of 1879 (an updated edition from his original 1869 volume) combined how-to instructions on making hairwork jewelry, guidelines for dyeing hair, and, as always, a way to order hairwork to be completed by Mark Campbell (or an employee of his). Courtesy The Winterthur Library, Printed Book and Periodical Collection.

for the jeweller," although in its first series of instructions, in 1850, *Godey's* was content to merely assure amateur workers that "the pattern will appear complete and ready to receive whatever clasp, snap, or slide it is thought proper to affix to it."[34] Mark Campbell, always the eager entrepreneur, suggested that because "all articles intended to be worn as jewelry, should, of course, be mounted with gold, and as this kind of work is not done in all jewelry establishments, I wish to say that my facilities for this branch of business is complete, and the work done is in the best possible manner. I guarantee satisfaction in all cases, let the style desired be what it may. In sending braids to be mounted, draw on paper, as near as can be, the style or design you want."[35] Another hair worker, Christopher Edwards, in 1857, directed his advertisement, "To Hair Braiders" to whom he "Respectfully announces to the public, that he continues to make Mountings for Hair Jewelry."[36] This was probably how most hair jewelry was finally finished.

In 1859, Emily Sargeant made for her friend Mrs. Nabby Walton a hair brooch simple in manufacture and material, yet deeply expressive of the ways some women lived out the essence of maternal doctrine. Emily Sargeant wrote Mrs. Walton:

> Jan 13–1859
> Dear Mrs. Walton,
> I have finished your pin at last so I will now explain it to you. The outside is your hair the end Daisies are Lorena's & Adella's the side ones Lilla's & Lissie's the center is Stella's the next two rows are Harriet's the next two Jemima's. I thought I would put in the childrens hair for the reasons one was I thought it would please them & the next it would please you & and the next it would add to the beauty of the pin. . . .
>
> Very truly yours,
> Emily Sargeant[37]

The pin Emily created for Nabby Walton was only two inches wide, but it still was able to contain eight individuals—Mrs. Walton and her children. Sargeant created miniature flowers of hair-wrapped wire, the same technique used in larger-scale hair wreaths. The various flower shapes were sewn onto a cardboard-and-satin backing. The entire circumference of the pin was bordered with a flat, looped wire wrapped in Mrs. Walton's hair. Mrs. Walton's maternal presence encircled and protected the hair—and thus, quite literally, the bodies—of her seven children. A material evocation of the otherwise ephemeral virtues of motherly love and care, the Walton family was (sans father) presented whole, unified by the mother's guidance.

Mrs. Walton's brooch powerfully iterated her own encompassing attention to her children and her own sacrifices for them.

Hair jewelry could also tie generations together. Mrs. Charles Stuart Foster's necklace likewise figuratively and literally wove together her children and her self. Her necklace is an example of a "bead" hair necklace. The hair is woven of two distinct shades of medium brown and blonde, and at the base of the necklace are three acorns delicately formed of the same blonde hair. The brown hair is of Eleanor Nevins McCool, Mrs. Foster's mother, and the lighter hair was that of one of her children.[38]

Mothers would often combine their own hair with that of their children, or weave their children's hair together to represent both familial and biological ties. For instance, the Cardoza brooch and watch fob set was made from the hair of two young girls in the 1860s. The watch fob was woven of one color of light-brown hair, and the two charms hung from it were of two distinct colors. The Cardoza brooch is an open-frame circle, and in the circle hangs a small heart, which has panels of woven hair on either side. The panels are of a light-brown hair, with a blonde shade woven into it to make a plaid pattern.[39]

The interwoven patterns in hair jewelry, such as Mrs. Foster's and the Cardoza pieces, were fashionable and worked well with the fabric styles and colors of clothing of the period, especially the brown-and-cream scotch plaids popular from the 1850s to the 1870s.[40] At the same time, plaid-patterned hair of light and dark made explicit the entwined nature of the relationships between mothers and children (Figure 13).

Mrs. C. A. Harper's fashionable hairwork brooch balanced its frivolous appearance with the bodily material of several individuals. The hair of three forebearers is combined to form a bow of open braid beads with a large cross pendant. Artificial pearls glued within the centers of the flowers provided the final decorative touch. The effect is multitextured and variously colored, and probably looked well against the heavy, often dark tones of a matron's dress.[41] In wearing her brooch, its owner augmented her own appearance and demonstrated familial ties within a sentimental context.

Physically, hair jewelry could combine individuals into one object and that collective activity was reiterated when hair jewelry was exchanged. A gift of hair jewelry represented and even created connections between individuals. In one family, women exchanged personal tokens such as miniatures and hair as a method of entwining individual members together. "One sister sent another 'a braid of her own hair to wear on you[r] wrist wear it and remember the giver.' "[42] Individuals proffered and accepted one

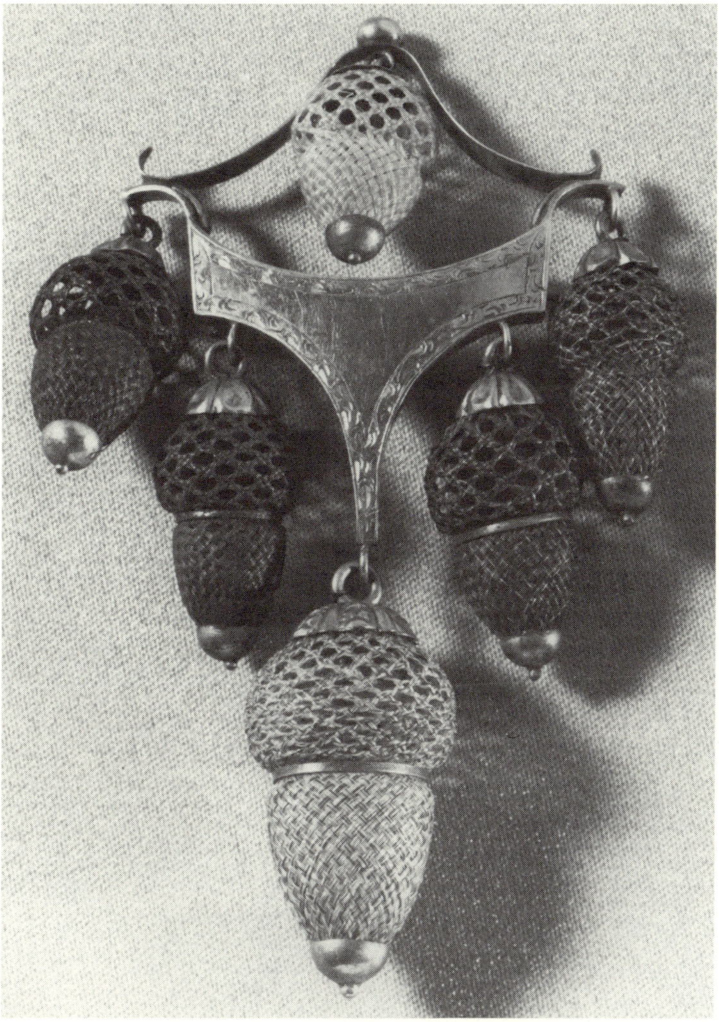

Figure 13. The hair of more than one individual was used to represent unity and closeness and to create a more pleasing piece of jewelry. These open-work braided acorn shapes dangle in an arrangement that makes the most of the contrast with light- and dark-colored hair. Fashion and sentiment were by no means contradictory. Courtesy National Museum of American History, Kenneth E. Behring Center, Smithsonian Institution.

another as they exchanged hair jewelry. Yet once again, hair jewelry represented no easy solutions to the dilemmas of sentimentality, of consumerism, or of self-representation.

Hairwork Albums

Hair did not have to be woven into a piece of jewelry, however. Often families simply exchanged locks of hair. In 1850, Sarah Rivers noted to her husband in a letter, "I received a letter from Brother Edward . . . he sent me some of his little boys' hair and in return I sent him a lock of our childrens and I have a little curl of Minna's [their youngest daughter] that was left that I will send to you as she is always telling me to write to you and frequently writes herself."[43] And at the top of the letter a small lock of hair was sewn onto the page.

Hair albums—that is, autograph albums that included hair—were popular until the end of the nineteenth century. Like a hair wreath, albums visually knit individuals together to form a single object. And, as with the hair wreaths, the relationships that surrounded an individual were replicated in the album. But the verses accompanying a lock of hair provided additional commentary, and often events outside those relationships appear. As Emma Egy prepared to marry Joseph Miller, and to move to Kansas, her friends inscribed their emotions in her album and presented her with locks of their hair. George Garber wrote,

In hours of calm reflection
In hours of social glee
If you should by recollection
Think of friends, think of me.
Geo. Garber[44]

Many of the verses echo George Garber's somewhat plaintive assumption that Emma was going to be surrounded by new friends, who might very well supplant her present acquaintances. For example, R. Garber wrote,

Forget me not when far away
When other friends you greet
Forget me not when with the [illegible]
in Social cheer you meet.
R. Garber

Much of the Garbers' concern over "losing" Emma was rooted in the reality of the difficulties of maintaining relationships over long physical distances, with only letters and the promise of very occasional visits serving as enduring connections. A departure such as Emma's from her circle of loved ones was an event of genuine sadness, as Debbie L. Garrett revealed in her verse in Emma's album.

This lock of hair to thee I bestow
When long I've loved with fervent heart
But still it grieves my soul to know
That we must part.

And further reiterating the sorrowful tone of the verse, above this somber verse rests a lock of hair nestled beneath a clumsily shaped black satin heart.

An impending marriage was the occasion for other albums to be started as well. In 1865, Virginia Catherine Persinger began her album.[45] Forty-three of Virginia's friends and family wrote entries and contributed locks of hair to her album. Her sibling wrote on August 30, 1865, "Jinnie in one week more shall have passed you will become the found [*sic*] and loving bride of the man who is first in your affections." Attached was a lock of hair.

In the same album, Virginia's friend James Aldophus Boswell (a future relation) wrote a lengthy entry. "Friendship is the gem that binds," he noted, "Mortal hearts in sweet fraternity. . . . Through motives of friendship pure, A ringlet from my brow, I proffer thee." Next to the handwritten line, "Friendship is the gem that binds" a thick ringlet of black and grey hair is sewn onto the page.

In Emma Egy's album, Elisabeth Shrontz included an elaborate verse to accompany an equally ornate, looped and braided lock of her hair. Shrontz neatly described why hair was such an effective means of communicating one's most intangible emotions.

Dear friend accept these lines
E'e[r] traced in friendship's hand
A token that love entwines,
Bound hearts with the mystic band.

Emma may our friendship ever prove
United both with truth and love.
Thus may we soar to realms on high
Heaven born friendship never dies.

Elisabeth's verse wove a complicated set of assumptions together into a powerful statement of emotional "truth." First, the inadequacy of merely writing one's thoughts is recognized when Elisabeth begged of Emma to "accept these lines / E'e[r] traced in friendship's hand." Elisabeth, however, offered an immediate remedy to the ephemeral "trace" of friendship when she followed with "a token that love entwines." The token was, of course, Elisabeth's own hair, wrapped, looped, braided and literally twined around a thin wire. Thus Elisabeth was assured that she has "bound hearts with the mystic band" of a relationship "united both with truth and love." Elisabeth ended by noting that "heaven born friendship never dies." Such enduring affinities were satisfyingly expressed through the abiding presence of Elizabeth's own hair.

The metaphor of entwinement to represent emotional relationships was common in the mid-nineteenth century. As discussed earlier, a mother's role was to entwine individual members into a family. In September 1832, Overton Bernard was traveling. Writing a letter to his wife Martha while sitting in a public tavern in Philadelphia, Overton wrote of his love for her and their family. "When my business is over of an evening I think and think again of my dearest Martha. . . . Our sweet and interesting little children are gathered by the minds eye into the endearing group, I fall asleep with them entwined around my heart. . . ."[46] In 1850, in a letter to her husband, Sarah Rivers wrote, "I enjoy as I learn your value I love you if possible more than ever and feel your absence more deeply. You have succeeded in twining yourself around my heart until I can feel no happiness unconnected with you."[47] To twine one's self about another was to create a dependency that allowed each individual to flourish.

While albums used hair as an emphasis on the emotional ties between individuals, the closeness and the intimacy hair symbolized was not always a comfort. While Emma Egy Miller's album was filled with affectionate verses, she also had an everlasting reminder of some of the tensions she was leaving behind in her move west. Here, the ties of relationships were less as bonds of affection than the sinews of obligations were strikingly revealed in one longer entry. Written the year of the Millers' departure from Pennsylvania, Nancy Wise, the wife of the Reverend Elder John Wise, wrote,

We have long been acquainted, and trying
to live together in a church capacity, As
a memento, I give this lock of hair. If you

outlive me, you will then remember me,
Your Sister. You will in the lock see some
grey hair, while yours is bright and fair,
When you are old and grey as I.
You will then feel you soon must die,
And then your heart with care be riven.
Your great desire will be for heaven.

Under this lugubrious free verse rests three locks of hair, each simply braided twists. Nancy's comment "trying to live together in a church capacity" reflected a certain unease, if not outright distaste, for Emma. The admonitory advice that the future holds gray hair, a riven heart, and a yearning toward death was within the sentimental religiosity of the mid-nineteenth century, although Nancy Wise phrased such sentiments far more bluntly than many would (Figure 14).

Hair albums, like hair jewelry, were portable emblems of entwinement. By making one's own hairwork, whether by laboriously weaving a piece of jewelry or by creating an album of verses and locks of hair, middle-class Americans during the 1850s and 1860s demonstrated their sentimentality, their stylishness, and their rejection of market-driven values. Similarly, hair wreaths and three-dimensional hairwork demonstrated those stances as well as a woman's artistic abilities. While jewelry, letters, and albums were nominally private, the public space of the parlor allowed for sanctioned display of a woman's private affiliations.[48]

Hair Wreaths

Hair wreaths were often quite large—some were up to four feet in diameter, but most were between one and two feet in diameter. Wreaths were rarely made in a circle, but rather, had a horseshoe shape. Their three-dimensionality required a shadowbox frame, and, because of their ornate appearance, the multiple shades of the hair, and their size, hair wreaths were usually intended for the parlor wall. As Mrs. Jones noted,

the formation of wreaths, bouquets, etc., for framing as house-ornaments has become exceedingly popular in the past few years. This mode of preserving the hair possesses many advantages, inasmuch as thereby a large collection may be made, and the hair of families thus preserved in a form not only pleasing and appropriate, but so lasting, as well; that it may be handed down from generation to generation

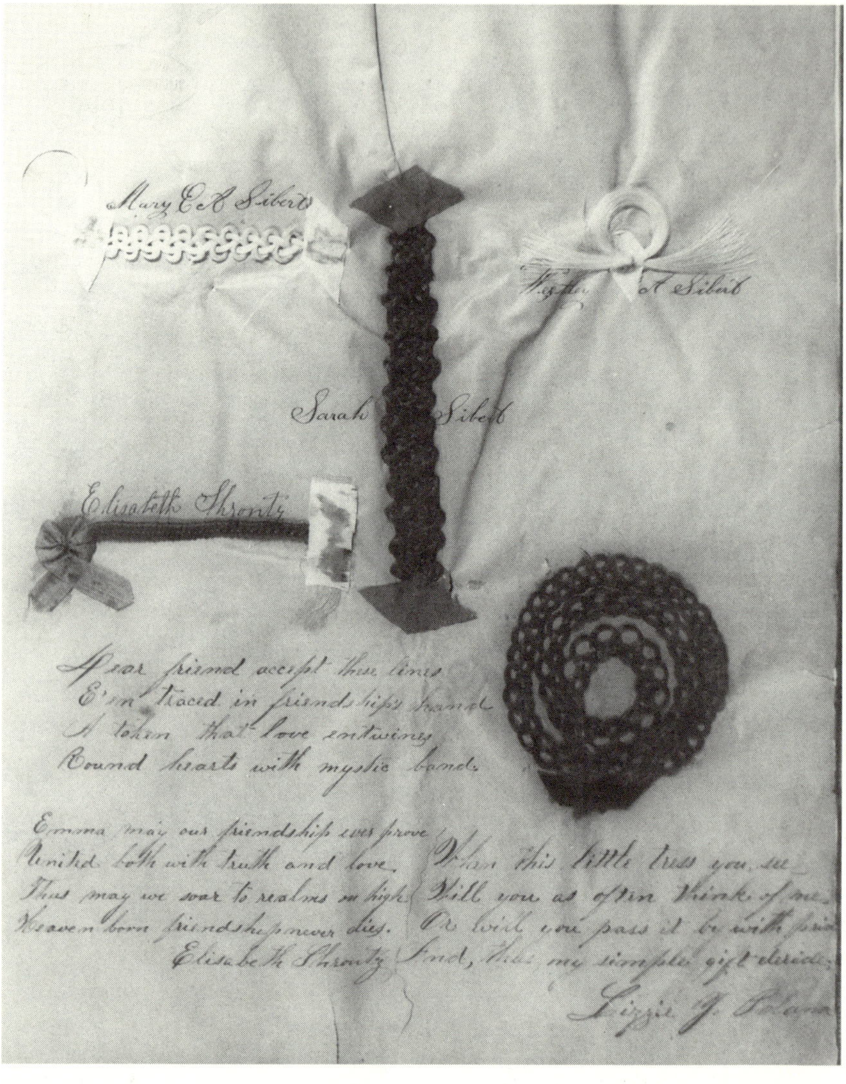

Figure 14. Emma Egy Miller's friends Mary, Hester, Sarah, Elisabeth, and Lizzie are presented in her album through their worked hair and signatures. Lizzie worked her hair into an eyelet braid and looped that into concentric circles. She wrote her "Dear friend" that this is "a token that love entwines." Courtesy Watkins Community Museum, Lawrence, Kansas.

as one of those "heirlooms" always valued and sacred as a "*memento mori*" of those gone before.[49]

Hair wreaths may have been large in size, but they were made piece by piece, flower by flower, and leaf by leaf. As Jones had suggested, each piece required only short lengths of hair, while almost all jewelry work required long lengths (usually up to eighteen inches). Thus, as Mrs. Jones remarked, a collection of family members could be gathered into one form. Women created an object that was the literal "circle of friends and home" so highly prized in middle-class culture. Used primarily to decorate parlor walls, family hair wreaths provided a visual focus for the ephemeral "happy home" and its ideal circle of family and friends.[50]

In addition, hair wreaths offered women the opportunity to create almost infinite variations of the theme of the flower. Hair colors could be combined to create varicolored flowers. Parlor hair wreaths exploited hair's ability to be manipulated into a world of naturalistic and fantastic shapes. By making a hair wreath, women created a decorative object, which in its variety of textures and colors was a suitable match for the visually dense styles of fabric and ornamentation of nineteenth-century parlors.[51]

Wreaths were made from hair worked into the shape of leaves, flowers, buds, and other floral forms and attached together, most commonly in a horseshoe or circular pattern. The human hair was either wrapped around or gimped between thin wires. The hair leaves and flowers often were augmented with glass beads, artificial pearls, and manufactured artificial flower parts, such as brightly colored stamens. The base usually was either wooden or metal, and all the elements were tightly wired onto this form. Finally, the completed wreath was mounted in a shadow box under glass and hung on the parlor wall. Because of the three-dimensional bulk of the wreath, most shadow boxes are three or more inches deep. Hair wreaths were substantial in size and appearance, and stood out even in the visually full space of the parlor room (Figure 15).

To begin a hair wreath, one needed, first, the hair. The required tools varied. Mrs. Jones listed mucilage glue, annealed wire (often called "hair wire"), round gold and pearl beads, and a few wire rings "such as are used for curtains." Mrs. Urbino required her readers to gather together the same, but also scissors, a pair of pincers, a piece of whalebone, and three different sizes of knitting needles. These tools could be purchased from catalog dealers, a local dry-goods dealer, or even a fancywork shop by the 1830s.[52] In the short story, "Taking Boarders," the Darlingtons, a beleaguered genteel

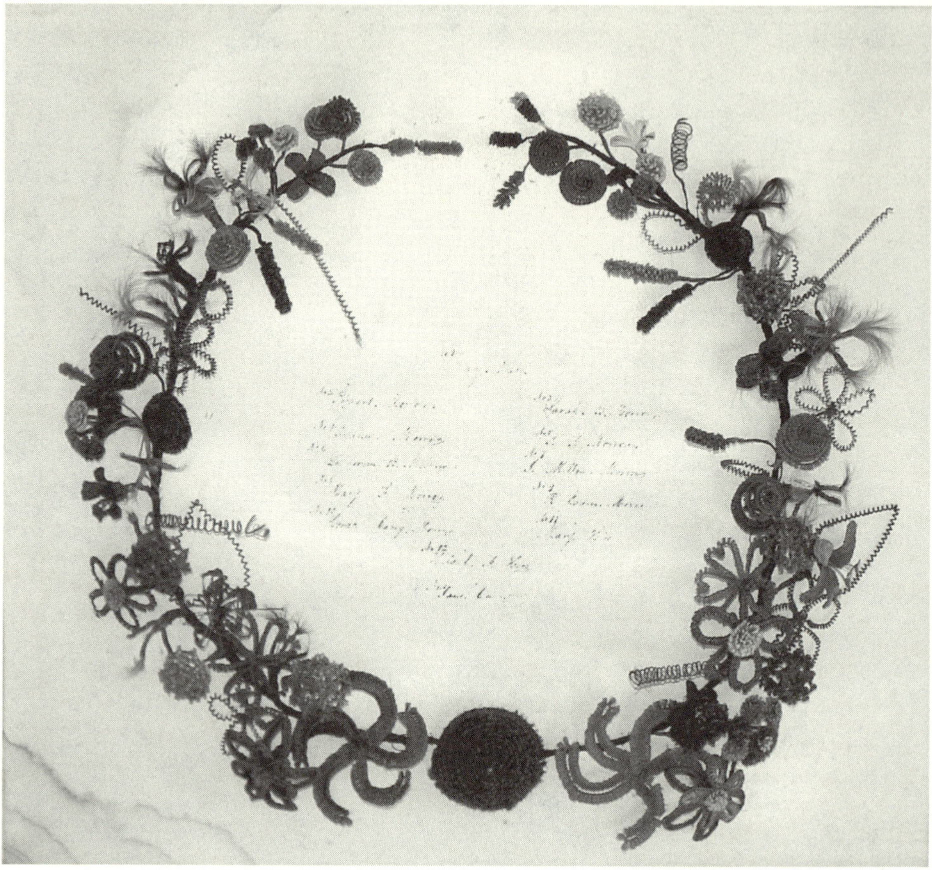

Figure 15. Hair wreaths often incorporated the hair of many individuals, evident in the various shades of browns and grays. In this way, a circle of family could be rendered visible and, at the same time, a woman's labor—usually so ephemeral and intangible—took on a physical form. This wreath represents thirteen individuals in one family. Courtesy Preble County Historical Society, Eaton, Ohio.

family, are advised by an uncle that "hundreds of women resort to keeping boarders as a means of supporting their families, when they might do it more easily, with less exposure, and greater certainty . . . in the keeping of a store for the sale of fancy and useful articles."[53]

In his wholesale catalog of 1886, Henry Bristow offered "hair wire in spools" for six cents each, and gum arabic for five cents a box. Materials like hair wire and beads and floral pistils were sold by craft-supply companies that specialized in artificial flower supplies. The 1885 Waterman and Hunt price list for wax flowers included wire covered in silk, stem wires, stamens by the bunch for sixty-five cents, "flower cups" (small molds that could cover the wire ends of the flowers), and chenille, all materials useful in any kind of artificial-flower making, including hair flowers for wreaths. In 1897, the Ladies' Art Company offered, among other novelties, the "Complete Tissue Paper Flower Outfit," that included "1 spool Hair Wire, 1 spool Cotton Covered Wire, 1 doz. Wire Stems, 1 doz. Wire Centres," and other materials. Such accessories as hair wire, cotton covered wire, stems, and "centres" (artificial pistils and stamens), were common in hair wreaths as were tissue-paper flowers.[54]

Two distinct techniques were used to make flowers and leaves of hair. Mrs. C. S. Jones's instructions were for the relatively simple "looped" flowers. Essentially her technique involved looping cleansed hair to form flower shapes. For instance, to make the basic loop, hair was attached to the wire, looped evenly, and attached again with the wire. The loops were arranged to form a flower shape, beads were attached in the center, and the stem was carefully wrapped.

Mrs. Levina Urbino and others preferred to make "gimped" flowers.[55] Gimping used the same materials of wire and hair as those used for the looped flowers. The two wires were crossed and twisted, a loop of hair drawn between the two wires and, again, the wires crossed and twisted. The result was a "gimped" strand of regularly looped hair on a wire base. These wire-hair lengths could then be bent into the shapes of leaves, flowers, and tendrils (Figure 16).

Both Jones and Urbino recommended that hair workers "take nature for your guide." Urbino suggested that "it is well to have a pattern. If you can not see hair flowers, take natural ones, and by fastening strands of hair to a wire, and binding with floss, endeavor to imitate nature."[56] One reason Jones and Urbino were able to set their readers loose on the world of nature was that both techniques for making hairwork differed little from other fancywork skills. Two examples, making flower shapes using thread wrapped on wire to make "lace" and crocheting flowers, demonstrated the way different kinds of fancywork blended into one another. Even crafts like feather work resembled hairwork techniques.[57]

In addition, wool-work, popular at the same times as hairwork, used nearly identical techniques for making flower shapes. The technique is only slightly different than Mrs. Jones's for hairwork. In fact, both crafts used a "thready" material (worsted wool or hair) on a base of wire and used beads

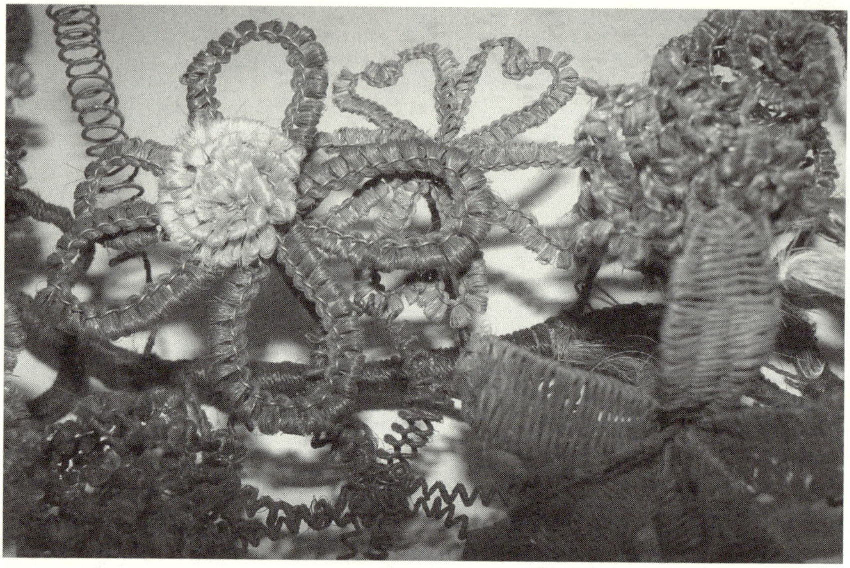

Figure 16. Wrapping hair around wire was a popular technique. The hair was fixed between two wires to create a string of loops, and the hair-covered wire could be bent into petal shapes, center buttons of concentric circles of wire, and, here, heart-shaped petals. Even the spirals are hair wrapped around wire. Courtesy Preble County Historical Society, Eaton, Ohio.

and artificial flower pieces, such as pistils, to ornament the flowers. In 1862, *Godey's* published directions on making worsted-wool flowers.[58] Wool offered the variety of colors, of course, and could be matted and shaped, but the results were similar to those of the flowers made of hair. In the 1870s, Louise Imig made a wreath of both materials. For the wool flowers, she wrapped wire with wool yarn and wound these lengths around a knitting needle to make corkscrew shapes. She also made several flowers of pompons of wool, a very simple wool-working technique.[59]

Most wreaths incorporated both looped and gimped flowers. The cautions regarding the challenges of making hair flowers were not without some foundation, for many wreaths represented more heart than hand skill. For example, the wreath of the Theyer and McMaster families is very messy, with loops of hair springing from their fastenings of unsightly brown embroidery thread. Despite the lack of finesse or skill exhibited in the wreath, the significance of the wreath was not undermined. Using the hair of several family members, the wreath—as awkward, gangly, and even clumsily fashioned as it is—succeeded as a family heirloom, and satisfied its role as an object drawing together various members of an extended family.[60]

In 1855, Mrs. Allison made her own family's hair wreath. Nearly two-and-a-half feet in diameter, the wreath represents forty-eight individuals. Each flower and leaf has next to it a penciled inscription written on the paper backing. While Mrs. Allison included the names of each of the forty-eight people, she did omit one individual—herself. Her presence is only noted in the inked inscription at the base of the wreath: "Made by Mrs. Allison, Lynchburg, OHIO, January 11, 1855."[61]

Wreaths, with their symbolic knitting together of individuals, did not always reflect familial affiliations. In 1893, Nida Bailey recalled in a lengthy account how, in 1864, she was "fired with intense ambition," as she characterized it. She set to work to create what she was sure would be the highest price getter in the St. Louis Sanitary Commission Fund Raising Fair. "For the sake of preserving family hair, I had learned a very delicate manner of weaving it, which had been much admired, and I had no doubt of being able to produce a beautiful wreath, if I could only get the hair—," she recalled in 1893. Her plan was audacious indeed, for she wanted to make "a wreath of flowers woven from the hair of President Lincoln and his cabinet officers and all the prominent officers of the army and navy." As she pointed out in 1893, this was no easy task under the best of circumstances, but, in 1864, "the parties whom I had to reach, were widely scattered and many of them constantly on the move, so that it was no easy matter to locate them all, and by the time I had obtained their addresses, I would learn from the newspapers that Gen. A [*sic*] had been relieved, or Gen. B had advanced or retreated or perchance been killed."

According to Nida Bailey's own testimony, she found far more success at obtaining hair donations when she appealed to the women in the men's lives. Grant's hair was received through a donation of his wife, who "kindly gave me a part of a lock which he had given her when he went to the Mexican war." Elmer Ellsworth's hair was provided by his grieving mother, who gave a lock of his hair, hoping, according to Nida, that "it might benefit the cause in which her darling son lost his life." In all, Nida was able to use the hair of over thirty men, from William Seward, then secretary of state in Lincoln's cabinet to Winfield Scott, then lieutenant general of the Union Army.

Nida, "after many weeks of patient toil" completed the wreath in time for the fair. She was (we hope duly) proud of the results: "It was indeed a 'thing of beauty' and as the donors of the hair were then in the heat of battle and one already killed who had a few weeks before sent his hair with an appreciative letter [the letter, of course, on display with the wreath], it was imbued with a peculiarly tender interest." Recalling her moment of glory in 1893, she described the display of her wreath: "Mounted in its beautiful gilt frame—richly embossed with the national emblem and garnished by a back ground of crimson drapery, with two beautiful silk flags floating over all, I think no one article in that great exposition attracted so much attention as did that wreath with its environments. There was always a crowd around it, and being mounted 8 or 10 ft. from the floor, could be easily seen by all." The wreath was raffled off for $400, and was bought by a "southern lady who, I was informed, prized it only for its beauty."

Nida's pride in her work, and especially in its public display, point to the ambivalence that characterized her wreath project from the start. Nida was by no means a professional hair worker, yet she made a hair wreath expressly for sale, albeit for a charity sale. Instead of entwining family and friends around herself, she created a wreath that literally knit together individuals who shared a common political and military enterprise. Clearly one reading of her wreath was that it represented a unified cause, that of the Union's. But her uniquely feminine and sentimental effort found a friendlier audience with women, at least in her efforts at securing the hair. And Nida mourned, apparently for the rest of her life, the "loss" of her wreath. As she wrote in 1893, "I did not know the owner's name or residence. In the excitement and confusion of that last morning when the Fair was breaking up, I had failed to do that last thing which might have enabled me to regain the relic. Thirty years have been a long time to regret so slight an oversight. With my regrets have been mingled those of my husband and children." It was not simply that their mother had played a "central" role in the Civil War effort, "but as the wreath was their mother's creation, it had for them, more than an historical interest." Emotionally, Nida had viewed the wreath as similar to her other hairworking efforts: as a gift for a family member. But the reality of its "sale" meant that the result of her labors was forever removed from her reach.[62]

Later examples of hair wreaths often used far more elaborate frames, perhaps in keeping with the increasingly ornate quality of parlor decoration.[63] A wreath made in the 1880s used a wood frame that itself was relatively simple, but the backing of gold satin that the wreath is mounted on was decorated with silk-twisted trim. Mrs. Annie Baker Gunhus's 1890 wreath is a simple horseshoe shape and rather skimpy in appearance. But its backing is of loose folds of ivory silk, with sides of the same fabric that are carefully seamed and drawn tight. The frame is elaborately scalloped, and stained to look like alternating bands of mahogany and ebony.[64]

In the 1880s or 1890s, Mrs. A. Jackson created a flat design of a female mourner, an imposing tomb, and a floating cherub. Rendered in hair and wire, her design hearkened back to memorial scenes popular a hundred years before, when William Dunklin's miniature had been created.[65] Most larger-scale hair mourning objects were not, however, in as pictorial a form. Most chose to symbolically represent individuals. When the Bjornsens lost their twelve-year-old daughter Hannah in February 1894, they had a wreath made (probably professionally) of her hair and that of her remaining three siblings and her parents.[66]

Once the hairwork—whether jewelry or a wreath—was completed, a woman had to consider how to best display the piece. Because public display was an important component of hairwork's value as a sentimental object, the choice of what was called "mounting" was important. Most women took their hairwork to professionals to be properly "finished." Thus, the commercial market was where hairwork was endowed with its final touch of fashionableness.

In 1863, a young wife and mother living in Pennsylvania, Rachel Bowman Cormany, found making hairwork could be helpful in times of economic need and also garner her some public attention. Rachel's husband, Samuel, served in the Union Army, leaving Rachel and their young daughter in unfamiliar surroundings. Soon after Samuel had unexpectedly visited Rachel after a months-long absence of serving in battles, Rachel began a new fancywork project. On August 17, 1863, she recorded in her diary, "This morning I got word that the case [a shadow-box frame] for my hair flowers was completed—P.M. I went for it. Its real nice. I asked him (John Hazelett) what the charges were—'Well Mrs Cormany—I admired your hairflower so much & I thought if the case would be acceptable I would make it for you if you would make me a boquet of hair flowers.'" Mr. Hazelett's offer was joyfully received by Rachel. She wrote that she declared to him, "O! Mr. H I shall certainly [d]o that if that satisfies you &c &c & thanked him for the case." Rachel welcomed the opportunity for bartering, for money was tight with Samuel gone.[67]

For the lonely Rachel, the attention her hair flowers garnered was even more valuable than the bartering. As she carried her case home, she wrote, "some 1/2 dozen or more ladies come running to see my flowers . . . those ladies of course were disappointed when they saw the empty case—All seem anxious to see the flowers."

After she brought the case home, Rachel still had to finish her hair flowers and mount them in readiness for others to look at them. The next day, August 18, she "worked at my hair flowers & completed the wreath & boquet for the centre." The next day she put the hair flowers in the case, noting it "looks pretty." And the following day, as promised, "Mrs McGowan—Mrs Sulenberger & Miss Rudy took tea with me—Had a nice little visit. . . . All admired my hair flowers very much."[68] By displaying her handiwork and, through that handiwork, demonstrating her close ties to other, absent individuals to her new neighbors, Rachel found a way to belong to what was formerly a closed community.

Chapter 4
Made to Order

The woven strands of hair that composed a piece of hair jewelry represented the various threads of a person's life. Parents, partner, and children could be braided together, and the unfathomable number of small interactions that constituted relationships could be physically represented in the complicated structure of a hair watch chain or necklace. Those same strands represented labor as well. Thousands of independent hair workers built careers by creating, one after another, beautiful, intricate pieces of hair jewelry. Even as large-scale companies began to dominate the hairwork market, the actual hairwork—smoothly woven hair watch chains, ornately patterned earrings of hair, or flat braids of bracelets—was made by human hands. Those hands were both symbols of the emotional and personal satisfaction the commercial market offered for its paying customers, and an image of the impersonal, cold, and at times dehumanizing effects of a market in which even a person's intimate relationships were subject to being valued and priced accordingly.

The market of hairwork production retained the basic structure that characterized it in the 1850s and 1860s; hairwork was produced by a mixture of small, independent producers and retailers, and some small-scale mail-order companies. But in the 1870s and continuing to the early 1900s, larger-scale distributors of hairwork coexisted with the independent craftswomen and -men. Customers expected that hairwork be made by hand and of the hair supplied by the customer. Thus, acceptable hairwork could not be mechanically or mass-produced. In the 1870s, several hair workers attempted to gain a national market, largely by advertising in national jewelers' magazines (and not, it is noted, to the general public). Their efforts were constrained by the nature of their product, the consistently low levels of credit available to them, personal vagaries of fortune and strategy, and shifts in the American economy that increasingly favored larger businesses and corporations, not individual craftsmen and -women. They were hampered from all sides: production of hairwork was limited by the demands of its sentimental appeal and the nature of its raw material; distribution could be conducted on a wider scale, but that would threaten the personalized aspects of the product; financiers favored larger corporations, not small businesses.

Who Were the Professional Hair Workers?

Despite the persistence of amateur hairwork crafting, in the 1870s and 1880s most Americans probably attained their hairwork jewelry from a local retailer. As in the 1770s to the 1860s, a customer, usually a woman, went through a local jeweler. Hairwork was custom work, made to order, very much like other products for women such as hats and dresses.[1] If the jeweler was also a hair worker, then the customer would explain what he or she wanted and the jeweler would create the item. More likely, however, the customer selected a style from a pattern book provided by a distant hair worker, gave the hair to the jeweler, and waited until the order came in. The local retailer was simply the intermediary in this emotionally laden business transaction.

Manufactories similar to Cooke's small eighteenth-century establishment persisted through the nineteenth century. But by the 1870s and 1880s, the small artisan workshop had given way to less personal "factories" where hair was worked by a variety of hands. And in another difference from earlier periods, hairwork firms often employed women to make the hair jewelry. The factory floors were themselves gender-segregated. Mark Campbell's catalog of 1867 depicts himself as *the* hair worker sitting straight and capable before his braiding table (Figure 17). In the same volume, however, Campbell's female braiders are pictured lined up before large windows, and on the other side of the room the male jewelry makers toil. The women sat behind Campbell at braiding tables, carefully moving weighted strands of hair to form the elaborate, twisted chains. Male co-workers created the gold mountings, the bands of rings, the clasps for the necklaces, and the hooks for the watch chains. This arrangement was not uncommon in jewelry production.[2]

Independent hair workers, that is, hair workers who advertised their craft without reference to a manufactory, were a surprisingly diverse group ranging from Northern European Americans to African Americans. Not unexpectedly, recent European immigrants, such as the Moutoux Brothers in New York, were among these artisans.[3] Hairwork, from ornamental hair-

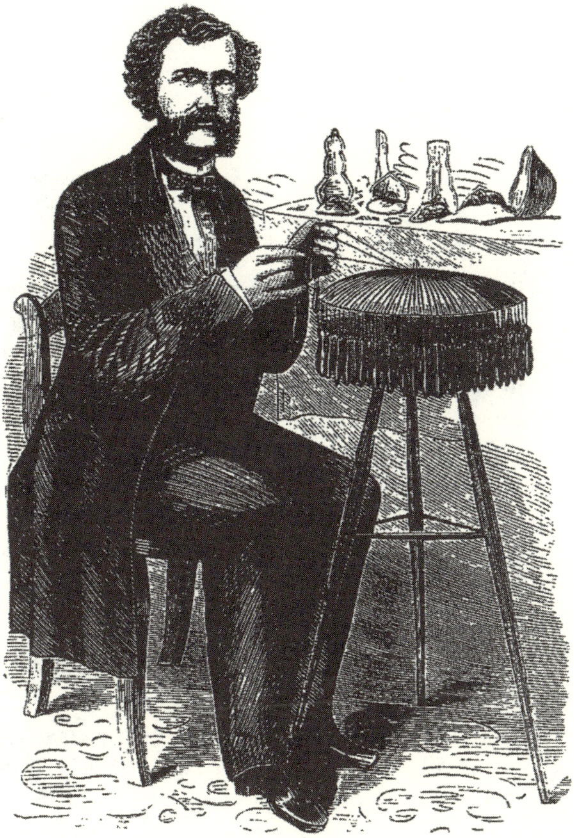

Figure 17. Mark Campbell pauses while working an extremely complex hairwork braid of perhaps forty strands or more. He holds three lengths of hair, each weighted with a lead bobbin, and the worked braid will soon emerge through the hole at the center of the braiding table. Behind him are displays of his finished work. From Mark Campbell, *Hair Manual, or Self-Instructor* (1879). Courtesy The Winterthur Library, Printed Book and Periodical collection.

work to hairdressing, was practiced by African American men and women.[4] In Chicago in the 1860s, for example, Adolph Ohswaldt offered hair jewelry. Despite his Germanic name, Ohswaldt is listed as a "col'd" man in an 1865 city directory. Other African Americans in Chicago, including Jared Gray, were also offering hair jewelry as well as wigs, toupees, and hairdressing. And in Philadelphia, at least two African Americans, George and Elizabeth Stewart, were making hair jewelry professionally in the same years.[5]

Hairwork had a key advantage for African Americans in the ante- and postbellum years: as in the eighteenth century, the craft required minimal stock to be on hand. Free African Americans, especially in the years prior to the Civil War, had little access to the capital and credit necessary to set up successful shops.[6] That was, in part, why hair working was also attractive to eighteenth-century white men recently released from their apprenticeships and what made hair working a career open to such a diverse group of workers in the nineteenth century. A hair-working business required very little start-up stock, no machinery, and very few, if any, employees. For women, especially urban white women, these advantages were even stronger. Hair working was mentioned as a possible "girl's" employment in a novel aimed at young women, along with "bee-keeping, librarian, telegraph operator . . . milliner, florist" and so on.[7]

One white Bavarian American woman, Katharine (sometimes Catherine, Catharine, or Katherine) Schmitt, had an independent hairwork shop from 1854 until 1900 in Philadelphia.[8] Her lengthy career demonstrates how some women were able to flourish in the hair-working field. Hair workers such as Schmitt described themselves as both artists and "mechanics" who provided hairwork of consistent designs to appeal to nineteenth-century customers intent on purchasing jewelry that was fashionable as well as individualized.

Throughout her career, Schmitt entered and won contests for "artistic creations" of hairwork, while she also created standard styles of hair jewelry to satisfy her less-adventuresome customers. She began professional hair working in the United States with a partner, Fredrick Stubenrauch (or Friedrich Steubenrauch). They created both hairwork and jewelry, a typical offering as hairwork alone could probably not support a shop.[9] Their partnership lasted until 1871 and, at that point, the former colleagues set up separate shops. In 1870, the two partners were doing about $5,000 to $10,000 of business annually, and were rated as a "fair" credit risk. As the sole proprietor after 1870, Katharine Schmitt had between $2,000 and $5,000 of business a year, but retained her "fair" credit ranking.[10]

In 1860, while the two were still partners, it was Katharine Schmitt who was interviewed by the Bureau of Census worker. She reported a real-estate value of $2,000, with her personal real estate valued at $1,000. By 1870, when she was interviewed for the manufacturing census, "Madame K. Schmidt" reported $10,000 invested in her business, a figure much higher than that reported to the Dun and Bradstreet investigators. She had four employees, all reportedly above the age of fifteen, and she paid out $1,196 the previous year in wages (a $299 a year income on average per worker).[11] It is impossible to ascertain if her employees (all women) were also hair workers. Katharine Schmitt was, therefore, a proprietor and an employer as well as a craftswoman.

Other women struggled to maintain small-scale hair-working businesses. Mrs. Hannah Schnepper started a shop in the Bowery in New York City, but she was never able to gain solid footing. In 1869, a Dun agent reported that she had been "in bus [business] some years and is regarded honest and respectable, but is not believed to possess much means." Three years later, Mrs. Schnepper was "not now living with her husband they are having difficulty and seperated. She is doing business on her own account and is a very reliable worthy woman of moderate means." Mrs. Schnepper persisted on her own, and in 1872 she gave up millinery and offered only hairwork. Despite an "active business," however, she could not "seem to get square," as the Dun agent feelingly stated it. Finally, in 1872 Schnepper maintained her hairwork business, but added what the Dun agent called a "Dollar Store." She ceased applying for credit the year after.[12]

The Hair Worker as a Mechanic and an Inventor

Hair workers were understood to be "mechanics," reflecting the trade's origins as an artisan craft. In the early 1840s, the Franklin Institute exhibitions included "fancy articles" for which prize competitions were held. In 1842, for example, F. J. Dressler was accorded a certificate of Honorable Mention for a case display of "fancy hair work."[13] The Franklin Institute was not alone in its recognition of what it termed the "mechanical" skill of hair workers. Other exhibitions, including the Middlesex Mechanic Association of Lowell, Massachusetts; the Metropolitan Mechanics' Institute of Washington, D.C.; and the Manufacturers' and Mechanics' Institute of Boston, included hairwork and other kinds of fancy articles.[14]

Katharine Schmitt, for example, entered artisan competitions and received awards for her creations throughout her long career. In 1854 and then again in 1874, she received medals from the Franklin Institute, and she included both commendations in her advertisements. In 1874, the institute commented that her "work is of the best character, very neatly finished, and of great variety and ingenuity of design." In 1877 and in 1878, she received "first premium" medals at the Philadelphia Centennial and, in 1881, she announced in an advertisement that her work had been awarded three premium medals (Figure 18).[15]

Some hair jewelers patented their innovations. In 1861, J. S. Palmer, a hair worker in Providence, Rhode Island, (and Providence was, of course, the center of the jewelry industry), patented his paneled bracelet. Its recessed panels provided "suitable plates containing hair work" or other sen-

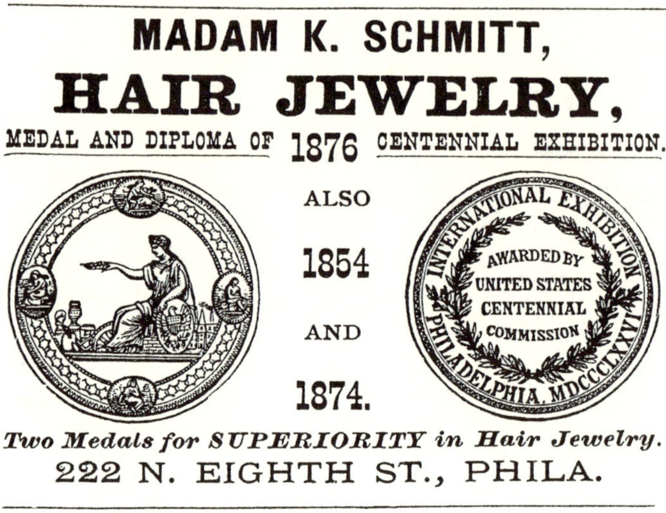

Figure 18. Katharine Schmitt touts her awards for hairwork in national competitions. In the hair-working business for fifty years, Schmitt not only supported her own family with her business, she employed several women as well. Hair working offered entrepreneurial opportunity in the 1860s and 1870s. Advertisement, *Gopsill's Philadelphia City Directory for 1881*.

timental objects such as painted miniatures.[16] In 1866, Lorenzo Sauter of Jersey City, New Jersey, touted in his advertisements that he was the "patantee and sole manufacturer of the Patent Revolving Rings" that could be found in other pattern books besides his own. His ring allowed the wearer to conceal the hair mounted in it by virtue of an outer casing that encircled the ring. It was clever; by sliding the outer covering completely around the ring, Sauter claimed that "the hair contained in the body [would] be entirely concealed, so that the exterior of the ring will be the same as that of an ordinary plain ring, and the hair will be protected from any injury which might happen to it if exposed in washing the hands or from other causes."[17]

Such inventions were not entered in the mechanical fairs, however. The kinds of hairwork submitted to these competitions were statements of artistic bravado that did not characterize a creator's typical work. In the 1853 New York Crystal Palace Exhibition, the Linherr brothers entered a most wonderful piece of hairwork artistry. As a parlor magazine exclaimed, "Just think of a tea set made of a lover's hair!" It was, the paper solemnly judged, a remarkable "show of skill and patience that has necessarily been em-

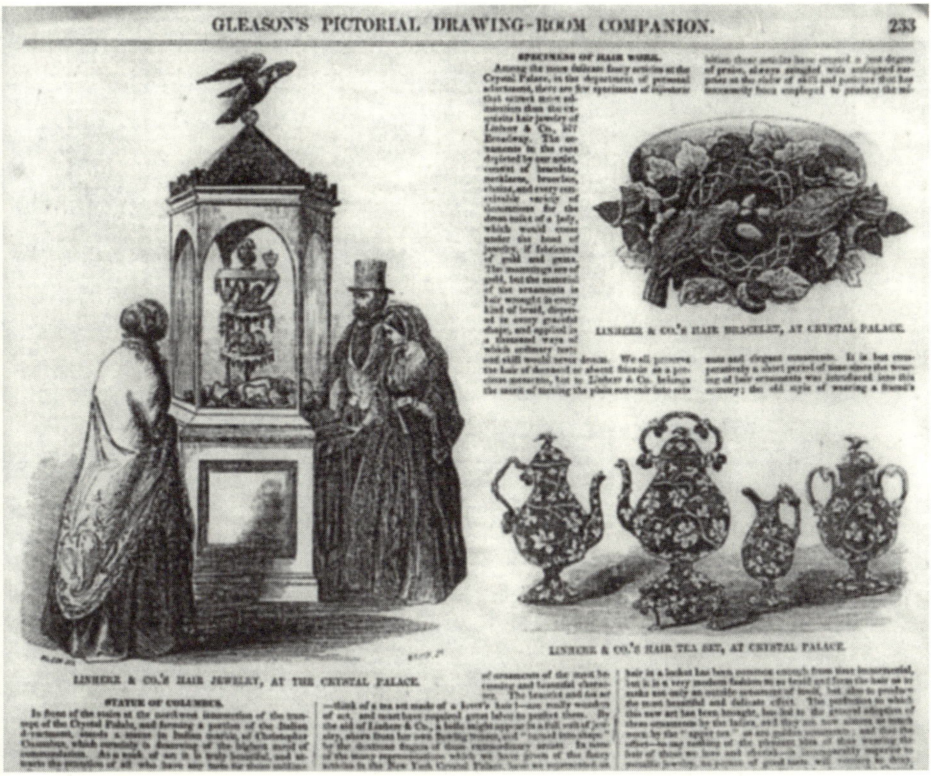
GLEASON'S PICTORIAL DRAWING-ROOM COMPANION. 233

LINHERR & CO.'S HAIR BRACELET, AT CRYSTAL PALACE.

LINHERR & CO.'S HAIR TEA SET, AT CRYSTAL PALACE.

LINHERR & CO.'S HAIR JEWELRY, AT THE CRYSTAL PALACE.

Figure 19. Little could compete with a tea set made of hair, created by the Linherr brothers. In a stunning display of hairwork virtuosity, both the tea set and elaborate bracelet impressed visitors to the 1853 New York Crystal Palace Exhibition. Hairwork regularly appeared in mechanics' fairs, state and county fairs, and exhibitions of commercial and artistic products such as this one. From "Specimens of Hair Work," *Gleason's Pictorial Drawing-Room Companion* 5.15 (Oct. 8, 1853), 233.

ployed to produce the minute and elegant ornaments."[18] And as we can well imagine from inspecting the accompanying illustration, the tea set was indeed a marvel. But the Linherrs, talented as they might have been, relied on standard hairwork to conduct their business. In 1859, Christian Linherr wrote a receipt to a young lady for a breastpin priced at $6.00. This was a typical price for one of the most popular forms of hair jewelry (Figure 19).[19]

Similarly, Katharine Schmitt, who won several medals for technical prowess at the mechanics' exhibitions, produced hair jewelry in the most common styles. The Smithsonian collection includes a lyre-shaped fob that was made by Schmitt and her partner, Stubenrauch, sometime between 1863 and 1870. The fob is a generic style, offered in numerous hairwork catalogs from the 1860s until 1900.[20] Schmitt's customer did not seek distinctive styles of hair jewelry. Instead, the hair itself was sufficient to establish individuality; the style was subordinated to that. In 1871, Schmitt's advertisements addressed these twin demands. She offered that she "keeps on hand, in her new store, 'HAIR JEWELRY.'" This suggested that Schmitt had examples of hair jewelry already made so that customers could inspect her handiwork in order to select a style for their own use. She also announced, "Articles of this kind are manufactured by the above in the most beautiful style of approved workmanship, and from the identical hair furnished by her customers." It was, as another commentator put it, "the real hair given." Selling her own handiwork but in generic styles, this assurance was indeed necessary for her customers.[21]

The Hair Worker as Retailer

Some hair workers were able to sustain their business and themselves by hairwork alone, but they were the exception. Most retailers who provided hairwork were either general jewelers who offered hairwork as one of many jewelry styles, or they were hair workers who offered an array of other hair goods, including hairdressing and wig making. Mrs. A. S. Rollo of Wilmington, Delaware, specialized in "Hair Jewelry & Hair Flowers a specialty, Switches, Wigs, and Natural Wavy Front Pieces."[22] The Misses M. A. Shaw and A. M Shafer in Springfield, Ohio, used a double-sided separate trade card to advertise their diversified business. First, they provided "Ladies' Hair Dressing and Shampooing" in their rooms at 18 S. Limestone Street. The back of the card described the pair as "artists in hair, also manufacturers and dealers in every description of ornamented hair goods." As "artists in hair," they were creators of sentimental hair art and also artificial hair workers. They also provided toiletries, a dandruff tonic, and cleaned kid gloves.[23]

All of these specialties, from beauty tonics, dyes, hairstyling, and even hair jewelry, shared a common role as personal ornamentation. One virtue of such dealers was that their activities in such a wide field of "ornament" accorded them a degree of professionalism and expertise.[24] Many of these companies and hair dealers offered a wide variety of goods, but such outlets are not the mass market. Historians have argued that "big retailing" took three distinct forms in the United States: mail-order businesses, department stores, and chain stores.[25] None of the previously discussed hairwork dealers could boast a national market of sales of a wide variety of goods. Some hairwork dealers used innovative marketing techniques to secure a place in the changing market of personal goods. But no national hairwork dealers could boast of being a "big business" in terms of saturation of market, plethora of goods, or even large retail units.

Instead, some hairwork jewelers advertised in national publications and functioned as "jobbers" for smaller, local jewelers. Traditionally, most jobbers purchased goods in large lots ("jobs") and sold these lots in smaller units to retailers who had shops. Goods transacted in this way included ready-made clothing, housewares, textiles, cleaning agents, jewelry, and other goods.[26] By the 1860s, 80 percent of the goods sold by retailers were provided by jobbers. Specialty and made-to-order goods could not be "jobbed" in the same fashion. But a local jeweler who was not trained in hairwork could still offer such jewelry selections by contracting with a larger house to fill any orders. In 1878, O. Schwencke informed readers of the *Jewelers' Circular*, a jewelry trade magazine, that he offered "fine hair jewelry" with "Solid Gold Mountings for Hair Jewelry, kept constantly on hand, and made to order at shortest notice." He made a special assurance to jewelers, "Orders from the country trade promptly attended to." The following year, a promotional note in the same journal advertised that Mr. Schwencke "has achieved a high reputation as a maker of artistic jewelry. . . . He is constantly producing the newest effects in hair work. Dealers who have special orders for device work, would do well to consult" him.[27] Schwencke's business, then, relied on retail jewelers who turned to him to create the hair jewelry for which they had an order.

The single greatest limitation on the development of a national-scale hairwork business was the nature of its production. Unlike other jewelry products that, by the late 1870s, were likely made using machine dies and cuts, there was simply no way to mass produce or even machine produce the product, mainly because of the emotional meanings of the product; there was little if any interest throughout the nineteenth century for hairwork that was not made of hair that the customer had an affiliation to. There was also the difficulty of customer choice. It is apparent from the consistent emphasis on the wide selections of style that customers expected to be able to order from a wide array of different styles, or even be able to sketch out a hairwork piece of their own design, and have it made of the hair that they provided. For this reason, there was no way to efficiently create the product except one by one, made to order, and by hand.

Not only did this hamper production, it limited the credit available to hair workers. Credit agencies such as Dun and Company specialized in providing credit ratings based on a business owner's reputation, the business's state of health, and the value of the business itself. Hair workers may have been honest, but their stock in trade was very difficult to measure. Thus, in 1877 one agent noted that John A. Linherr was difficult to rate "as his stock in trade is of very uncertain value it is impossible to make an accurate estimate." He was deemed "good" for only small amounts of credit. Two years later, Linherr was "getting behind for some time, and on account of non-payment of rent was obliged to vacate the premises and is presently out of business." Whether his lack of credit led to his business's demise we don't know, but it certainly did not help him to have no credit extended to him.[28]

Other goods were made in similar fashion, but as the nineteenth century progressed, these were the most luxurious or most expensive goods available. Hairwork, though, was a middle-class phenomenon whose retail prices reflected that position. Other decorative goods that were not easily mass produced were often batch and custom manufactured. Fashion textiles, apparel, furniture, and other "small goods" were batch produced in small lots by innovative factories that were able to quickly fill small orders from large retailers. Likewise, custom work built each item per individual order and, while findings and fasteners such as the mountings or chain clasps were mass produced, the items were individually produced. Few firms survived on custom work alone; most relied on a mixture of batch production and individual orders.[29]

The few hair workers who aspired to a national market advertised in national trade magazines in an effort to "job" for small jewelry retail stores where the owner presumably did not make hairwork.[30] These ambitious hair workers advertised in national to-the-trade jewelry publications, published pattern books for retailers and catalogue houses, and tended to also invent and patent designs in hair jewelry. Despite these efforts, most of these "national" hairwork houses remained small businesses with limited capital and stock and very limited growth potential.

F. J. Loeper, in his own pattern book of the 1880s, carefully explained the process of securing hairwork from a dealer. Addressing himself "to the Trade," Loeper assured that "orders are filled within from 6 to 10 days upon receipt of Hair." Loeper accepted loose combings (that is, hair gathered from a hairbrush) or even "a very small quantity of hair" for some items—an instruction that would have surprised amateur hair workers, who were often cautioned not to underestimate the amount of hair needed for hairwork. Of course, Loeper was not addressing customers, but retail outlets who may have been less concerned with thoughts of how a full hair chain might be made from a few wisps of hair.

In 1879, Charles Theodore Menger (or rather, his family) advertised in the nationally distributed business publication, *The Jewelers' Circular and Horological Review*. Located in New York, Menger offered to "send a large Pattern Book and Price List, containing all the latest design on receipt of 50 cts. . . . I also fill orders taken from any other book upon advice of name and number of design." His willingness to copy the designs of other dealers was a savvy and aggressive sales technique. However, in 1875 a Dun credit investigator had found that Charles had actually died in 1873, and his widow and son continued to "run the old business under the old style."[31] The business survived for awhile; in 1885 a different Dun investigator found Charles' wife, son, and now, daughter, were busy. "They manufacture hair jewelry for the trade and mainly upon orders." It was a small-scale business, with only a "small amt. invested in Machinery + Tools + carry but little Stock."[32] By 1888, the Mengers were finally out of business.

Lorenzo Sauter was also ambitious. In the 1870s, he advertised frequently in *The Watchmaker and Jeweler*, a trade publication.[33] As noted earlier, Sauter also patented his innovative hair jewelry designs, and of course touted such patented products in his advertisements to the trade. In 1880, Lorenzo Sauter announced to the readership of the *Jewelers' Circular* his new "Pattern Books containing 300 designs of the most current articles." As Menger's family did, Sauter sold his book of design for fifty cents. Like Charles Menger and the Menger family, Sauter filled orders for the trade. A Dun agent praised Sauter as a "very prudent, economical man doing a small business . . . manufactures considerable hair jewellery on orders as well as carrying a small stock of rings, etc."[34] Sauter, who had patented some of his hair jewelry designs, released a pattern book of three hundred designs in the early 1880s.

Hairwork dealers, such as Mark Campbell in Chicago, emerged. From the 1860s to the late 1870s, Mark Campbell tried and failed to create an empire built on hairwork. His company, headquartered in Chicago and with an office in New York City, published catalogues and instructional manuals, was a national mail-order business, and acted as a jobber and repairer of hair jewelry. In addition, Campbell ran a hairdresser's shop and made artificial hairpieces. His triumvirate of business efforts as publisher, ornamental hairworker, and artificial-hair dealer represented the multiplicity of the commerce in hair in the nineteenth century. His failure at all three endeavors stems from the economic challenges to small businesses in the post–Civil War years. Campbell appears to have been caught between larger economic trends that favored larger-scale business and the reality of hairwork: it was always hand-produced on a small scale, with each individual product a singular creation.

Campbell's own promotional material exploited the idiosyncratic character of his product. In 1862, in a local mugbook (these "histories" of a city profiled local businesses using effusive language and were actually a series of paid advertisements), the author waxed eloquent over Campbell's products. "Who that has gazed upon the hair wrought in many a strange and artistic device—secured from the wavy ringlets of some beautiful girls, or the brow of the loved or the lost, but will cherish them as *gems of the beautiful* forever?"[35] That was in 1862, when Campbell's business was largely retail. So sentiment reigned, because that was the motivating factor for consumers.

Campbell was ambitious, and had visions of having a nationally renowned manufactory of hairwork. In 1867, he published his *Self-Instructor*, which provided everyday people the "secrets" of hair working. But he was also soliciting hair-jewelry business, and thus emphasized the manufacturing prowess of his enterprise in a circular promoting his new book: "I manufacture and sell, at wholesale and retail, hair jewelry and gold mountings for hair jewelry, of every pattern and device, to suit the fancy of my patrons. I have given years of study and practical experience to this branch of my business, and have so perfected and enlarged my MANUFACTURING FACILITIES as to feel confident of being able to give entire satisfaction in workmanship and price."[36] The reality of Campbell's business differed from the perfect and enlarged factory he described and depicted in his advertisement. In fact, he did not even have an actual retail store at the time. Because of his ambitions, Campbell had petitioned the R. G. Dun Company to rate his credit. In April 1868, the Dun agent noted that Mr. Campbell told him he owned the lease on the building next to his and was planning on using the money to put up a storefront. The agent, checking up on Campbell's story, was assured by "parties who know a great deal abt [about] his affairs that his statement is not out of the way." The agent noted that Campbell wasn't all talk; "he does a larger bus [business] than all others in the trade in the

City . . . is a vg [very good] enterprising man + no doubt good for all he wants."[37]

Campbell did fairly well for several years, but, in June 1871, he faced a downturn in business and prospects. This year, the agent reported that Campbell told him "Bus. [business] has been very dull for past year . . . [and] he says hard up just now but business is picking up." Campbell had moved his business from Clarke Street to State Street, but, while the move to the higher profile street front helped, his overhead escalated. The Dun agent noted sourly that Campbell "could not save much as his style of living has long been extravagant. His new store cost him as he admitted [a high rent] . . . his store is fitted up in a first rate manner + it is not that the trade will increase much if any by the change." In fact, the agent found after checking on Campbell's story, that Campbell was "behind with his rent, which is a bad feature. It is admitted by excellent authorities that he has branched out too largely for his means that great care should be exercising large credit." Dun never found a need to visit Mark Campbell's business again, and he ceased listing his business in the city directories. Campbell, did, however, persist in his business efforts, publishing editions of his *Self-Instructor* in 1875 and 1879, and continuing to tout his hairwork business long after he had applied for a credit rating.[38]

In 1872, another hairwork dealer in Chicago was also struggling to keep his business afloat and his ambitions alive. Jared Gray (sometimes referred to as Jacob or John) was an African American man with a hairwork business that eventually branched out from the simple offerings of hairwork and hairdressing to toiletries, wigs, and other hair accessories. He had started hair working in Chicago in 1859.[39]

The credit firm of R. G. Dun was never very positive in its comments about Mr. Gray, and often quite harsh. In the assessment of Dun and Company, Mr. Gray was consistently in debt, rarely paid his bills in a timely fashion, and was not worth the risk of credit. The agents often found him difficult to deal with, in that he appeared forthcoming in his answers, but when they checked up on his comments, they often found he had lied to them. For example, in 1869 the agent visited Jared Gray at his business at 77 Clark Street, just down the street from Mark Campbell's competing business. The agent confronted Gray about rumors of large debts, but "he denies it and says he owes altogether abt. 200." But the agent found upon questioning other sources, "It is suspected however that he has either mtge [a mortgage] or made over his ppty [property] to E. [unidentified individual]." In 1870, Gray had "no credit in this city or with anybody who has had dealings with him."[40] Gray had an excuse for this state of affairs, or at least for his inability to pay off his outstanding debts. His stock orders from Europe were not arriving on time, so figuring that the orders simply would never arrive, he reordered supplies from another house. Then both orders arrived, and he then had two orders to pay off instead of one. The Dun agent sourly noted that whether this was the case or not, Gray had a debt repayment plan that stretched over six years and was carrying a heavy mortgage. He simply was not a good credit risk.

In 1871, Gray endured even more setbacks for the business. Jared Gray had suffered losses in the Chicago fire in October of that year and, with his son and wife, he was attempting to regain his lost business trade. It is unclear when Jared married, but his wife was a white, foreign-born woman whose race and family resources helped steady Jared's business attempts. Still, when the Dun credit agent checked in on the Grays in mid-1872, he found their business in disarray. Having "lost everything his insurance was bad and . . . his old matter are still unsettled."[41] The Grays were conducting the business under Mrs. Gray's name, a common practice for small businesses. By sheltering the business under the woman's name, the debts incurred under the man's name were nominally left unpaid.[42]

In 1873, Gray placed a lengthy advertisement in Midwestern papers. Gray's business was described as "the old house" which, prior to the fire of 1871, was doing $70,000 to $80,000 of business a year (a gross overstatement if Dun's credit reports are correct). Gray had, according to the advertisement, been traveling throughout Europe buying quality hair, and also learning the various "manipulations" of the hair trade.[43]

In 1875, the Dun agent found the situation much the same. The business was still under Mrs. Gray's name, Jared (referred to as John here) had outstanding judgments still to pay. But Mrs. Gray's European ties were paying off for the family. Jared Gray told the agent that "his wife's friends in Europe gave her a start and she has a stock of . . . [text unclear] all from Europe and paid for." This news helped persuade the Dun agent to look more favorably on Mr. Gray himself. He is, the agent noted, "a colored gentleman with a white wife and have a good reputation before the fire." But the struggle to survive as a business was evident, for the agent also noted that "his stock is very small and we cannot get any information here abt him, but would recom'nd caution."[44] The next year Mr. Gray filed for bankruptcy.

Jewelry Wholesalers, Mass-Market Retailers, and Hair Workers

Aside from individual dealers such as Campbell, Gray, Loeper, and others who attempted to reach retail owners throughout the country, larger companies also sought to fulfill hairwork orders. These larger companies, however, never specialized in hairwork. Most often, if Mark Campbell received orders from his advertisements in national jewelers' trade journals, it was from these large companies. Clapp and Company, the J. H. Purdy and Company, the S. H. Clement Company and the A. C. Becken Company were jewelry wholesalers who offered retail jewelers enormous selections that included hairwork made to order. It was these wholesalers who likely offered individual hair workers the bulk of their business. Wholesalers also offered repair services that were likely also contracted out to independent hair workers.

Wholesalers could braid the hair given or provide mounting services for hair already braided. In 1888, Clapp and Company offered hair-chain mountings for $12.50 and $14.00 each, and there was "allowance made for Hair furnished braided." J. H. Purdy and Company listed in its repair price list a "Two-Strand Hair Chain" for $2.00, and "Hair Chain Braiding" for $1.50 each. In an undated commercial dealers' resource book, one-strand hair-chain braiding was listed at $1.00, and two-strand hair chains for $2.00. In 1889, the S. H. Clement Company of Chicago offered "braiding hair vest chains" for $1.50, and hair-bracelet braiding for $1.50 to $2.00 each. The S. H. Clement Company attempted, as did many other wholesalers, to accommodate itself to the vagaries of jewelers' needs and, by extension, the consumer's desires. S. H. Clement Company would, as noted above, braid hair. "When mountings are bought of us, no extra charge is made for putting together," claimed the company. Furthermore, the company emphasized its willingness to complete all kinds of hairwork, not just hair chains. "Hair braiding for pins, ear rings, lockets, rings, neck chains, etc. made on short notice and at lowest prices." A similar "package" was offered at the beginning of the twentieth century by the A. C. Becken Company. The company advertised its "Gentlemen's Real Human Hair Vest Chains" with rolled gold plate slides, bars, and tips. At the same time, in its repair price list it offered "Hair Chain Braiding" and noted parenthetically that "when mountings are bought of us we will fit to chain without extra charge."[45]

As discussed earlier, it was *Godey's Lady's Book and Magazine* that dominated the early years of the direct mail-order hairwork. *Godey's* practice, however, waned and by the 1870s, they were filling fewer and fewer orders for hairwork. By March 1870, the magazine listed no hairwork in its "Philadelphia Agency" notes. This does not suggest that hairwork had declined in popularity—indeed, the 1870s was a decade in which hairwork was extremely popular. Rather, subscribers were no longer turning to *Godey's* to purchase hairwork.

Instead, it was the mass marketers who gained most of the mail-order hair-jewelry market. Both Montgomery Ward and Company, founded in 1872, and Sears, Roebuck and Company, founded in 1886, offered hair chains and hair fobs. In 1894, an option for men's watch chains was "hair chains made to order." Wards instructed customers to "send us the hair and we will braid in style." The company offered hair-chain styles, and also offered to sell mountings at an extra charge. In addition, Wards offered a substantial watch chain for $1.15 and a "sensible, practical hair vest chain. Just the right length; elegantly mounted with gold-filled mountings" for $1.50.[46] In 1880, *Ehrich's Fashion Quarterly*, a periodical published by a large department store, began to offer hair jewelry. Because of the "great increase in the number of orders forwarded us for goods of this description," the company was able "to increase our facilities for manufacturing, and consequently to effect a marked reduction in prices." The lower prices applied to "Our Hair Jewelry . . . in the first-class style of workmanship." The catalogue offered ten kinds of hair jewelry, from a "Very Rich Bracelet" for $8.50 to an anchor charm for $3.50.[47]

A lower price for customers could only come at the expense of the hair worker. Because hairwork had to be handmade, one of the few ways to lower costs was for the hair workers to simply charge less per item. Another way to lower costs, of course, would be for the hair worker to make the items ahead of time, using human hair purchased from hair dealers who more often provided the raw material for ready-made wigs, falls, and curls. Obviously, hair workers began to do this, and wholesalers began to offer retail jewelers hair vest chains by the dozen rather than singly. The Jewelers' Wholesale Supply Depot in 1883 offered a standard selection of hair-chain mountings that would have been used by hair workers or even a retail jeweler interested in mounting customers' amateur hairwork.[48]

The following year, the same company offered the same selection of vest chains with one difference. Instead of hair vest chains by the dozen, the company now offered the hair chains singly—for $3.00 each. Instead of a thrifty $27.00 a dozen, or $2.25 each, the cost to retailers was 75 cents more.[49] Not only does this reveal the painfully low value accorded to the hair worker's labor, it suggests that retailers—or, more likely, customers—were not ready for depersonalized, ready-made hairwork.

Professionally Made Hairwork as an Insincere Product

The arguments that this commercial market posed a threat to the sincerity, authenticity, and meaning of hairwork persisted into the late 1800s. Mrs. C. S. Jones, for example, writing in 1876 echoes the language used in the 1850s. She wrote,

> The professional hair-manufacturers can doubtless perform this work more artistically, and bring it to a far higher degree of perfection than the mere amateur; but when we take into consideration the liability of having the hair of some other person substituted for that of our own cherished friend, or that careless hands have idly drawn through their fingers the tresses which it appears almost sacrilegious to have even looked upon with a cold glance, the thought is repugnant. The ability to so arrange and secure each strand of the sacred treasure, becomes an accomplishment truly valuable, and worthy of all patience and skill required in its performance.[50]

Jones's comments suggest how the effects of the commercial market had intensified since the 1850s. The great skills of the professional hair worker were acknowledged, but those advantages were supposedly outweighed by the sentimental requirements of sincerity and authenticity. In the 1850s, *Godey's* had promised that its instructions would allow any woman to "manufacture" her own hairwork; in 1876, Jones used language that distanced even amateur creations from the market. In Jones's words, instead of manufacturing hairwork, amateur craftswomen were to "arrange and secure each strand of the sacred treasure." Hair working was now a ritualized sacramental act wholly apart from the cold hands of the professional hair worker. Clearly there was reason to worry about those cold hands. The National Artistic Hair Work Company, in its catalog that provided detailed instructions on making one's own hairwork and offered hundreds of designs of hair jewelry that they could make for the customer, pointed out to its prospective customers that "the public can have their valuable hair work done at their own homes where they may feel satisfied that their hair will be made up to suit them, in the place of sending it away to some large city by a jewelry dealer. Nine chances out of ten they throw the hair away and supply other in place of it, which is already made up."[51] The images Jones presented, of menacing hands coldly riffling through the pieces of one's beloved's body, and the National Artistic Hair Work Company's description of hair simply being tossed out, and even *Godey's* and Campbell's sketches of the horror of never knowing for certain if the hair in one's piece of jewelry was really that of a loved one, were well-calculated for their audience. Middle-class Americans faced an uncertain market of several dimensions. Of course, the market of goods was rapidly shifting out of sight, relocated to sites unknown. Instead of patronizing a local jeweler, many women who wanted hairwork done were faced with sending the hair off to an unseen and unknown worker and dealer. But this was only one side of the market. Middle-class Americans were also coping with an uncertain social world in which, it was feared, individuals could fake their sincerity and character. Even one's social and economic position, seemingly so stable, was built on the shaky foundations of an ever-changing, heartless market. Promoters of amateur hairwork promised certainty, authenticity, and a way to remain fashionable while circumventing the market of mass production, and addressed larger issues than simply how to create one's own hairwork.

Hairwork existed within the context of increasingly dominant machine production and manufactured commodities. And hairwork was a particularly curious commercial product in both its production and circulation. Hair, seemingly the most authentic of materials, became a doubtful substance when it was worked over by the market. Throughout the nineteenth century, advertisers, dealers, and magazine writers expressed concern over hairwork's authenticity. At issue was not only the credibility of hairwork but the validity of sentimentality. The position of the emerging middle class, and the individuals within it, rested on the utility of sentimentality. Sentimentality's effectiveness, in turn, depended on a balance between naiveté and fashion, between naturalness and artifice. Hairwork as a sentimental consumer good offered a way to wed these disparate priorities and to satisfy simultaneously contradictory requirements of both (Figure 20).

Nineteenth-century Americans valued machine-produced goods for their ability to transform materials into something with the appearance of another thing. Artificiality was prized as an emblem of the technological innovations of the industrial era. It was what has been termed a "culture of imitation." Underlying this celebratory attitude was unease with the implications of a shift toward mechanized production of goods. One response was to glorify the technological possibilities.[52] Yet those artificial results of

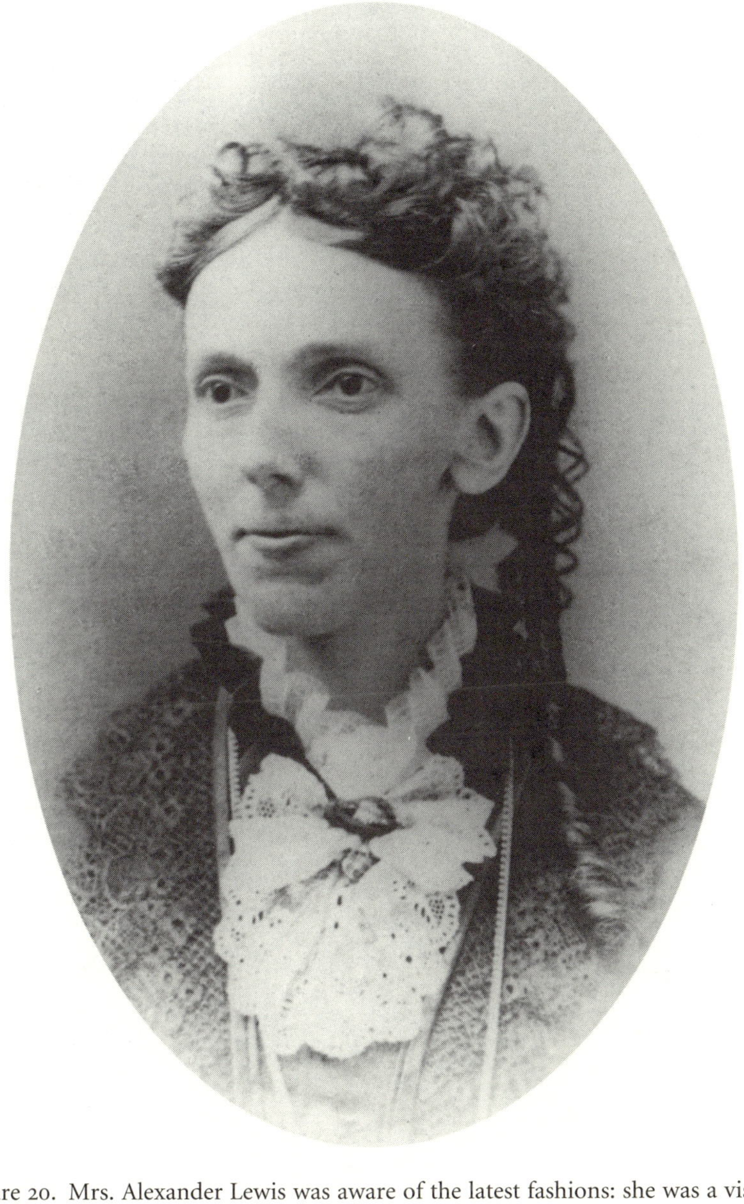

Figure 20. Mrs. Alexander Lewis was aware of the latest fashions: she was a vision of ruffles, curls, and lace. Her seeming frivolity was tempered by her brooch made of hair, which anchors her neck scarf at the base of her throat. With such jewelry, she could be both fashionable and unquestionably sincere. Courtesy Kansas Collection, Spencer Research Library, University of Kansas Libraries.

the machine were also viewed as lacking some fundamental quality of "realness." So at the same time that American culture was touting the extraordinary benefits of technological change, it nostalgically mythologized a more "natural" state of being, whether that naturalness was expressed as material simplicity or as political ignorance.

Hairwork was both a craft of imitation and a statement of authentic presence; it was artificial and natural at the same time. By the late nineteenth century, it appeared that almost everything could be manufactured, and everything could be faked. For example, even the rarest jewels and metals could be manufactured by workers in a factory.[53] And this artificial world had its twin, it seemed to many, in a dishonest, hypocritical social world in which even one's character could be faked. Hairwork's substance and manufacture promised to alleviate these concerns by demonstrating honesty in its material of the body and integrity in its origin of a product of the human hand. It was irreproducible and produced, authentic and yet the product of a transformative process in which raw materials (hair, metals, thread, and twine) were changed into a valuable commodity of the market and of the heart. This was in part why hairwork was so prized by nineteenth-century Americans. It was in many ways the perfect product of the market, satisfying emotional as well as social needs.

Chapter 5

Fancies of the Heart

For many middle-class Americans in the nineteenth century, hairwork made by their own hands was one of the most honest, true, and sincere objects they could own. Although it was readily available from the market, hairwork could be made at home inexpensively, if not always all that easily. The cost of amateur-produced hairwork was in the time and labor of the women who made it. Hairwork represented emotional as well as physical work for the middle-class women who created it for themselves, for their family members, and for posterity.[1]

Hairwork was fancy*work*—when a woman created a piece of ornamental hairwork, she invested innumerable hours making a decorative object that combined her own labor, her own emotion, and the hair of those she loved. There were all kinds of fancywork, from needlework to featherwork to shellwork, and, yes, to hairwork. Women created fancywork in the nineteenth century for reasons that ranged from personal creativity to a material expression of being a woman, especially a middle-class woman, in nineteenth-century America. Fancywork was prescribed to women as an appropriate, *feminine* activity in fiction, women's periodicals, instructional manuals, and educational institutions. At the same time, however, some women embraced the pleasures and the tedium of fancywork. Above all, fancywork, usually unpaid, usually tedious, and purposefully difficult to complete, was *work*.

Fancywork made tangible the ideology of separate spheres of men's and women's lives. It demonstrated women's noncalculating capacities that contrasted so fittingly with men's supposedly natural competitive natures. At the same time, because fancywork was made by middle-class women whose work was to produce effects (a happy home, a carefully decorated parlor, well-mannered children, a sympathetic marriage), fancywork's laborious qualities were consistently remarked on. At times, fancywork was calculated in terms of economic, abstract values. This was understandable given the increasing dominance of a market of commodities and a cultural world that reflected the abstracted values of labor and tangible production on nineteenth-century middle-class Americans.

Fancywork had multiple functions within the tenets of domestic ideology. Innocuous as it may have appeared, fancywork effectively enforced a discipline onto the women who performed it. As they followed elaborate rules and directions and were involved for hours producing often extraordinarily complicated objects, women not only learned the craft but crafted themselves as proper women. While writers of domestic manuals, and especially those of fancywork instructional books, lauded the moralistic and beneficent aspects of home crafting, they also remarked on fancywork's valuable position as a tangible product of a woman's activity. A happy home was the product not only of a woman's gentle, loving hand but also of her careful husbanding of the family's financial and social resources. To embark on a fancywork project was to demonstrate one's ability to integrate heart and money, for fancywork was a product of a woman's selfless love for her husband and family as well as evidence of her frugality and her understanding of the demands of the market.

Because it was made of the body of the family members themselves and often made of the woman's own hair, hair fancywork brought all these issues to rest intimately in the self. Hairwork was intensely private yet was meant for public display. Middle-class white women created wreaths and albums for display in their parlors and for public competitions such as fairs. Hair fancywork exemplified their adherence to the dicta of separate sphere ideology in which women functioned within the domestic realm and hairwork simultaneously accomplished the public displays required of sentimentality and middle-class identity. Yet fancywork was, as its name reveals, fanciful, and thus provided an avenue of self-expression for many women. Indeed, prescriptive literature suggested fancywork to women as a creative activity because it balanced confinement within rules with freedom of self-expression.

Hairwork in the World of Separate Spheres

Nineteenth-century middle-class Americans saw an ideal partnership between a wife and husband to be one of separate spheres. Women were to be wives and mothers, concerned with the domestic life of the family, while men were husbands and fathers, soldiering on in the marketplace. As a poem of 1860 instructed women readers, "Be gentle. 'Tis for you he toils /

And thinks, and strives to gain / Home comforts and home happiness: Don't let him strive in vain."[2] Two separate yet joined worlds, the argument went. While historians have found that actual lives were more often the exception to this "rule," that does not mean that nineteenth-century Americans did not use the ideas constantly in their discussions of proper women's and men's roles. Key to both spheres was an economic relationship. In ideal terms, men made the money, and women used that money to create a domestic life that made the men's coldhearted labor worth performing. Again, historians have found that so many families were exceptions to this ideal that it functioned as an idealized goal rather than reality. But the rhetoric used by advisers was that of the separate spheres.

Nineteenth-century domestic advice books used a neat metaphor to make their argument. It was the difference between a "house" and a "home." Men, it was argued, "built a house," that is, provided through their labor in the market the means to create the skeleton of the residence. This image influenced how everyday people viewed their own lives. Thus, in 1860, Samuel Cormany, who was busy building a home for himself and his intended wife, wrote, "Completing the Cage for my Bird goes on slowly." Once a man had finished building the house, a woman ornamented the physical surroundings.[3]

"You are to make a home," Henry T. Williams commanded his female audience in 1878. Williams, publisher and sometime author of a mini-empire of domestic instructional manuals, had pinned his own economic fortunes to women's desire to "make a home." He argued that when a "man shuts his door behind him and carefully locks back all the day's perplexities and cares; what is he to find when he opens the *other* door, and his own bit of life is reached; when the one fragment of day he may call his own dawns down upon him? House-wife, 'house-mother' you are to answer. You are to make the home."[4] It was a world of spheres marked by the physical door. In Williams's scheme, when a man walked through the door of his *house*, he entered his wife's *home* and he could then commence "the one fragment of day he may call his own." A man's as well as a woman's true life began in the home. The woman was "to build it [the home] *within*"[5] [emphasis in original], wrote another adviser. A true Home-Maker, still another domestic adviser suggested, "talks with tender humility of "Our Home"—recognizing within the material structure, the building not made with hands, but eternal in the hearts of those who have been borne, each a share, in rearing and beautifying it."[6]

To add beauty to the home was not simply to preserve the fitness of the man within it, but "again, a Home, in village or country, where Beauty is created, possesses a higher market value."[7] However, that was not meant to suggest that the harsh valuations of a market economy were acknowledged as central to a middle-class household (even if they were). "There is a world of difference between a house and a home," argued Julia Cowles near the end of the nineteenth century, "and the difference is not measured by money." A house and home were instead "measured by the heart interest of the home-keeper, to whom no work is trivial which affects the pleasure or comfort of those who share her home."[8] Thus, the monetary value of domesticity was transmuted to that onto which no value can be placed—the presence of true heart and emotion. The economic language reveals, however, a contradiction at the heart of that home. Women's lives were about money, even if the rhetoric argued that their lives were about heart.

Women's proclivity to excel in matters of taste distinguished men's and women's work from one another. Indeed, the highest praise heard of a woman was, perhaps, when a man remarked, as he looked on the bleak government quarters assigned him in the course of his job, "Well, it *does* look frightfully, but it will be all right when my wife comes; *she* could create beauty and a home, out of a fragment."[9] In 1874, the Reverend John A. Anderson, president of the Kansas Agricultural College, argued that women were actually more endowed with perceptive capacities, for while "the construction of a bridge, or the alignment of a road-bed, is simply a mathematical problem," other tasks, such as "fitting a dress or shaping a mantle is more a matter of imitation than computation; trimming a bonnet is a question of form and colors, that is, effect." Men were inferior; "no man can arrange the furniture of a room as tastefully as a woman of equal education; or give the final pull, push or puff to another woman's dress; while, in the matter of back hair and frizzing, the vacuous incapacity of man amount to sheer sublimity!" Thus, argued Anderson, young women should be encouraged in their development of what he called "wifely" skills and formally trained to meet their natural, bodily predilections.[10]

In his 1885 manual, George Peltz argued, "There is a realm of decorative possibility where the wives and daughters of our homes reign supreme. Their skillful fingers and exquisite taste work wonders of ornamentation. The internal fittings and furnishing of a house are but the framework on which those who love and brighten home display their choice embellishments."[11] Anderson and Peltz inscribed a world of womanly self-expression that was not a vast expanse of opportunity. Women "reign[ed] supreme" in the home. This dominance was gained through work and not simply proffered. Women, through the labor of "their skillful fingers" and their acceptance of the dicta of femininity (as evidenced in their "exquisite taste") could decorate and hence, effect real change in the home. Peltz echoed the ideological division between the masculine enterprise of physically building the house and the expectation that women would decorate such space. This reflected the more limited, and hence more confining, role allotted to women.

In the rhetoric of nineteenth-century domestic ideology, it was women—not men—who enjoyed a seamless life of self-expression. Women were able to "make for one's self a *home*" where beauty and utility "form a perfect pair, (and united), a perfect whole."[12] Another domestic adviser argued that housework was "not vulgar: it is a fine art; it grasps with one hand beauty, with the other utility; it has its harmonies like music, and its order like the stars in their courses."[13]

While women experienced a harmony between beauty and utility, men were doomed to a peripatetic life between home and work, which was only made a "perfect whole" through the active presence of women. Women and their domestic realm were vital in cohering men's otherwise disparate and disjointed lives. Without doubt, this was a form of work, albeit a gentle counterpart to men's recognized and monetarily compensated labors. *Godey's Lady's Book* deliberately contrasted the two sexes' rewards by reminding women to "think of the toils, the anxieties, the mortifications, and wear that father undergoes to secure for your comfortable homes, and [you should] compensate them for their trials by making them happy by their own firesides."[14]

Women were not exempt from the market. In fact, women's work was, in part, to create a home by selecting and often making the multitude of objects nineteenth-century, middle-class Americans deemed necessary, from furniture to the "softening influences" of pictures, drapery, carpets, and fancywork. "It is woman's peculiar province to supply this need of beauty in the home, to cover the hard facts of life with something pleasant to look upon—something to refine and elevate."[15] For Williams and others, a true home was one that reflected the "moral, intellectual, spiritual and social point of view" of the wife.[16]

This moral mission to decorate homes legitimated the purchase of household goods such as furniture, framed prints, and other kinds of accessories.[17] Henry T. Williams characterized a true woman as a person of spiritual and moral integrity who needed to exert discipline about money matters. It was a woman's duty, Williams advised, to possess "both judgement and discrimination to carry out the entire scheme of household arrangement and embellishments in a manner so chaste and delicate that it cannot offend the critical eye." Thus a woman's influence over morality was evidenced in her taste and through her ability to discern tastefulness in "this day of cheap decoration and vulgar display."[18]

Despite the infiltration of vulgarity in society, Williams noted that "cheap luxury *is* easily obtained in this day by any woman who possesses the use of hands and head." In another book, Williams explained further what he meant by "cheap luxury." "To live simply, to master and control our expenditures, is a sore need. . . . SIMPLE LIVING! That is what the necessities of the times demand, and when we have once commenced to reform our households to the code, we shall wonder that we ever allowed ourselves to be slaves to such customs and fashions [of vulgar spending]."[19] Only when a household conformed to the "code" could a house become a home. As another domestic manual advised, "If good housekeeping builds up the walls of Home, good taste, a thing closely allied with good housekeeping, gives them the finishing touch and makes the Home beautiful."[20] And good taste was, of course, the "cheap luxury" ideal of Williams. For Williams, "cheap luxury" was found in crafting items for the home. By creating products themselves, women could attain luxury that superseded any "cheap" market value.

Although women's housekeeping, decorating, and entertaining was not understood to be "work" in the conventional sense of wage labor, the language of waged work consistently appeared in discussions about the domestic responsibilities of women. Marriage, the home, and fancywork itself were the products of a calculus of heart and money that safely framed a middle-class woman's proper role in a changing economic system. In Julia McNair Wright's domestic-advice manual, *The Complete Home*, a character, Aunt Sophronia, presented an elaborate mathematical proof of the relationship between marriage and business. Aunt Sophronia assured her niece Miriam that "possibly you may discover that you are a larger capitalist than you thought!" Aunt Sophronia explained that Miriam's capitalist bent could be seen in her intended marriage to Mark, which was "sound in body and mind, [thus] you have at once a very large portion of that capital needful for upbuilding a happy and long-enduring Home."

Miriam's duties in this incipient partnership were carefully distinguished from those of Mark's. "That Home, Miriam," advised Aunt Sophronia, "you are to build up within, while Mark build[s] without." His "business knowledge" provided the financial capital for this enterprise (the structural components, as it were) and Miriam was to "build" the interior dimensions. Thus, both individuals played an economic role, although Miriam's, as with other proper middle-class wives, was constrained within the bounds of home.

Aunt Sophronia cautioned, "You must know *how* everything should be done, even though you may not have to do it yourself." This was "a true ability for housekeeping, a masterly knowledge of it, [and] one of the finest capitals a woman can bring into a marriage partnership," Aunt Sophronia continued. "I should set it against any large cash capital which her husband had, as without it his capital would be likely to be wasted." Aunt Sophronia imagined a woman's mastery of the demands of housekeeping to be that by which a man's base capital can increase.[21]

It is here that nineteenth-century "fragmented" men and "unified" women met at Williams's door between the work world and the home. "If we cultivate Beauty in the Home, we produce there greater care and better and more cheerful spirits, consequently better health, and therefore less outlay for sickness, beside having more effective working-force," argued Wright.[22] In part, Wright acknowledged the desperate economic weakness of women within the middle-class separate-sphere ideology. Without a man, a middle-class woman was literally adrift with no real economic role, little opportunity to earn a subsistence wage, and very few options. Thus, while Wright relied on a sentimentalized vision of Beauty wafting through the home as if clean breezes were chasing ill winds away, she also—ever so gently—reminded her female audience of the necessity of the work they performed within that house. That work, while positioned as solely for others, was ultimately for the woman's own good.

Within this space, women explored the "realm of decorative possibility," and thus created an interior space of harmony, domesticity, and happy self-expression through their relations to others while fulfilling their biological destinies. There was at work, then, a dual control in the promise of "reign supreme." A woman could express herself, but only within the confines of "her" home and only in relation to others. Only through others' approbation did a woman find her "true self." And, of course, no proper woman need fear such judgment if she had the appropriate knowledge of "exquisite taste" (a natural outcome of her biologically predestined fate) and if she acted to her fullest capacity as a woman.

Self-expression was liberation within confinement and the source of influence, if not actual power. Only through their attentions to others would women's lives and selves amplify. Fancywork could help women accomplish this task. Thus, in 1886, "Madam Worth" noted that "the fair and fanciful creations of the needle have exerted a marked influence over the homes and hearts of mankind."[23] By making objects that decorated the home, adorned family members, and signaled a family's allegiance to its middle-class identity, middle-class women unified "the homes and hearts of mankind." And simultaneously, by exercising "her inventive powers," a woman created a fuller, more extensive, more satisfying self whose meaning and value was derived from those she served and aided.

The parlor became, by the mid-nineteenth century, the focus of women's efforts to express themselves through material goods. Women were to perform a balancing act between the "fancy" goods of the market and the "fancies" of the heart that could ameliorate the worldliness of those required market goods. The parlor was where market and heart met. "Make the parlor the outpost, the window of your home!" exhorted one author. The parlor was the public face of the family and usually was the woman's sole venue for reaching outward from the confines of the home while remaining safely within its boundaries. By displaying purchased items that demonstrated good taste and handmade articles that expressed sentimental attachments, a woman created a haven for her family. Hence, the parlor was thought of as a "kingdom of great possibility" for women that composed "the shrine to which their [women's] deepest devotion is paid, and on which their choicest offerings are laid."[24] It was where women could best demonstrate their selflessness and service toward their families.[25]

As one author wailed, however, it was "such bondage, such thankless service to enter!" Without the addition of handmade fancywork, it was an impossible task. A woman was supposed to be able "to gather together combinations, rich and rare, throughout chamber and hall; things new, and things old; things curious, and things commonplace—each filling their own niche of ornament or usefulness, and each expressing the individual taste of the owner."[26] But as this author pointed out, no one except the wealthiest had those kinds of funds, nor did many women have the time to devote to such meticulous decorating.

Making fancywork; selecting furniture, draperies, and carpets; planting flower gardens; and building indoor gardens—all these manufactured the refinement of the "cheap luxury" that Williams argued was so important to a happy home. Fancywork, as the act of creating decorative objects, was perhaps the ultimate production of household beauty that, while seemingly so trivial, held such import to a woman's economic well-being. Fancywork provided the heart-capital that ensured a woman's livelihood through her husband's comfort and happiness; it was indeed "of immense value" to the women who performed it, the men for whom it was nominally done, and the children of a woman's household.

Rhetorically exalted as fancywork may have been, its demands often appeared inane and even, perhaps, a bit wasteful of a woman's time and energies to its most adamant advocates. Criticism began in the 1850s and continued until the end of the century. The maven of fancywork instructions, *Godey's Lady's Book and Magazine*, wrote with concern, "We have often felt regret, when watching the different work-table occupations of our fair lady friends, to remark how little of the truly useful seems to attract their attention."[27] In 1883, Laura Langford decried the waste fancywork could represent. "The time spent in making trash in the way of so-called fancy articles is immense, and the homes made unattractive with the varieties of tidies, mats, foot-rests, rugs and other fancy work, are far too numerous." She derided fancy needlework and the sewing of finery such as ruffles and flounces. "The price paid for finery by too many of the sex is dyspepsia." Despite her criticism, however, Langford was all for sewing and crafting, but she warned that "it becomes a cross when the tyranny of fashion demands too much."[28] And then she demonstrated her belief that fancywork and sewing could be redeemed, by providing instructions for such in her book.

Like Langford and *Godey's*, Henry Williams recognized that fancywork could be onerous. But he was quick to assure his female readers that "there is something in the most disagreeable occupations of life around which a woman can twine pleasant fancies, from whose outgrowth an honest pride can be developed." Williams and others were careful to link the necessity of domestic duties, truly one of "the most disagreeable occupations of life," as he admitted, with an opportunity to create a better self around which "an honest pride can be developed." "Home is the soul itself," intoned Charles Sargent in 1900, and it was argued that women were blessed in their opportunity to do this intimate form of "soul-work." This work of soul and heart could be accomplished through domestic duties that included the creation of innumerable objects of fancywork. As Madam Worth claimed in 1886, because "a woman's highest bliss [is] to minister to the wants, the convenience and the pleasure of those she loves," a woman will contrive to the "early and active exercise, in the fabrication of articles calculated to accomplish those desirable aims." Such suppression of selfish desires to the subordination of others' pleasures was difficult, but in the end promised to be rewarding. Mary Terhune advised, "It is when she binds thought, strength, and sentiment down to slavish toil, over and beyond the obligation to keep her house clean, comfortable, and tasteful, that she comes short of the queenly office of Home-Maker."[29]

Hairwork in Fairs and Exhibitions

While middle-class women were ideally isolated from the marketplace (even while arbiters of domesticity acknowledged that women were enmeshed in the market) and from the realities of paid work, their expertise at fancywork was sometimes recognized in public. For example, amateurs competed in making hairwork in local fairs and exhibitions. Fairs were one of the most explicitly public arenas in which women's domestic productions, including fancywork, were displayed and judged. However, even this might not secure a housewife public acknowledgment of her work. For instance, in the 1830s in Oneida County, New York, awards were proffered to the male heads of households, and "even prizes for needlework went to men on the grounds that a domestic manufacture was any item 'produced in the household of the owner.' "[30] Later in the nineteenth century, at least in Kansas, this did not hold true. For instance, the Kansas State Fair in 1873 (a good four decades after the New York fairs) awarded prizes under women's own names or their married names for fancyworks such as lace making, tatting, and "work in hair."[31]

Although the degree of recognition might vary, state fairs, county fairs, and national expositions usually included displays of women's domestic work in competitions. By the 1850s, many fairs included fancywork categories of competition.[32] In 1871, a woman selling an engraving of General Grant at a fair in San Jose, California, took a break from her sales work. She wrote in her autobiography that she "attended the Fair as a spectator, not as peddler. . . . I stopped to examine the needle-work, wax-flowers, and paintings."[33] Such fancywork exhibits often included hairwork. In Kansas, a Mrs. I. S. Bellingham of St. Joseph, Missouri, was awarded a prize for "best sample of work in hair" in 1873, and other women garnered similar awards in the following years.[34]

In 1874, Mrs. Mary T. Gray, superintendent of the exhibition and prize committee of the fine arts category of the Kansas State Fair, defended criticism about the fancywork that was included in her category. She wrote to the state board of agriculture that her guideline was that famous dictum, "the most beautiful things in the world are the most useless." She argued that, while the expense and apparent frivolity of artistic creations (including photographs, oils, and the women's section of needlework and fancy works) may have seemed out of place, "if art is worth anything, its best use is to bring the beautiful in form and color home to the household, and to mingle its subtle influences with the whole framework of social and family life." Therefore, she continued, the state fair committee should offer monies for women and children to improve their artistic expertise. Why not, she wondered, offer incentive "to girls to execute squares, triangles and parallelograms in architectural and linear and perspective drawing upon paper, in place of those in calico upon bed-quilts." "If [I were] not aware that your Board personally do not belong to the class, little to be envied, in whose hearts the charities of the imagination lie dead, I would never even ask this of you," she assured the Board.[35]

Gray needed men's charitable imaginations to spring forth, for she was suggesting the very thing people feared that the public display and recognition of women's work would foment. The Reverend John Anderson's arguments to the nascent Board of Regents in Kansas for the proper course for educating women were delivered in the same year Gray proffered her own course of education to the Agricultural Board of Kansas. Anderson, of course, suggested that women were best suited for decorative effects, and he believed they were deficient in matters of computation, causation, and adaptation. In fact, Gray's logical leap from quilt squares to executing geometric figures was precisely what Anderson and others in the state were hoping to avoid. Anderson, however, advised educating women in those areas believed to be specifically useful in their future lives, such as "[in] the proper care of the sick, . . . in the art of cutting and making her own clothing tastefully; in the art of cookery; in that of setting a table, brightening a room, beautifying a garden; . . . the art of making home brighter to the little ones than streets, more attractive to its adults than saloons."[36]

Anderson firmly reestablished where women's work was best performed—in the home and its confines. Gray's argument that women were already participating in the "manly" fields of practical knowledge such as geometry would find little acceptance in the public sphere of masculine activity. Women's work could be displayed and acknowledged in legitimate arenas such as state fairs, as long as it was understood that these forays outside the home were merely for the betterment of that home. Gray's suggestion potentially would have placed women outside of that proscribed arena. Anderson's more conservative suggestions were those most likely to be adopted—geometry and other mathematical principles were in fact not included in the "woman's course of study and of life."[37]

Hair Wreaths and Hair Albums at Home

Middle-class women's lives were, in the 1870s and 1880s, to be spent within the domestic world of home and family. For many women, this was a deeply satisfying world but frustrating in its lack of recognized value. Fancywork was one way for women to gain public acknowledgment of the hard work of making a house and home, while still attesting to the ways in which the domestic world could not be valued as the public world of competition. Hair albums and wreaths provided a way for middle-class women to fulfill the expectations of domesticity while offering tangible evidence of that work and allowing them to create objects of deeply personal significance. The discipline of hairwork—the endless gimping of hair and wire, looping minute strands, arranging flowers and leaves, coordinating entries into an album—did not diminish the sentimental and emotional aspects of the completed object. Indeed, the extraordinary skill and time demanded by such wreaths and albums derived in part from their creators' acquiescence to those disciplinary prescriptions.

In a short story of 1885, Mary E. Wilkins Freeman explored the various meanings of hair wreaths.[38] For Nancy Weeks, an older woman in the story, the wreath she created represented her family, her skill as an artist, and the necessary domestication of her otherwise impersonal new parlor. Having saved her money over the years, she finally was able to furnish her parlor with the newest styles of furniture. Her completed hair wreath now hung in a parlor decorated with new wallpaper, a Brussels carpet, red plush furniture, lamp mats, vase mats, and fire rugs. "Who made it?" asked a visitor, and her sister responded, "She made it." "'Why, you don't mean it! How could you ever have had the patience? All those little fine, beautiful flowers are made of—'

'*Hair*. Yes, every one of 'em. Jest look close. Thar's rose-buds, an' lilies, an' pansies, an' poppies, an' acorns, besides the leaves.' . . . Even Nancy Weeks's mild nature could not hinder her from straightening herself up a little out of mere self-respect as she gazed at her intricate handiwork with her admiring guests." Nancy listed each of her relatives who were included in the wreath, all deceased except for the originator of the red hair flower.

Her friend concluded, "It's such an ornament, and apart from that it must be such a comfort to you to have it."

In the story, the wreath also represented two fundamental misappropriations. After Nancy died, her husband Thomas quickly remarried. Her sister, Charlotte, felt that the wreath, made as it was of her and her sister's family, was rightfully hers. She stole the wreath and bullied Thomas into surrendering the rights of ownership to her. The wreath, made by a woman of her own, matrilineal family, was by rights her sister's property, not that of her widower husband (much less the property of that man's new wife!). The second mistake of ownership was the aberrant red hair. Nancy lusted after just the right accent of red, so her sister Charlotte stole the lock of red hair from her own daughter's bureau. It was the hair of the young girl's beau. Once he saw his token of love ornamenting the aunt's wreath, he left town, believing the daughter to have used him immodestly. The young girl, learning of her mother's theft, quickly wrote the young man, who then returned, declaring, "It's all right about the hair."

The story eloquently outlined the issues involved in hair wreaths: the preservation of family members; the expression of "true artistic instinct, and delight in work," as Freeman states; the decorative aspects of these parlor ornaments; and, finally, the fact that the wreaths were women's property. Made by women for the decoration of women's spaces in the home, and made as testament to women's emotional lives, wreaths could be mocked but their importance to the women who made them could not be negated or stolen.

Most women who crafted hair wreaths and jewelry were unacknowledged creators outside the walls of their own homes. Hair wreaths were simple to make but complicated in their details. Most wreaths used the hair of many individuals, and the women who constructed these decorations tried to record the individuals represented in the flowers and leaves. Ironically, the women who created the wreaths rarely included their own hair. For example, the Luke family wreath was made by a sister of Harry Luke's of the hair of his children between 1880 and 1883. The wreath incorporates the hair of Lewis, Emelia, Nettie, Alvina, Harry, and one other child.[39] The dating is ascertained through the fact that Alvina (Luke) Peffer is born in 1879 and is represented in the wreath, but Henry W. Luke, the youngest Luke child, was born 1883, but is not included.[40]

The creators of hair wreaths who omitted their own hair, did, in fact, demonstrate their presence because it was through the creation of the wreaths that such women disclosed their lives. They were, in effect, at the center, which the individual components of the wreath encircled. By demonstrating her relationship to a variety of other people, women wreath makers demonstrated the composition of their true selves. Despite the obligatory self-effacement, no amount of rhetoric could erase the creative, active presence of women who made these hair objects.

As Mrs. Luke discovered, the inclusion of so many individuals required careful record keeping. At the time of its making, it was unlikely that anyone would mistake Mrs. Nettie (Luke) West's hair for that of young Alvina (Luke) Peffer, but it was often acknowledged that hair, despite its ability to reveal the true self, required a bit of narrative aid similar to what the fictional Nancy Weeks provided when she recited the relatives whose hair composed her wreath. Mrs. Allison, as we have seen, chose to pencil in the names on the paper backing her wreath, going so far as to draw lines between the name and its specific flower so that there could be no confusion. Other women found various methods of keeping the hair and individual aligned. Some merely singled out more prominent personages for individualized identification, such as when Carline Markee notes that the "white hair is from Betsy Webster, cousin to Daniel [Webster]."[41]

More often, though, women were egalitarian in their notations, giving all those present their due. In Waukesha County, Wisconsin, one woman attached sixteen tiny numbered paper tags to the wire base of each separate leaf or flower. She then listed on a separate card the number and the name of the corresponding individual.[42] The Tuttle family's wreath maker relied on the same numbering system, but she incorporated the list of numbers and names into her object of display. She surrounded the horseshoe wreath and its central bouquet with five small cards on shelf paper, on which were listed the numbers and names of those represented. Thus she created three concentric circles, each gradually widening outward.[43]

The Sackett family had a three-dimensional tree of hair-wrapped wires instead of a more common parlor wreath. Thus, the family's hair—the genealogical tree—could form a literal tree of hair.[44] Its maker was faced with the arduous task of not only bringing together the hair of fifty family members and friends but also keeping the relationships between the hair and each individual stable. She used two separate cards to list each member and, as other women did, attached tiny numbered paper tags to each element of the tree.

Often the record-keeping dimension of hairwork determined the form of the wreath. Many times, wreath makers chose to create the distinct parts of each flower with different colors of hair. So, for instance, one Wisconsin woman made each petal of each flower out of three concentric loops of hair-wrapped wire, and each loop was of a different individual's hair. Her notations demonstrate her method. On one flower she noted, "the gray Father Stephen, darkest Emily Wesley, Sam Smith and boy." Another flower with an outer ring of petals of dark brown hair and a center of light blond hair was labeled "the lightest Stella Stephens." Twenty-four individual names are listed.

As carefully as she recorded whose hair was where, the wreath maker arranged the hair according to color rather than any discernible familial relationship. Usually the "accent" colors of blond and red form the center of the flowers, with the ubiquitous brown nearly always functioning as the larger, outside border of the petals. Here, the decorative impact of the contrast of hair colors superseded the emotional and sentimental significance of using that hair to illustrate relationships in a tangible form.

Mrs. A. Jackson created a frame presumably to surround a photograph of the person whose hair she used to create her design. With hair-wrapped wire (the same technique used in making hair wreaths), Mrs. Jackson made a flat design of a female mourner, an imposing tomb, and a floating cherub. Rendered in hair and wire, her design hearkened back to memorial scenes popular a hundred years before, when William Dunklin's eighteenth-century miniature had been created (see Figure 6).[45]

Most larger-scale hair mourning objects were not, however, unique in form. While there are certainly examples of hair wreaths made from only the deceased person's hair, more often women chose to bring together the deceased and the living. The Bjornsens lost their 12-year-old daughter Hannah in February 1894. Hannah left behind her three siblings and her parents. A memorial wreath, combining the hair of Hannah with that of her family, contains several different shades of hair.[46]

Hair albums were another way for a woman to display her private affiliation. Albums were often family albums that served as a tactile map of kin relationships. Usually with little narration and sometimes with no identification of the hair locks by names, there are, however, telling patterns of arrangement of family members in the album. Usually a woman assembling a hair family album arranged family members on a single page, with parents or married partners placed toward the top of the page. In Adelaide Dickinson's album, for instance, she used braided and sometimes looped hair to denote each member and she systematically arranged each grouping according to gender. Throughout her album, Dickinson placed the male to the top left and the female to the top right, thus replicating the traditional gendered spatial arrangement of male-female pairs.[47] Such an arrangement was common for this type of family album.[48]

In an album by another woman, the top-left hair entry was labeled "father" and its counterpart, "mother." Here, the entire family group was neatly arranged in rows, with father and mother at the top, and each child below. Each name was accompanied by a tiny (one-half-inch) braid sewn onto the commercially lined notebook paper. Just as with some of the autograph albums, this genealogical album was amended after its creation, for under John T. Miller's entry is the added caption, "dide 1875."[49]

Hair albums were popular throughout the nineteenth century. Plain albums that included hair and perhaps a caption changed little during the century. By the Civil War, though, and especially by the 1870s, the availability of cheap lithographed illustrations led to the popularity of scrap albums. These albums were created by gluing scrap images onto pages. Usually the pages followed a theme; for example, a page might include several dozen images of rabbits snipped from calendars, magazines, trade cards, and books. A woman would comb through all sorts of printed materials in search of appropriate scraps. In March 1862, Rachel Bowman noted that she had "commenced pasting my scraps into an old magazine to make a book of them. . . . Such a litterary looking room as we do have, scarcely a spot of carpet can be seen for the refuse papers strewn over it."[50] In the 1870s, *Harper's Bazaar* offered detailed instructions for making "a pretty scrap album for a drawing room."[51] Scrap album making, then, was a craft proscribed by the market but also was a creative expression of a woman's taste.

Some women included hair with their scraps to create uniquely personalized albums. These functioned a bit like the modern scrap album. Although there are commercialized elements to them, such as the lithographed scraps, the inclusion of hair heightened the autobiographical character of the album. Viewing a hair scrap album from the nineteenth century could be an intensely intimate experience, because the maker's personality and life is laid out so clearly on the album's pages.[52]

In 1883, a young Salome C. Flanagan created her self-titled "Hair Book, Presented as a Keepsake From Salome C. Flanagan to her Sister Ursula F. Brown at Pottsdam New York Brid[ge]port September 11 1883." Salome's album reveals how one young woman combined consumerist activity and the more intimate models of sentimental culture to express her own unique perspective.

The album is wholly handmade, with hand-sewn paper pages enclosed in a carefully constructed cover. Most pages have various commercial lithograph scraps accompanied with handwritten inscriptions and hair braids that are looped and fixed onto the page.[53] The first page of the book has a commercially produced scrap of a phoenix paired with two imposing figures of Lady Justice on either side. There are ornate cutout borders of green paper, commercially printed with fleur-de-lis and braid patterns. And, not commercially created, are two braids of human hair. One braid is coiled like a snake and sewn onto the paper page, while the other is looped, tied with a tiny blue velvet ribbon, and likewise sewn onto the page. Handwritten initials appear beneath each hair braid.[54]

On another page, Flanagan placed the lock of hair within the tight grasp of a lithographic image of a hand. The page is bordered with a lower edge of a black band bookended with two upright coffin shapes. Flanagan combined images that were familiar and comforting to most nineteenth-century Americans. The hand shape is a familiar motif of memorialization, found on innumerable grave markers of the period, and represented the dead reaching toward the living, or God or heaven welcoming the dead.[55] Such imagery would have offered condolence in its representation of the close relationship between the living and deceased members of a large family.

The human hair placed in the curled-over fingers of the hand of the lithograph scrap is a useful metaphor for Flanagan's creative mining of the traditional and the newly commercial. That which was impersonal by the nature of its mass production and marketing—the lithographed scrap of the hand—was transformed into an object of undeniable, enduring individual meaning when Flanagan glued the human hair into the hand's grasp. Including hair of her family in the grasp of the commercial hand makes this album a testament not only to the creative activity of a young woman but also to the growing presence of a market of sentimental goods. That same mass market of nominally impersonal goods was rendered intimate and personally meaningful when integrated into the emotional world of Flanagan's album.[56] While her amalgamation of sentiment and morbidity, of the market and the self, may appear strikingly original, it is likewise evident that Flanagan remained within an "idiom of domesticity," that vocabulary of women's handicrafts that effectively restrained the more fanciful elements of her creative expression (Figure 21).

Hairwork was supposed to be fashionable, sentimental, sincere, public, and private. It was a product of a market of personal goods, but it was also supposed to represent that which could never be truly marketed: personal relationships and emotion. Middle-class women were, in similar ways, supposed to be unconcerned with the market of goods and competition. They

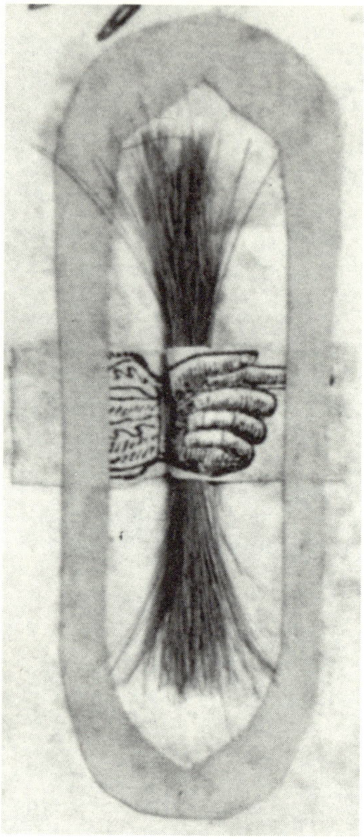

Figure 21. A wisp of hair is grasped by the mechanically reproduced hand. This detail from Salome Flanagan's scrap album presents us with the commercial world (in the form of the printed hand) and the sentimental world of hand manufacture, evident in the uneven edges of the circle and the hair itself. Courtesy private collection of Leila Cohoon and The Hair Museum, Independence, Missouri.

were to be engrossed in domestic life, children, and family. These were the ideal expectations for women, never to be truly fulfilled. Middle-class women were deeply concerned with the realities of paid work, of political realities, and of public affairs. But they were *supposed* to be isolated, even protected from that harsh world.

Creating hairwork and other kinds of fancywork allowed middle-class women to be involved in a market of goods; at the same time, crafts asserted the persistent value of hand labor, of the home, and of being self-sufficient. Taking heart in hand, women created objects that garnered public acknowledgment of their acceptance of womanly ideals even as they participated in the world of market goods and of fashion. They created objects that were understood to be altogether feminine in character, while they engaged in an exercise of public display.

Chapter 6
A Man's Precious Talisman

Hairwork was feminine. Its associations were feminine: emotion, sentiment, memories. Its forms were likewise feminine, with elaborate braiding, flower forms, and beading. But this does not mean that men were somehow uninvolved with hairwork. Hairwork, especially the watch chain, was a popular gift to men from women. Evidence of letters, diaries, and museum-collection notes suggest that most watch chains, for instance, were gifts from women to men. These could be familial—from a mother to a son, or a sister to a brother—or romantic gifts from a woman to a man. Men were not exempt from sentimental expression, either. They preserved hair as mementos, for example. But the sentimentality that hairwork represented was most often expressed by women, and very often in the form of the gift of a watch chain to a man. Hairwork highlights accepted women's work roles of domesticity, and men's hair jewelry was tied to men's work roles as those developed in the nineteenth century.

The Gift of Hairwork to Men

Hairwork was not only an acceptable gift but a desirable gift for men who worked in the heartless realm of the market. The feminized tenor of hairwork was in part what made the gift so fitting. Men's emotional relationships with women—whether familial or romantic—were a balance to the work world they were preparing to excel in. Hairwork was a reminder of that "other world" of emotion and relationships that validated the competitiveness of a man's professional life.

For a typical middle-class, young, unmarried man, his relationship to his mother was the most intense emotional connection he had.[1] Hence, it is not surprising that hairwork was an appropriate gift from a mother to her son. Hair jewelry in the forms of watch fobs and small objects such as bookmarks offered mothers a way to extend through time and space their attentions to their sons even as the young men entered adulthood. Indeed, gifts representative of a young man's newly attained status as an adult could help them through their transition from youth, which often had been characterized by a constant and intimate relationship with their mothers.

This intimacy was buttressed by a cultural ideology that legitimated it. Nineteenth-century mothers were expected to devote themselves to the moral guidance and nurturance of their children and, in the case of young boys, to ameliorate their masculine "natural" predilection toward violence. The effect of this gendered structure of childhood meant that men were thoroughly educated in understanding the sexes as quite distinct, with women as dependent and caring, and with men as autonomous and powerful.[2] While maturity was a necessary move into that wider world of masculine adulthood, young men often paradoxically yearned for the comforting safety of their childhood and their formerly intimate relationship with their mother at the same moment they were actively distancing themselves from that haven.[3]

Hairwork made of a mother's own body could mime the sustaining relationship between mothers and their sons. Thus such mother-to-son gifts were provocative because they physically represented an intimacy at once physical and emotional. At the same time, because the watch fob symbolized adult manhood for middle-class Americans, a young man expressed an adult identity apart from, yet still close to, his mother and his family.

In 1875, a mother gave her son John a watch fob made of her own hair braided into a standard twist with a clasp joining the two lengths of brown hair. The clasp is faced with six flattened sides, and engraved on four of the squares are the words "Mother–to–John–1875."[4] Here, the woman is subsumed into the all-important and generic role of "mother," and the son stands as a marked individual, "John," as well he must within the nineteenth-century ideals of self-made manhood. In the 1880s, Jacob Hengen's mother and brother sent him a commercially printed bookmark with his mother's brown and gray hair sewn on its front. Adorned with their mother's hair, Jacob's bookmark is a gift from both his mother and brother in Germany.[5] The hair is accompanied with a commercially printed poem:

To a Mother

Dear Mother,
Let thy tender care
Be graven on my head;
May God for

years thy life yet
spare,
Averting death's
rude dart,
now gratefully
feel thy worth
Oh Mother!
How I love thee!
May joy await thee
here on earth
And heaven smile
Above thee.

The poem tells of lasting effects of maternal influence: "Let thy tender care / Be graven on my head." Tones of mother-worship are aptly emphasized by repeated exclamation points. The inclusion of the mother's hair reiterates the commercially produced and printed verses, individualizes the rather high-flown commercialized sentiments for both son and mother, and helps counteract the anonymity of the bland title, "To a Mother."

Many men also maintained close relationships with their sisters well into their adult years. The brother-sister pairing of two young adults of the opposite sex had the advantage of being sexless and still deeply emotional.[6] The absence of any acknowledgment of sexual tension made such relationships safe for both the brother and sister. A man's tie to his sister also offered a safe venue to test out assumptions about women's adult behavior. In either intent or practice, however, these brother-sister "partnerships" were not meant to act as surrogates for heterosexual, romantic relationships, but instead were venues for maturation for both young men and young women.[7]

When it came to sisters, even the most conservative of men could blossom with tolerance and could, at times, encourage behaviors they expressly did not desire in romantic partners. Young men would audition various ideas about their expectations for women's behavior through their relationships with their sisters and would turn to their sisters for empathetic condolence and encouragement. Thus, the connections formed during a shared childhood often served as an emotional lifeline for many men and women as they moved into adulthood. In this context, Daniel O'Connor's prize possession of a fob made of his sister's hair was not surprising. Daniel's sister, Anna O'Connor Bruce, in the form of his watch fob, accompanied Daniel as he traveled from his home in Lowell, Massachusetts, to Virginia, and, finally, to St. Paul, Minnesota, where he lived the rest of his life.[8]

As a young boy moved into adulthood, a man's relationships with his mother and sisters formed the basis for his aspirations in heterosexual romantic partnerships.[9] Heterosexual romance promised young men self-fulfillment but with an attendant risk and arduous effort. Romance could allow men to reach a "utopia" of emotional satisfaction, but their success was never guaranteed.[10]

It was not simply a way to become familiar with one's potential partner (although the dilemmas of self-exposure were integral in romance); it was also a method to learn about one's own self. Romantic love promised to amalgamate various elements of individuals into a whole that, in turn, would form the seamlessly unified middle-class family.[11] And the family was the foundation of society itself, it was argued.

The dichotomy between work and home was sharply drawn for both men and women, and romance was firmly positioned in the realm of home and heart, far distant from the competitive world of work and ruthless effort. Indeed, romance promised to wed the disparate worlds of female privacy and masculine public life.[12] In the matrix of such complicated emotions, and with the underpinning of gendered roles, which argued for women's economic incapacity and men's economic activity, courtship and marriage posed particularly difficult challenges for the individuals involved.

In the eighteenth century, courtship and marriage had been largely public actions that displayed the social connections of the couple. But in the nineteenth century, emphasis increasingly shifted to private rituals. For instance, engagements were publicized through personal channels rather than community-wide notifications. To mark the newly private character of engagements, tokens such as rings were used to signify the relationship.[13] In place of public announcements of impending marriage, middle-class couples used jewelry to suggest the newly formed alliances in a manner acceptable to the public and private demands of sentimentality.

A short poem written in 1855 describes some of the ways engagement hair jewelry could represent the pungent combination of individuation and subsumation, public display and private emotion, and the underlying economic realities. The narrator proudly rejected the appeal of "fancy" rings, which she argued were redolent with false emotion and artificial love. Instead, she claimed,

And this, my bonnie, braided ring,
Enwoven of his hair,
Shall be the proudest ornament
My heart shall wish to wear.

Our young women did look forward to the day when the "real" ring arrived, but

Until my finger set,
A golden ring shall shine,
And all the world shall know me his,
And Allan will be mine![14]

Here we see how hair jewelry could, at least within the rhetorical confines of this poem, satisfyingly resolve a variety of issues romantic engagements posed. The female narrator delineated between the "private" expression of love, the hair ring that is "the proudest ornament / My heart shall wish to wear," and the more public statement of the golden ring that "shall shine / And all the world shall know me his." Hair jewelry was for moderated, public statements of nominally private sentiments, while gold—a well-recognized commodity of impersonal value—represented the more extensive announcement of their partnership. The two rings signaled the ideal pattern of development in a romance: first, quiet, private nurturing of the relationship, capped with a second, bolder, more openly social pronouncement.

The hair ring was well-suited for its more confidential role, as it contained the hair of her fiancé and was worn on her body, and thus echoed the unity their incipient marriage would bring. And hair's ability to convey true emotion and sincerity contrasted with the glittering ostentation of richer gems. Certainly those with empty hearts might value expensive gems, but those of true sentiment recognized the superiority of the gift of self that hair jewelry represented.[15]

Hair jewelry negotiated the public and private worlds of middle-class Americans because romantic love was no more isolated from the market than were the individuals involved. In fact, the "utopia" of soulful connections between men and women was a site where individuals intersected with the market. While romantic love was idealized as separate from the market, in fact for many nineteenth-century Americans "the experience of romantic love was translated into economic practices and . . . in turn, economic practices were translated into a structure of feeling."[16] Marriage in the nineteenth century, as in any other time period, was at its heart an economic arrangement. Romance entailed recognition by another person of the value of one's self—a value that was, ideally, considered apart from the market, and was instead a measure of one's "true" worth. But a marriage was also a formal economic relationship between a man, who was supposed to labor for money to create the household, and a woman, who was to create the home of family and comfort. Economic language crept into romantic discussions, often providing an oblique way for men and women to negotiate the terms of their personal relationships. Hair jewelry physically represented the positive valuation of self found in successful romantic relationships while providing a way to seemingly resist the economic realities underpinning heterosexual, romantic alliances.

In 1870, Blanche Butler and her fiancé, Adelbert Ames, began what would be a decades-long series of letters exchanged during their life together.[17] First they faced a long-distance engagement. As they used gifts to solidify a relationship that developed during their separation, they outlined the nature of their future marriage and partnership. Their discussions about their gifting reveal the ways that at least some middle-class Americans negotiated the economic disparities and emotional "work" of men and women. Gift exchanges are extra-monetary trades. People give one another gifts to exchange goods of value without the calculation of profit. Thus, gifts often play an important role as a romance develops and matures, because the gift exchanges argue that the relationship is *not* an economic one (even as the two partners establish their economic relations).

At the beginning of their engagement, Adelbert was in Washington, D.C., serving as a U.S. senator, while Blanche continued to reside with her family in Lowell, Massachusetts. His first gift was dangerously close to egoism. He wrote Blanche, "I found in the passageway between the Senate and the House a woman selling photographs pasted to the bottom of the ordinary globular glass paperweights—among them was mine, which I bought and will send you by express. It is the one you liked best, and which, as it is through the glass, is a very good picture. Tell me how you like it."[18] Adelbert's status as a war hero and his service as a senator from Mississippi warranted adorning souvenirs with his visage.[19] In choosing a public image of himself for a private audience of one, Adelbert neatly united the public world of masculine activity and the private sphere of emotional and familial life.[20] Souvenirs themselves fall into these two categories. First, there are the public souvenirs that are purchasable and market-produced. Then, of course, there are the private souvenirs that trace an individual's life history. Adelbert managed to produce a gift that answers both meanings.

Adelbert was careful to balance the self-glorification evoked through the image of his leaning over a table of trinkets to select one decorated with his own image when he told Blanche that he had carefully chosen "the one you liked best." Thus Adelbert personalized his selection, suggesting it was

Blanche's prior preference that guided his actions. In a deprecating tone, he added that "as it is through the glass, is a very good picture." Finally, to give to another an image of one's self, no matter how depersonalized (for example, a tourist souvenir), was to subject one's self to scrutiny. Recalling Sarah Folwell's uneasy display of photographic images of herself to those around her and her earnest "which do you like best?", Adelbert asked Blanche, "Tell me how you like it."

Blanche was silent about how she liked it, although she briefly noted to Adelbert that "the paperweight comes to me nicely." In fact, Blanche was more concerned with her own gift. Like Adelbert's, it was an image of herself, but unlike Adelbert's image of himself as a man of public activity, her gift was markedly private. It was a locket that hid a photograph of herself and a lock of her hair. For Blanche, the worrisome issue was not the photographic image but the inclusion of her own hair. She wrote Adelbert, asking, "Now shall I send you the locket? Through the mail or by express? I do not know which would be best . . . I am now debating in my own mind the propriety of putting a lock of hair opposite the picture. If it were any other color than red I should not hesitate. But red is so unromantic. What shall I do? I might dye a little piece—it would be my hair all the same—or perhaps it would be better not to have any put in."[21] First, Blanche positioned her gift as intimate. She questioned the propriety of including her hair, especially, as she teasingly noted, her *red* hair. "Red is so unromantic," and the locket, of course, was meant as a romantic, private gift.[22] She suggested a subterfuge—she could, as a coquette might, dye her hair. Artificially colored or not, it would, of course, "be my hair all the same," for nothing can change the fact that the hair was of her own self. To encase a piece of her self within the confines of a locket also evoked the sexual dimension of their evolving relationship.[23] In fact, Blanche's suggestion that she might dye her hair acknowledged that even hidden in a locket, her gift of two different images of herself was a public gift, intended to be displayed, and was her own tangible acceptance of Adelbert's proposal. Her teasing comments about her hair color only clarified for Adelbert that for her to give the gift, and for him to accept it, was to reiterate the public aspects of their heretofore largely private relationship.

Adelbert's response outlined the appeal of hair as a gift between lovers. Adelbert excitedly wrote, "dear Blanche, I was very glad, happy, to receive your beautiful token—not beautiful, that is secondary—it was dear and precious. Your sweet face and a lock of your beautiful hair. Your hair seemed to bring you very near me. I thank you, Love, for the locket, the picture, and the hair. I shall always wear them. I shall suspend the locket by my watch guard. I love you, and feel so grateful to you for your love token."[24] Adelbert correctly gauged what component of the gift was the most significant: Blanche's hair. First, he demoted the notion of beauty and its sometime corollary, superficiality, arguing that it was the token itself, not its apparent beauty that was most valuable. Second, it was Blanche's hair that received the accolade of beauty that was withheld from the locket itself. Her hair garnered this praise because of its active quality, for "your hair seemed to bring you very near me." Blanche's hair effected her physical presence, and thus was of the greatest value.

Although Blanche's gift was nominally private, she had noted to Adelbert that it was also public, and Adelbert did not question this. The locket was meant to be worn, and wear it he would: "I shall suspend the locket by my watch guard."[25] Later, Adelbert elaborated on this public display of the locket, writing, "I shall attach your precious locket to my chain. Yes, *chain*, to hold you fast. As yet I have not been to any jeweler to have it done, but shall do so before I leave for Lowell. It will make a very beautiful ornament."[26] Adelbert responded to Blanche's gift by repeatedly noting the need to *attach* her gift to his body because a gift such as a locket or an irreproducible image of one's self could always be lost, just as the emotions of the relationship could dissipate.[27] The fact that the locket was a *gift* of self, freely offered, signified Blanche's acceptance not only of Adelbert but of her role as companion and wife.

Both gifts—Adelbert's photographic paperweight and Blanche's locket with its photograph and lock of hair—transformed the couple into objects to be longed for and possessed. Indeed, by transforming themselves into physical objects (a paperweight, a locket), Adelbert and Blanche made themselves into "objects of desire."[28] Each gift represented the self made physical in the exchange of photographic images. And both gifts acted as souvenirs—Adelbert's explicitly related to the tradition of the public souvenir, and Blanche's "love token" was a private souvenir. Blanche's gift was, however, the more personal and, therefore, the more treacherous. She presented herself as an object of desire—and her locket of hair echoed her body. It was a preliminary act of the bodily consummation their marriage promised. Blanche had presented herself unadorned and, yet, encased in gold. Adelbert's gift presented him as the masculine object of desire—a being of public enterprise, recognized for his actions, successful in the public world.

That this bond was one forged privately but was for public consumption was made clear a year later, after their marriage. Adelbert, traveling (as he did for much of their marriage), began a conversation with a young couple, and apparently bragged about the beauty of his young wife. To prove his point, Adelbert wrote to Blanche, "I showed them your picture, as it is in my little locket."[29]

Sentimental Men and Hairwork: An Odd Fit

Most nineteenth-century middle-class men were immersed in work and in the public sphere. Masculinity itself was increasingly defined by how a man earned a living.[30] Men were supposed to prosper in the public world of commerce, competition, and work. While many nineteenth-century Americans honored the ideal of the autonomous male, such a figure posed certain worries as well. While men's competitiveness was rewarded socially and financially, there was a moral cost that appeared to threaten men's character.[31] Women, their capacities for emotion, and the feminine world they inhabited, could counter the negative effects of the market men were thrown into as adults.

For other men, sentimentality offered consolation for the vagaries of life. Whether those trials were work related or not, sentimentality was not considered incongruent with manhood. In 1828, Walter Mason Oddie, a landscape painter living in New York, sat alone and mused. He wrote, "1828 Feby 19 This day, three years ago, 1825, I was married to Julia. During this time I have been liberally blessed with the sweets of matrimony—. . . The love and adoration by which I was governed when I offered my hand and heart to the lovely being who was the constant object of my thoughts has remained an inmate of my bosom—Time has had no effect upon my affection, but in cementing more strongly the tie by which they were bound."[32] With that, he folded the lock of hair back into its small paper envelope that was marked "Julia's March 1824."[33] Sentiment was intended to reiterate and intensify the emotional resonance of a relationship, and the lock of hair, carefully saved from their courtship, served as a physical talisman of his emotional ties to Julia. Such reminiscencing was deeply sentimental in its attempt to evoke emotion without a promised resolution. The token of hair was the physical reminder of an ongoing emotional experience that Oddie willingly sustained, for as he noted at the end of his entry, "Time has had no effect upon my affection." In fact, Oddie's remembrances served the purpose of maintaining his affections, not resolving them.

Oddie's sentimentalism was undeniably private, although he recorded it in the potentially public form of a diary. Private acts of sentimentality, though, were safer than public ones, for when men ventured into the sentimental arena—the realm of women—they risked failure. Even male reprobates, the "outsiders" of sentimental culture, sometimes attempted (with little success) to redeem themselves by appropriating sentimental language to explain their actions.[34] In "bachelor sentimental fiction" (novels and short stories that presented never-married men wistfully imagining the happiness of a home life that they had not secured yet) men were especially likely to be presented as sentimental fools.[35] Other short stories and novels persistently depicted hapless men who were flummoxed by the craftiness of the market, the illusive appeal of sentimental consumerism, and the insincerities of sentimental expression that was "bought and paid for." Fictional accounts repeatedly suggested that while women might be able to navigate the treacherous waters of such a world, men were likely to flounder, and eventually, to drown.

In a short story of 1844, "The Blond Hair," a doctor recounted his own near suicide. He showed his friend the sentimental token that had saved him from the act of jumping off a bridge, and that in turn he has treasured in a locket-ring. It was a blond hair that he had found clinging to his coat just as he began his aborted leap. Retelling his story, "The doctor carefully closed his ring, after having pressed to his lips his precious talisman."[36] The doctor had carefully analyzed the single hair and decided that its original owner was a woman of true beauty and delicate temperament. Alas, in the end the doctor discovers that this hair came from his charwoman's elaborate blond wig. Ideally, a man's attempt at sentimentality should connect him to true and sincere feelings, and thus acceptably affirm the integrity of his character. Here, a man's fumbling attempts go awry, and his sentiment renders him clownish. He ruefully continues to treasure the hair despite its commercialized, artificial origins. He hopes that the hair *could* be from a beautiful woman's head. Key to the misunderstanding was that the hair is his charwoman's hair—a woman of the lower classes. Sentimentality was the marker of someone attuned to the emotional resonances of life—a person of middle to upper classes. A charwoman was excluded from this sensitivity, it was argued, and therefore her hair could only be ridiculous.

In the story of the Coopers presented in Chapter 2, it was the husband's sentimental expectations that, when indulged, went terribly awry. It was Mr. Cooper who "was decidedly sentimental; . . . had an unexpected vein of romance hidden under his careless manner." Having read a tale about an armband woven of hair, "he liked the fancy very much, and had spoken of it several times." Mr. Cooper's sentimental desire, however, required his wife to turn to the market. As he tells her, "Only I should want you to braid it yourself, he said," in one of those lover-like outbreaks. "It would destroy all the poetry to have it go through the gum and bobbins of those hair-workers."[37] In order to have the hair mounted in its requisite gold band, however, Mrs. Cooper must resort to a commercial jeweler. That turn to the market was disastrous, for as manufactured by the market, Mr. Cooper's romantic vision mutated into a grotesque of sentiment. As Mr. Cooper noted, the result looked more like a dog-collar than a romantic armband. "The bracelet was a heavy hoop of gold, something like those so much the fashion for ladies' wear."[38]

In fiction, when men encroached on the feminine purview of sentimental consumerism, they were invariably rebuffed. They proved themselves inept at making the requisite connections between the purchased object and the sincere affections it represented. The doctor found, to his chagrin, that a wig was the source of his savior. Mr. Cooper's romantic sentiment did not find satisfaction in the professionally made bracelet. In fact, male attempts at sentimental consumerism could make men seem effeminate because such immersion in the market of goods was relegated as women's work. The jeweler translated Mr. Cooper's armband into a female accessory, a bracelet "something like those so much the fashion for ladies' wear."

The disadvantage was not only one's gender but one's class. In Alice Carey's 1852 novel, *Clovernook*, a young working-class man fails miserably in his attempt to appropriate the necessarily sincere, implicitly middle-class appearance he desires. At a parlor gathering, the female narrator was introduced to "a pale, slender young man. . . . His flaxen hair hung in curls down his shoulders; he wore his collar reversed, and a sprig of cedar in the buttonhole of his vest, which was of red and yellow colors."[39] This dandified creature was the local cooper earnestly attempting a fashionable exterior and romantic interior. The young cooper is a fictional representative of the widespread impact of the Romantic movement on working-class clothing, with his waistcoat, long curls, and jewelry.[40] His costume was completed by a "gold chain attached to a silver watch, and a bracelet of hair on the left wrist, fastened with a small tinsel clasp, [that] evinced that his tastes had not been cultivated with much care, though his face attested to some natural refinement."[41]

The discordant elements of his costume (gold and silver, a bracelet rather than a more appropriate watch chain) were the most tangible evidence that his character is flawed. This young man exhibited all the pitfalls that male sentimentality threatened. First, he was anything but sincere, and his gaudy clothing was only the most obvious hint of this. His feminine bracelet made of hair demonstrated his poor taste and his inability to successfully negotiate the challenges of finding tasteful, truthful, sincere sentimental goods. He wasn't inherently silly, the narrator acknowledged, as "his face attested to some natural refinement," but his true character was obscured by his poor attempt to act the middle-class man. His attempt to masquerade failed because he was both uneducated about the protocol and unable to select the necessary accessories.

The reasons these fictional men failed in their attempts at sentimental expression related to gendered assumptions about sentimentality, social class, and consumerism. All these men mismanaged the tension between the private, sincere, heartfelt experience of sentimentality and its necessarily public demonstration. They resorted to marketed goods to accomplish the public display, but, having done so, lost the authenticity of their sentiments.

Masculine expressions of sentimentality were appropriate only within certain parameters that were defined, in part, by the ways men and women were themselves defined. Men were considered naturally better suited to the competitive world of work and public life, while women were granted a supposedly natural apprehension of the realm of emotions. The market of goods was considered the purview of women, whose abilities to decorate, refine, and adorn led to the selection of tasteful and appropriate goods. Sentimental consumerism was a minefield of possible missteps for many men. But women, it was argued, were very well adapted to treading that path.

Hair Watch Chains Go to Work

Watch chains made of hair worked as sentimental consumer goods for men because they were both sentimental and practical. Bracelets and armbands were too close to the feminized character of sentiment, but watch chains, used to attach the masculine timekeeping instrument to men, were safely ensconced in the world of manly activity. Hair chains allowed men to display their adherence to two tenets of middle-class masculinity: loyalty to work and fidelity to one's family. At the same time, hair watch chains were intimate statements of identity and neutral testaments to one's status as a middle-class man. Men used hair jewelry made of their loved ones to personalize their appearance, to individualize the act of looking at one's watch, and to represent their embrace of the masculine role of provider and father. The competitive field of work was where a man was to create himself, as it were, by denying indulgences, disciplining his activity, and becoming his work.

Harry Pinkney's photograph from the 1880s is a typical, almost generic image of a nineteenth-century middle-class man.[42] Mr. Pinkney posed with one hand resting on a studio prop and his other hand angled behind him. His sack jacket, part of a loosely cut, ready-made suit, is spread open across his torso. Clearly visible between the gaps of his jacket is his watch chain made of hair.[43] The watch chain was the most visible and appropriate jewelry accessory to a middle-class man's work uniform (Figure 22).

Pinkney identified himself as a male, middle-class worker through his clothing. A business or work suit like Pinkney's was a recent development in men's fashions. The men's suit of the second half of the nineteenth century had its roots in the frock coats and breeches of the eighteenth century. By the 1870s, longer frock coats, with roots in aristocratic English gentry styles, never again became fashionable. Rather, the more economical, spare, and more closely cut suit coat had taken its place.[44]

The proper suit of the 1870s and 1880s was worn with a waistcoat. The waistcoat, or vest, had a small pocket on its front to hold a pocket watch. The watch was secured to a buttonhole on the vest with a "fob"—a ribbon, chain, or braid of silk or hair. This style of wearing a pocket watch was so prevalent that pocket watches were also known as "fob watches." In the early nineteenth century, the fob was usually a flat, short piece of ribbon, attached to the waistband of a man's breeches. Another way to wear a watch was to slide the watch into the flat front pockets near the pants' waist.[45]

By the 1820s and 1830s, though, men's pants styles had changed. In the late eighteenth century, men's breeches were very tight, knee-length, and worn with stockings. But by the 1820s, men's pants reached their ankles (never since rising), widened, and became the trousers so familiar in the late twentieth century. With this style shift, the watch fob narrowed and elongated into a chain. The new vest watch chain (sometimes also called an "Albert chain" in honor of Prince Albert of Great Britain), as one historian has aptly described it, "spread across the stomach from one waistcoat pocket to the other." Still retaining its older name of fob, the watch chain was one of the most acceptable forms of male jewelry.[46]

Pinkney's ready-made suit coat perfectly suited the new mode of rushed, constantly timed work. Having moved work and labor away from

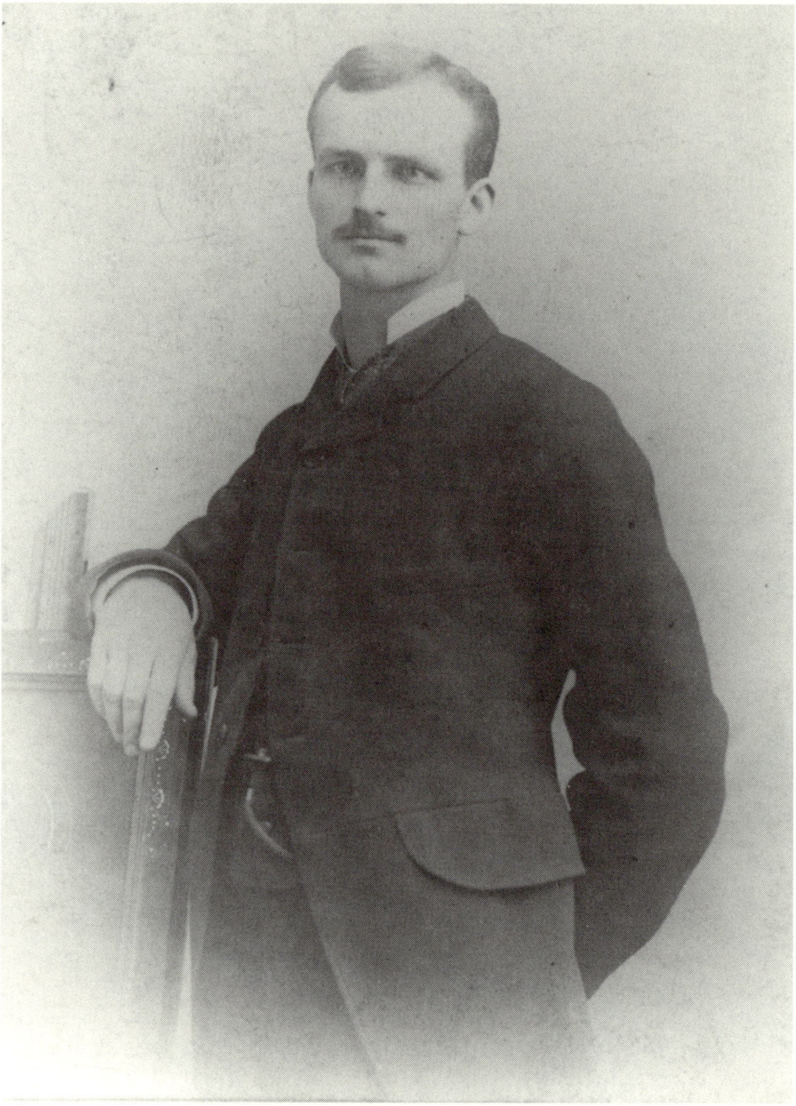

Figure 22. Harry Pinkney is a young man well on his way to success in 1880s Lawrence, Kansas. He stands confidently in his business suit, with his watch chain made of hair looped through his waistcoat with the watch tucked into the pocket to the side, under his jacket. With his hair watch chain prominently displayed, Harry embodies nineteenth-century manhood through his sentimental attachments *and* attention to business life. Courtesy, Kansas Collection, Spencer Research Library, University of Kansas.

the home, most middle-class and working-class men labored under the eye of the clock. Time was all-important in measuring the worth of a person's labor, and wages earned were relative to the value of one's work conducted in a given amount of time. Every minute counted and, for many wage workers, every minute was literally calculated at a specific monetary value.[47] "Good work" was increasingly defined in terms of time saved and time carefully "spent" on producing useful work, so a watch was a necessity.[48]

Pinkney's portrait asserted his fulfillment of the tenets of nineteenth-century middle-class manhood. He was a man willing to discipline himself in order to reach his goals, and the watch communicated this.[49] While time-keeping represented employers' increasing ability to valuate a worker's time, individual time-keeping pieces, such as a pocket watch, offered individuals the ability to control their own time within those circumstances. Pocket watches "were probably the only example of a clearly industrial machine carried close to the body."[50] Portable watches brought the rationalizing effects of the market literally close to home.

A pocket watch so perfectly embodied the desired characteristics of manhood that boys often received a watch as a present to mark their passage into adulthood. In an 1874 novel, a young adult man arrived home from his world travels bearing gifts for his family. His nephew opened his gift as his uncle exclaimed, " 'For you, Felix! because you are your father's namesake.' . . . For once, the gay youth was speechless with emotion when he beheld a neat watch—gold, with a hunting case, his initials engraved on the inside. 'I could not give it to the son of a nobler, purer, more righteous gentleman!' subjoined the donor, emphatically."[51] Felix's time piece gave him the sheen of what his uncle teasingly called his "manly beauty." In fact, Felix had become a man, invested with a man's responsibility to solemnly draw out his pocket watch to check the passage of time.

By 1874, when the account of Felix's watch was published, cheap, readily available pocket watches were an essential accessory for a middle-class man. The Civil War had encouraged the development of inexpensive watches and, by 1865, companies such as Dennison Watch Company found the majority of their sales in their least expensive styles. By the early 1880s, most pocket watches sold for three to five dollars—not inexpensive but worth an investment on the part of most middle-class and many working-class families.[52] Advertisements and catalogues of the 1870s and 1880s reflect the demand for watch chains made of hair. By the 1880s, jewelry catalogues and mass marketers offered hair watch chains along with gold and silver link chains. G. M. Hansen Novelties Company (circa 1870s) offered the entire gamut of possible materials, from silver and gold chains, wide ribbon "chains," and a hair chain with gold trimming. Prices ranged from $4.00 for coin silver chains, to $1.25 for gilt-covered silver or for a hair chain. Edwin Creer, advertising his wares in London in 1887, offered an Albert guard of hair with gold mountings.[53]

The *Busiest House in America* catalogue of 1888 offered hair mounts by the dozen. The simplest styles cost a jeweler as little as one dollar each (wholesale), while the most elaborate styles of chased gold cost eleven dollars each. Each "hair mount" was a fob finding set, and included the bar, clasp, and ending (Figure 23). In 1899, J. H. Purdy and Company's *Twentieth Century Catalogue of Supplies for Watchmakers, Jewelers and Kindred Trades* offered hair mounts as pieces. A jeweler could buy, for instance, one dozen rolled plate bars for two dollars, and gold octagon-shaped clasps for as little as $2.25 a dozen. J. H. Purdy and Company also offered hair-chain mountings as a set for as little as $8.00 a dozen for rolled plate, engraved mounts. Other companies limited their offerings to complete sets of mountings. In 1900, the American Consumers' Alliance (Inc.) carried hair-chain mountings ornamented with garnets and "brilliants" for $1.45 to $4.50 each. In 1904, the styles of hair-chain mounting varied from the very simple and inexpensive to the elaborately expensive. By the end of the century, mass marketers such as Sears, Roebuck and Company, and Montgomery Ward and Company, offered hair chains, jewelry mountings, and repairs. As Sears, Roebuck urged prospective customers in 1902, "BE IN LINE. Everybody is wearing a Fob." Montgomery Ward's catalogue argued that they offered a "sensible, practical Hair Vest Chain."[54]

Often, the hair used in a man's watch chain was that of his fiancé or his wife. Sarah Heywood, as we saw earlier, had a watch chain made of her hair for her fiancé Samuel Folwell. Blanche Butler placed her hair in a locket for her fiancé, Adelbert Ames, and expected he would attach the charm to his watch chain, which he did. Dr. H. W. Youmans, a physician in Mukwonago, Wisconsin, in the 1870s, wore a watch chain made of his wife's hair. His son had woven the chain in the 1860s, during service in the Civil War.[55]

For others, watch chains made of hair were doubled souvenirs that commemorated public events as well as personal affections. For instance, Rose Evans took advantage of her tour of the Columbian Exposition in Chicago to have a watch chain made of her hair for her husband.[56] And for many men, their watch chain of their wife's hair was a treasured and often-worn accessory. For instance, the Reverend Charles Hendley wore the watch chain of his wife's hair for years, as both his family reports and the gently

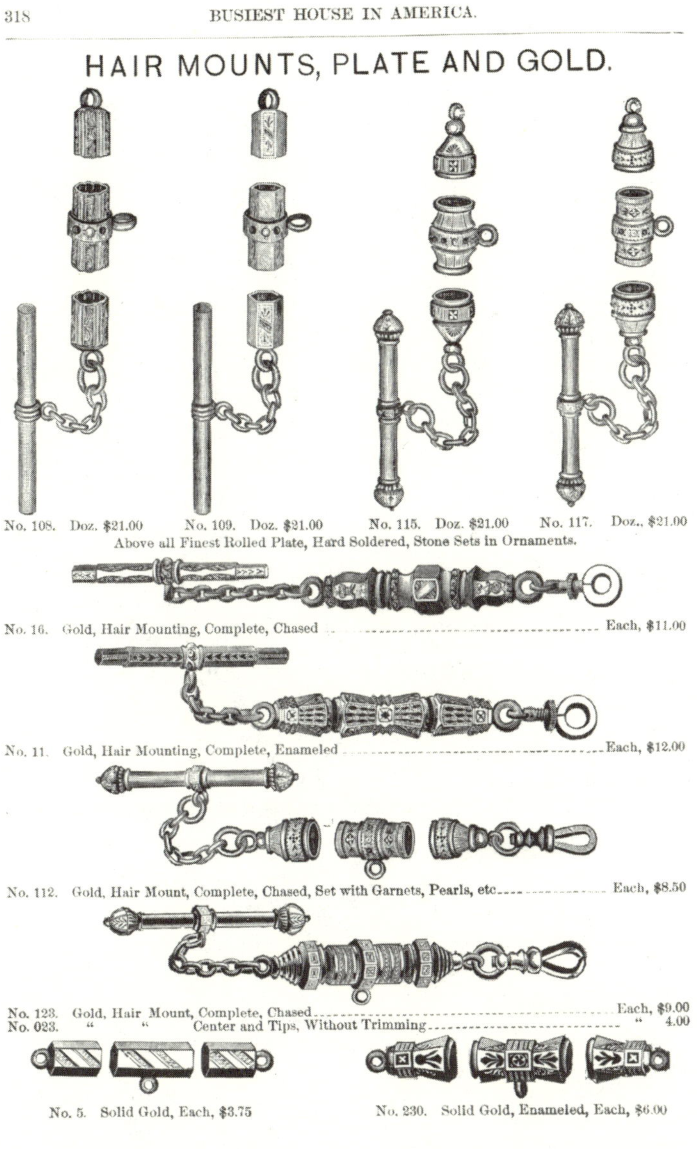

Figure 23. These hair mounts were sold to retail jewelers and hair workers throughout the country during the last half of the nineteenth century. The gold mountings were some of the more upscale designs available, but even they formed part of a watch chain most middle-class men could afford. From *The Busiest House in America,* Chicago, 1888. Courtesy, The Winterthur Library: Printed Book and Periodical Collection.

frayed ends of his chain attest.[57] William Hawtin's watch chain, made of his wife's hair, also appears to have been consistently used throughout his lifetime.[58]

Hair watch chains represented a tension more complicated than the neatly divided rhetorical arguments of separate spheres ideology. Separate spheres ideological arguments suggested that hair watch chains were created by women to remind men of the dependents that men's labor supported. This interpretation is a partial explanation about why hair watch chains were so popular among middle-class men. But men's jewelry made of hair legitimated the male work space: the work world made possible the domestic world. At the same time, though, its practical consciousness of the demands of the work world dangling at its end disciplined this sentimental expression. Such visibly sentimental and feminized symbols as hair watch chains evoked the physical, iconic wife and alluded to the benevolent intentions of the business world. Hair watch chains, then, can be understood as critiques of the male work space that without the presence of women and children would be dehumanizing.

In 1878, Henry T. Williams wrote, "The daily toil on the farm, or in office, store or shop is perhaps cheerfully endured by this father of the house; the work carefully, even willingly performed, but it necessarily brings weariness." More than a decade earlier, *Godey's Book and Magazine* had sounded the alarm, arguing that men's activities outside the home were indeed treacherous. A man "travels [the road of life] in pursuit of competence or wealth," but it was not an easy road. "On the contrary, it is a rough and rugged path, beset with 'wait-a-bit' thorns, and full of pitfalls. . . . After every day's journey over this worse than rough turnpike road, the wayfarer needs something more than rest; he requires solace and deserves it." The remedy lay in the consoling confines of the home. Men's relief was found, as *Godey's* suggested, in their wives' "warm greetings" and "fond glances" and their childrens' "welcome shouts." "These tokens of affection and sympathy constitute the poetry which reconciles us to the prose of life." Indeed, throughout the nineteenth century, most middle-class working men lived their lives within families, whether that of their birth or of their making.[59]

While the author used the term "tokens of affection" metaphorically, many middle-class men treasured actual tokens of affection and clearly understood, as well as participated in, the feminized realm of sentiment. Such tokens could metonymically embody those "warm greetings" of the happy home, and could be carried in tangible form by a man into the harsher world of market competition. By expressing emotions on the familiar ground of the patriarchal role, men ameliorated the deadening effects of commercial life.

After all, a married man worked not only for his own success but for the benefit of his family. The fortunes of an entire family rested on a middle-class man's ability to succeed within the demanding world of work.[60] A man had "the power to determine the place of his wife and children in the world. In other words, the self-made man of the nineteenth century made not only himself, but his family as well."[61] A great deal, then, besides one man's fate was represented by his pocket watch. Hair watch chains linked men's worlds of home and office, and they represented the ways that the home—the domestic sphere—made a man's work life imperative.

Even corporations adopted domesticity to cushion the competitive nature of work. From the 1870s through the 1930s, many corporations adopted domestic decoration, for example, because it offered the ability to recreate a patriarchal family structure that wedded authority with caretaking.[62] Domestic-like spaces such as executive offices—richly carpeted, adorned with carefully selected art, and comfortable furniture—may have contradicted the increasing rationalization of work life, but it served to individuate those surroundings.

The use of maternal images to emphasize the benevolent, kindly character and solid foundations of businesses began in the 1850s. Insurance companies, intent on developing reputations for "care-taking," found images of women particularly useful in promoting their own stability and their unique promises of fair treatment of customers.[63] Of course, the appropriation of images of women to serve purposes often quite distant from women's own interests was not new.[64] But by the 1850s, some corporations adopted the image of the stately female to provide a particularly feminine touch to their otherwise masculine enterprise.

Men, as discussed earlier, were revered when they exhibited a devotion to the self-denying life of work, yet that immersion in a masculine world threatened the basis of middle-class life: the family and the domestic sphere. Men were so identified through their work that it seemed they might lose their connections with their families. Men had to be reminded of their ties to the world outside of work, apart from other men. Wedded to the masculine work uniform, hair watch chains represented in their braids the ideally intertwined male life. This was no isolated renegade; rather, this was a steady, hard-working man whose efforts were not only to better himself but his family. This was a man firmly linked to both his work and his home. The hair in the watch chain bound the man to both his workplace and his heartplace. And, by wearing the constant presence of the home, a man's work was not a heartless undertaking but a necessary and welcome activity performed for the benefit of the entire society.

Throughout the nineteenth century, sentimentality was used to balance the capitalist work world. In a hair watch chain, this sentimental critique of work life was carefully controlled. The sentiment took the form of a watch chain. Its purpose was practical, and utilitarian, in that it attached a fundamentally useful object, the watch, to the worker. At the same time, men's watch chains made of hair integrated public life (symbolized by time and the time-keeper) and the private sphere of sentiment and affiliations. In this way, the challenge of sentimentality was defused and brought to accommodate the rationalizing goals of competitive capitalism.

Thus, hair jewelry for men and women not only took on different gendered forms but had specifically gendered meanings. Women's hair jewelry positioned women in a network of affiliations, often weaving together several different individuals and representing a woman's role as sister, daughter, wife, and mother. Women used the market of sentimental goods, and the plethora of hair-jewelry styles, to assert their position within a world of others.

Men's jewelry, however, was nominally practical, and its sentimentality subordinated to its utilitarian, masculine role. Hair watch chains linked men as individuals to others and acted as a bridge between work and home. Men's public role of provider was affirmed through the watch chain's association to time and work, and thus attested to the indelible bond between men and work. Hair jewelry, made of the natural material of the body, tangibly reiterated the ideals of middle-class, nineteenth-century American gender ideology. The naturalness of the material and the smoothness of hair jewelry's weave suggested the stability of the rhetoric, and represented the fundamental basis of a middle-class culture built on naturalized gender and class difference. The premises that lent hair jewelry its power as a sentimental consumer object seemed in little danger of becoming "untangled."

Chapter 7
The Only Manufacturer Remaining

They did not recognize it at the time, but the skilled, independent practitioners of hairwork had their heyday in the 1870s and 1880s. The 1890s was a period of decline for hairwork. It must not have seemed that way to hair workers themselves. There were still individual hair workers, but more often, large jewelry houses offered hairwork repair and just a few styles of hairwork jewelry. At the same time, the sentimental expression that gave hairwork legitimacy in middle-class culture waned. Hairwork, always poised between sincerity and artificiality, became the target of criticism. By the end of World War I, hairwork was no longer the desirable commodity it had been since the 1700s.

The trade of hairwork changed after the 1880s, and these shifts in the market of goods, and in the popular acceptance of sentimental expression, practically ensured the end of hairwork's popularity. In the 1880s, large jewelry houses entered the hairwork market. In some ways, they had the advantage: retail jewelers could have almost all customer orders filled by the same house, from gold rings to hairwork watch chains. A retailer did not have to search out a skilled and reliable hair worker; a jobber could contract the work out. And this practice continued through the 1890s. As always, a customer could go to a local jeweler, select a design from an illustrated catalogue, hand over the hair of the loved one, and return in several weeks to receive the completed piece of jewelry.

This practice of individual, custom-made production seemed quaint and a bit wasteful, however. In the 1880s, jewelry often incorporated a blank space for engraving an initial or a personal message, or even included an initial or a name. This was an effective way to produce jewelry in large batches but still with some personal attention. In its 1888 catalogue, the large wholesale dealer The Busiest House in America offered "hair chain mounts in various styles" and "Real Garnet Initial Pins" that were "furnished only on positive orders, in ten days' time."[1] The initial pins were apparently made to order. Jewelry catalogues abounded with personalized, or easy-to-personalize, articles, such as the "coin silver rings" with large front flat spaces that Clapp and Company offered in 1888.[2] Another company offered "friendship rings" or "bangle pins." The inexpensive jewelry (only fifty cents each) came with engraved discs. Customers provided the names and wore the jewelry to exhibit their friendships with others.[3] Cheap personalized jewelry allowed individuality even when paired with the lower costs of mass production.

The Moutoux Brothers: "Modern" Artisans

Independent hair workers persisted well into the twentieth century, but they struggled to compete with cheaper and more easily produced jewelry and with the waning of the sentimentality that lent hairwork its meaning. The Moutoux brothers, Emil and William, were traditional hair workers. Born in Germany, they arrived in New York in the mid-1850s.[4] The Moutoux brothers excelled in pictorial hairwork, where hair was worked to form miniatures or full-sized pictures of weeping willows, tombstones, and landscapes. William Ernst Moutoux was more prominent than Emil in the craft of hairwork throughout the second half of the nineteenth century, but both had long careers in jewelry and hairwork. Like other independent hair workers, William Ernst Moutoux won awards for his hairwork designs, such as the American Institute for Design Award in 1870.[5] He applied for credit and, in 1873, the Dun credit agency noted that the bulk of William's business was in working for the trade.[6] William gave up the hairwork business in the 1890s, having held out "until the time when the taste of the public had changed so much that he could not work profitably in his trade of converting human hair into different objects."[7]

In 1879, William placed a lengthy advertisement in the trade publication the *Jewelers' Circular and Horological Review*. He characterized himself as "the only leading personal Artist in Hair in this country," an honorarium that would have surprised and displeased the hundreds of hair artists throughout the country. William could claim this position because he had accrued medals, but he also argued that other hairwork dealers in the country used his designs. His place of business, he claimed, was a "factory and office." In some ways, he was continuing the older tradition of a hairwork "manufactory." He could offer "designs of the most complicated description"; he was able to render "Short or Baby hair made in the finest designs in your presence" or make "Portraits, or copy of noted paintings, made of family hair. . . . Lessons given in all branches," or you could write for "Large pattern books for the trade free."

What makes William Ernst Moutoux's career in hair working so interesting is that he survived with one foot in the older tradition of the artisan–hair worker and one foot in the new model of less personalized, more efficient production of hairwork. He continued the family craft, created innovative designs, offered lessons in his trade, and filled retail orders (designs finished "in your presence"). But in the new rapidly industrializing 1880s, he introduced new methods of selling hairwork. In 1884, Moutoux offered retailers "Wholesale prices for Hair Chain Braids in Assorted Colors, by the gross or dozen at half of book prices. Devices made at half of book prices if necessary."[8]

In the world of hair jewelry, this was a shocker. It was one of the first public admissions of what must have been a practice of less reputable houses: offering ready-made hairwork for the retail market. Throughout the nineteenth century, and especially from the 1860s on, there were concerns that, as one critic of the commercial hairwork world said, "The hair sent shall be that actually used."[9] The implications of William's advertisement to the trade was that, in fact, no, the hair was *not* the "real hair given" to the jeweler by the customer, but hair chains ready-made, far more convenient and profitable for the jeweler than custom-made work.

William Ernst Moutoux was in business until the end of the 1890s. In 1897, after almost a decade of not placing advertisements in trade publications, he paid for a brief listing in the *American Jeweler*. In very large letters he announced "HAIR + JEWELRY" and noted he was "the only manufacturer remaining in the United States."[10] In fact, Moutoux's claim might well have been true. He may have been the last large-scale jobber of hairwork in the country, but even more likely was that William felt alone and stranded after a career of competition and displays of finesse and skill that had garnered him not only a comfortable living but esteem from other craftsmen and craftswomen. In 1900, a U.S. census taker recorded that William Ernst Moutoux lived with his wife, four children, and a servant. He owned his house free of a mortgage, and was a "retired artist." His son, William Ernst Moutoux II, managed a jewelry store. The first William had apparently retired: the last hairwork manufacturer had ended his long career.[11]

Despite William's claim, other hair workers were addressing a national audience. In 1900, five New York City ornamental hair workers were listed in a national business directory.[12] In Philadelphia, Katherine Schmitt continued listing her business as "hair jewelry" until 1901, when she ceased listing at all.[13] By this point, only a very few professional hair workers remained in the entire country.

Jobbers and the Mass-Market Retailers: The New Hair Workers

One problem for independent hair workers was that jobbers, the companies who supplied hairwork to local retail jewelers, began in the 1890s to offer hair chains ready-made. To continue in the business, most professional hair workers would have to begin buying hair in bulk and creating hair chains to sell to the jobber by the gross or dozen. But meeting these demands of the market undermined the relevance of hair jewelry itself.

What had been the exception became the rule. Most jewelry wholesalers offered ready-made hairwork jewelry in bulk. In *Our Salesman* (1891), the company offered a three-strand hair vest chain by the dozen for $36.00, or a two-strand chain for only $24.00 a dozen.[14] A retailer could also have hair jewelry made to order. The company offered to braid a hair vest chain for $3.50, and hair chain mountings would add $2.00 to $9.50. A repair job would be done for $1.50. Obviously, for a retailer, it was far more economical to use ready-made hair vest chains, as those cost no more than $3.00 each if purchased by the dozen.[15]

The A. C. Becken Company offered nine different styles of hair vest chains, which appear to be offered ready-made. Elsewhere in its catalogue, under its repair list, the company announced its ability to make hair chains.[16] In 1899, the evocatively titled *The Restless and the Sleepless Standard Price List* offered basic jobbing materials, such as gilt hooks in five sizes, dozens of hair-chain mountings, and, on a page titled "Gents' Silk and Hair Vest Chains," four vest chains made of "real human hair" for $1.50 to $2.75.[17] The C. R. Hetter Jewelry Company also offered an array of vest chains, including three ready-made hair vest chains.[18]

It was still possible, of course, to have hair jewelry made to order with the hair supplied by customers. Surprisingly, some of the largest retailers were also the ones who maintained the older traditions of sentimental hairwork. In 1894, Montgomery Ward and Company offered four different styles of hair vest chains. Two were already mounted, but two chain patterns are shown without mountings. Under the two loose chains, the company instructs customers that these are "Hair Chains made to order Send us the hair and we will braid in style. . . . Mountings extra."[19] What the company was saying to customers reveals the state of the hairwork jewelry trade at the end of the century. The company offered hairwork made to order, or customers could select one of two ready-made hair vest chains.

Other large mass retailers hewed closer to the traditions of hairwork. Sears, Roebuck and Company began offering hair chains in 1896, and, in 1902, the company provided six different mounting styles and two different braid chains. Sears instructed customers to "Send hair to us. We can braid it in style" of those depicted on the page and offered a "fancy woven hair vest guard . . . with very fancy gold filled mounting @ for $1.35." The company warned customers that "we are not in position to quote prices on this guard made to order," a confusing notice. It suggests, in fact, that Sears was not able to provide the vest guard made in hair sent; rather, customers bought a vest guard already made of human hair. In the same catalog, Sears did offer "hair chain[s] made to order, in two pieces like [those pictured] above." Sears depicted two distinct braid styles, and five different mounts for the braid.[20]

In 1908, Sears signaled what may have been the death knell for hairwork. Rather painfully fulfilling all the concerns regarding hairwork as a mail-order product, Sears offered "Best quality rolled gold plate, gold filled and solid gold mountings, for gents' and ladies' hair and silk vest chains." No. 4K0666 was a "Hair chain braided to order . . . requires about 1½ ounces of hair combings to braid a chain. Is made in two pieces, and together with mountings is 12½ inches long. We do not do this braiding ourselves. We send it out; therefore we cannot guarantee same hair being used that is sent to us; you must assume all risk."[21]

Sears openly acknowledged that the *perception* that commercial hair marketers were uncaring was not a groundless concern: it was true. And by pairing the economic language of risk to the wholly natural and intimate material of a loved one's hair, Sears rendered hair like other unstable commodities. One of the nineteenth century's developments had been a commodities market that valued raw materials before they had been produced. So, for example, one could buy and sell, lose money, or make a profit from a wheat crop that had not even been planted. For many nineteenth-century Americans, this was immoral. The function of the futures market, such as the future of wheat crops, was to abstract value, to displace worth from the physical reality of the commodity (that is, the ton of wheat) and to hide the productive activity of farming itself. By characterizing hairwork as "speculative" (customers had to "assume all risk" just as market speculators gambled), Sears introduced a similar taint of groundlessness to hairwork. That which was a product of the human body and of the heart was rendered an abstract element of dubious value.[22]

Sears compounded the error of judgment when, in copy appearing just below the advertisement for hairwork, it offered a "Fancy woven three-strand hair vest guard . . . with very fancy rolled gold plate tips, slide bar, and swivel." However, the company cautioned, "We will not quote prices on this guard made to order, as the braiding is machine work."[23] Once again, Sears disavowed the "made to order" trade and, in doing so, misjudged the basis of the popularity of hairwork. Hairwork was sought after not because it was "fancy" and stylish (although, as we have seen, these were certainly implicit aspects of its popularity) but because it revealed the owner as criticizing those characteristics. Machine-made hairwork was just another fashionable product, without an aspect of individuality and sincerity.

Sears's comment, crass as it was, reflected a larger trend in the manufacture of jewelry for middle-class and working-class customers. One reason Sears was in the business of selling jewelry at all was that since the mid-1800s the production costs of jewelry had lowered as machine production took hold.[24] Acknowledgment that similar market forces meant that even hairwork was machine produced forced customers to accept that the dreaded "careless hands" of the market were combing through one's loved one's hair. But Sears was a *retailer* whose audience was customers. Sears's revelation was more significant than Moutoux's because while Moutoux was revealing a trade practice to the trade itself, Sears was informing customers about the otherwise hidden practices in the hair-jewelry market.

Was hairwork often made by machines? At least until the 1900s, it is unlikely for several reasons. First, the meaning of hairwork was entwined with its status as a product made by human hands and invested with human emotions. Second, the labor cost of hair working was minimal, and it is unlikely that individual hair workers such as William Ernst Moutoux or Katherine Schmitt, both of whom apprenticed in the 1850s and had independent shops into the 1880s, would have shifted to machine production, both for reasons of cost and for issues of professional integrity. Third, no evidence exists of actual machinery used to create hairwork. There are no patent applications, for example, which list hairwork manufacture as their goal. There are, however, patent applications for machines that produced products that appeared similar to popular forms of hair jewelry.

For example, in 1875 W. W. Alden of Providence, Rhode Island (a prominent jewelry manufacturing town), patented his "Improvement in

Braided Jewelry" that produced openwork woven earring drops.[25] But the material to be woven was wire, and the interior form was paper that was then burnt out from the center, leaving the open-weave drop to be mounted.[26] Of course, a manufacturer may have experimented with using hair as a material in his machines that wove the silk ribbon vest chains that were so often pictured next to woven hair chains in suppliers' catalogues.[27]

Hairwork persisted through the first twenty-five years of the twentieth century, but most jewelers' suppliers offered only a few standard hair vest chains and repair services. The S. F. Myers Company was typical. In their 1901 catalogue of wholesale jewelry, they urged retailers to note that they could repair and job practically any kind of jewelry need, "Everything in Watches, Watch Cases, Gold Jewelry, Diamond Jewelry, Hair Jewelry, Silver Ware," etc.[28] Other companies that offered repair services in the first decade of the twentieth century were A. C. Becken and C. R. Hettel.[29]

Sentimental hairwork had always coexisted, albeit uneasily, with a commercial trade in human hair. Hair jewelry retained a sentimental meaning insofar as it was understood to be distinct from the market-driven world of the hair trade. Throughout the nineteenth century, the two worlds of commercial hair—the hairwork industry and the artificial-hairpiece industry—had remained separate. But in the last decades of the nineteenth century, the artificial-hair market drew increasing attention. The narratives about the artificial-hair market, as seen in stories that appeared in women's and general-interest periodicals and in fiction, heightened the difference between the two worlds of hairwork, but it also suggested the possibility that sentimental hairwork was not all that different. Paired with changes in the production of hair jewelry, sentimental hairwork began to lose its luster.

The Hair Trade: Using Dead Hair

Louisa May Alcott's story of Jo's hair sale, discussed earlier, reminds us that mid–nineteenth-century Americans were aware that people could, and did, sell their hair for money. Beginning in the 1870s, periodicals and newspapers ran regular feature stories about women who sold their hair to be made into wigs and other kinds of artificial hairwork. In her patent application of 1869, Louise F. Shaw reflected how such stories were accepted by many readers. Shaw's patent was for artificial hair made of thread, a product for which there is a crying need, according to her. "It is well known," Miss Shaw proclaimed, "that the trade in human hair is enormous, and that the high price that the same commands, has induced unscrupulous persons to resort to measures for obtaining the same, that are detrimental to public health and morals."[30] It was also common knowledge, she continued, that "in many instances the hair is cut off the heads of the most loathsome and degraded women. . . . [and] it is well known to the trade that large quantities of hair are constantly put on the market that have been taken from the bodies of dead persons, that have been disinterred simply to obtain the hair, and this fact is frequently demonstrated from the roots of the hair remaining upon them as they have been pulled out of the putrid, decaying flesh of the dead."[31] With beliefs such as these accepted as truth, the taint of the commercial market of hair was clear. Sentimental hair jewelry functioned as a desirable good as long as it was understood to be distant from this world of girls and "loathsome" women selling their hair, or from the dead bodies dug up and the hair yanked off of them.

At the same time, hair-jewelry suppliers faced the perception that they often substituted ready-made human hairwork for the hair sent in with an order. Of course, hair jewelry was meaningful only if its integrity was assured. When a woman opened her package, she examined it. Was this the hair that had been sent in? If it was, the hair jewelry did indeed represent intimate emotions, but if it was counterfeit, insincerity was the result. And insincerity negated sentimentality.

One reason for all the attention paid to the international hair market was that the popularity of artificial hairwork and wigs begged explanation as to where all that hair originated from, since it was not from the heads of those who wore it. Because the hair used for wigs came from all over the world, stories about the market touted the virtues of global trade, the appeal of the exotic, and also the disturbing and politically sensitive issue of the influx of "others" into the United States. In addition, the hair market had always been a challenge to the producers of sentimental hairwork. While almost all hair that was "on the market" was used in artificial hairwork such as false falls, there was the constant specter of so much hair literally floating about the country. What if some of it, even a tiny bit, ended up in one's own hair brooch with one's mother's hair? The discussions of the hair market emphasized the vanity (and hypocrisy) of women (both those who wore artificial hair and those who willingly sold their own hair).[32] Given the international character of the hair market, and especially the supposedly high importation rates of hair into the United States, national stereotypes and racist ideas were aired in the course of describing the market itself.

In the 1860s, the *New-York Times* alleged that the "importation of human hair to this country involves the expenditure of upward of one million of dollars per annum."[33] There were only six major hair dealers in the country, the article continued. The imported hair came from France and Germany where, it was explained, "Peddlers in those countries, go from one town to another and purchase from the peasant girls their superfluous hair, paying them in peddlers' goods a trifling sum."[34] The article suggested that the hair "dealers become so expert in handling hair, that they are able to tell what part of the country it comes from, and in some instances, the exact town and family." The hair market was carefully structured around national categories: black and dark brown hair was from Spain, France, and Italy; light brown and chestnut shades came from young women in Germany; blonde hair from Sweden, and red hair from Scotland. There was, the article detailed, a nascent domestic market of selling hair, but "American women take too much pride in their natural head-covering to part with it readily."[35]

In the 1880s, the same newspaper described the yearly hair harvest in France. Conducted by the "lower order of trades" such as peddlers, the hair harvest was a mass hair-cutting festival that took place in May. Young girls, tempted by "his wares and shining coin," allowed the peddler to cut their "silken coils." Such was the beauty of these naive girls that "one can almost imagine that he can yet see the hand of the virgin's lover on its waving brilliancy."[36]

This story of French country girls selling their hair was a fixture in American newspapers and periodicals throughout the nineteenth century.[37] In 1900, *Wide World Magazine* ran a story, "The Human Hair Harvest in Brittany," written by an author who purportedly barely escaped with his life from the angry vendors of the hair.[38] The reporter went to a provincial town in June to observe for himself the hair harvest. It was a dangerous enterprise, remarked the reporter's friend, "for both the merchants and their customers are perfect savages, jealously guarding the secret of their queer traffic."[39] Our author bravely persevered. In the end, the story he tells is one familiar from the reports of the 1860s. Peddlers arrive loaded with feminine goods, which they traded with the town's girls. Now indebted to the peddler, when the hair shearers arrived the girls docilely allowed their beautiful hair to be shorn. It was, in this reporter's eyes, a poor bargain because "the cunning dealer manages to get out of the silly woman the entire commercial value of the shawl, thus obtaining her beautiful hair for nothing—hair which brings in at least fifty francs per kilogramme to the rascally merchant. Moreover, later on, when sorted and 'manufactured,' it is worth thirty times that sum."[40]

In the end, the Breton girls were subjected to the withering gaze of the male reporter. Referring to an accompanying photograph of the proceedings, he asked the readers to "notice on the right the unintelligent face of the peasants. So long as the country folk remain in their present condition of ignorance, this strange traffic will continue."[41]

Perhaps his article did enlighten the villagers. Only six years later, the *New York Daily Tribune* announced to its women readers, "'Coupeurs' Confront a Famine in Tresses, as Peasant Girls Refuse to Part with Them—They Want to Look Like Other Girls." A tradition dating from the Middle Ages had ended, according to the paper. Disposing of the traditional women's costume of black dresses ornamented with broad white caps, young girls also rejected the selling of their hair because without the cap their shorn heads were obvious and embarrassing.[42]

In 1913, Julius Price wrote of the fashion of Paris and London up to 1912. He sketched the familiar outlines of the trade in false hair in Europe, providing yet another version of the hair harvests with their requisite young female lambs shorn for other women's vanity. He made a point, however, of assuring readers of "a fact that will upset a popular fallacy: hospitals do not supply the hair used for wigs or chignon making. No hair cut after death is of any use to the wig-maker or coiffeur." In other words, it must be live hair, otherwise, he argued, it is brittle and cannot be curled and adapted into different shapes. And he asserted the feminine character of the enterprise, for "masculine hair has no value whatever, and is useless for even making mattresses."[43]

These descriptions of the European hair market, and thus the source for imported American artificial hairwork, reinforced the validity of sentimental conceptions of womanly virtue while they critiqued the hair sellers' failure to uphold those standards. The severed hair could reveal one's town or even one's family. The hair still radiated the presence of a lover's hand caressing it, even as that hair lay on the dirt of the village square. Girls yearning to possess trinkets and shawls forfeited their greater treasure of their own hair.

In addition to the growing awareness of the human hair trade were the racist assumptions revealed in discussions of that market. Hair was traditionally used by Western cultures to create markers of supposedly inherent racial and ethnic differences; inferiority was revealed in non-Caucasian hair. The market of human hair, already suspect through its trade in the human body, was viewed as a potential entry point of nonwhites into the white world. There was a racial hierarchy of hair sources. In 1874, the *New-York Times* announced in a headline: "Human Hair Supplies: An Impending Crisis in the Market."[44] While the story nominally warned of the decline of the international market of hair, it was an exposé of the "real" nature of hair collection. Italian hair, the article argued, was the mainstay of the hair trade. But Italy was building a national sewage drainage system that would endanger the supply of hair used to make the falls and other pieces worn by American ladies.

In Italy, the article alleged, women threw their hair into the refuse piles, which were then dumped into the open gutters of the towns. Then "the scavenger appears on the scene, . . . and like another Neptune, trident in hand, wades through the gutter, and hooks up every floating tangle of hair." This hair was separated by small children employed for the task. "It is said that, of late years, many hundred-weight of these heads and tails, grimly characterized as 'dead hair,' . . . [make their way] to our more northern centres of civilization." Those civilized countries like England "where existing systems of drainage present inseparable obstacles to the retention and utilization of refuse coils of hair," were in desperate need of the sewage hair of Italy. Sophisticated sanitary technology, then, was tied directly to the supply of wigs and falls. The most technologically advanced countries had the direst need for human hair, for they had no reliable source of material. As the "lower" countries developed, civilized countries would have little recourse. As this article points out, there was no alternative known to replace the Italian hair, as Japanese hair had a stubborn "wire-like rigidity" that made it impossible to work.

In a similar "from-the-gutters" story, Coles's *Dictionary of Dry Goods* discussed the various uses and sources of hair. Having surveyed the sale and use of animal hair, such as horsehair and its use in mattresses, the *Dictionary* noted that "the most valuable hair is human hair."[45] The best false hair, the article asserted, was from France, and it mentioned the famed Brittany hair harvests. But "the major portion of this wavy merchandise is obtained from the *rag-pickers.* These busy searchers of ash heaps and garbage barrels collect every day in the cities of Paris and London alone at least a hundred pounds of hair which some hundreds of thousands of women have combed out of their heads during the preceding twenty-four hours."[46] The hair was then carefully cleaned and sorted.

Asian hair was even more suspect than Italian hair fished out of gutters. In 1877, the *New-York Times* praised the Chinese merchants who "had a genius for trade, and in nothing do they show their mercantile aptitudes more clearly than in the readiness with which they meet every passing demand in the market." The most recently emerged demand met by the Chinese was the enlarged market for hair in Europe.[47]

Asian hair was consistently denigrated as the trade in such hair increased throughout the 1880s and 1890s. The terms echoed the obsessions of the most fervent American nativists of the period.[48] In 1893, the *New York Daily Tribune* announced, "Eight cars loaded with human hair arrived in Paris recently" from India and China.[49] This occurred despite the well-known fact, the article continued, that "this traffic . . . is the cause of the introduction of many diseases to Europe." "The hair is cut from persons after death in China, and . . . it often carries the germs of the disease," alleged the paper. Implied was a protectionist stance; Europe could import foreign hair if it wished to, but the United States should bar such dangerous products from entry. In the same fashion, the "Chinese Exclusion Law," as it was commonly referred to, had been enacted in 1882 to bar the Chinese people from entering the United States.[50]

In addition to imported human hair, horsehair was sometimes used to make hair-jewelry forms. In 1863, Harriet Smith wrote in her diary that a neighbor woman offered to make her a head dress of horsehair for five dollars "and for a whole set she asked fifteen dollars, that is earrings, breast pin and head dress, all made of horsehair. she said that she paid ten dollars to learn how, that she learned in Keokuk, Iowa. I would have liked to have seen a set but she had none made."[51] At least one commercial business specialized in horsehair jewelry. In the mid-nineteenth century, J. Fletcher offered "Horse Hair Jewelry . . . in sets of bracelets, ear rings, breast pins and necklaces, also guard chains, &c., in great variety of designs."[52] The horsehair was decorative, not sentimental, and there was no concern expressed over its use.

The End of the Popularity of Hairwork

In 1885, an English journal announced that hairwork had ended as a fashion. The death announcement was premature for England as well as for the United States, where the availability of commercially prepared hairwork was at its height. Nevertheless, the article, titled "Hair-Device Workers," portrayed a fleet of sad, desperate former hair workers. Hair devices, as we saw earlier, were the flat discs of worked hair popular in the eighteenth century. The article's author, writing in the late nineteenth century, conflated both palette-worked and braided hairwork, and blamed the excessive sentiment both forms of jewelry represented for the current distaste. As the author stated, the "hair-device worker does not precisely charge Byron with ruining his trade. It is we who, with the full conviction of it, do it on his behalf." The poignancy of the decline was sharpest when contrasted with its former immense popularity. The author asked his audience to consider, for example,

> if there was not once a time when your companion at dinner, your partner in the waltz, your *vis-a-vis* in the railway carriage, your neighbour at the *table-d'hôte*, were all hung with chains, were all decked with bracelets, with brooches, even with earrings formed of the hair of departed relatives and friends, finely woven memorials of almost every one they had lost. . . . And where are they now, those snakes and crosses and delicate globes of hair? Where are the mourning rings, the Albert chains, without which no gentleman was once complete? They have been slashed and torn and rent to pieces by Byron. They are unwoven and unravelled by him as surely as though he had done it with his teeth.[53]

The results of Byron's popularity, apparently, was the fulsome acceptance of hair tokens, which then became pointless assertions of individuality in the face of their common use. The result was pitiful former hair workers cast adrift in a world that now valued efficient production. The author depicted one hair worker who "carries specimens of her skill in a crumpled paper bag, and in the front sitting-room pours them trembling out on the table . . . her broad and honest face flushing at the thought of an order that has come at last."[54] Skilled hair workers were left with the leavings and scraps of careers.

Hairwork persisted in all its overwrought glory, but, by the 1920s, it had all but disappeared from the marketplace. Jewelers ceased to offer hairwork, retailers no longer listed hair chains and brooches in their catalogues, and the business was left to a couple of nameless jobbers. In an undated catalogue from the 1920s, the Graf Brothers offered several styles of human hair chains, including an exceptionally long "ladies' chain." The chains were sold by the dozen at very low prices (a single strand chain with elaborate weaving style changes was only $2.50 a dozen, and a flat woven braid was $7.00 a dozen). These chains might very well have been machine woven, as they were illustrated as having very tight braiding and elaborate varieties of braid patterns. The company noted, "Gray Chains made to order." Ironically, the Graf Brothers' principal business was in supplying wigmaker and hairdresser supplies, including "nitting" machines, wig stands, weaving cards and frames.[55]

In 1921, Wendell and Company issued a *Book of Designs* to select retailers that included an entire page of hairwork designs. They offered one style of vest chain, five rings (including one that closely resembled W. C. Peckham's 1868 design of a ring with a band that hid the hair underneath), two pendants (including one in the fashionable letter initial form), and a brooch. Prices ranged from $4.50 for the braiding only of the vest chain, to $60.00 for the brooch. The Company did not explain why it was offering jewelry that other jewelers had ceased offering by 1908. However, on the same page as the hair jewelry was a note that the company could repair enamel jewelry. "Master Enamelers and Enamel Patiners who worked for New York and Newark manufacturers during the period that Enameled Flower Jewelry was the rage are now in our employ. . . . Ours is, therefore, practically the only concern in the country at the present time that can promptly and satisfactorily handle this class of work."[56] Perhaps the hairwork was offered in the same spirit of providing other anachronistic styles in order to be a comprehensive supply house. Whatever the goal, the company did not offer the hairwork or repairs the following year (Figure 24).

The final commercial-trade word on hair jewelry was issued by Otto Young and Company, a large jewelry wholesaler that had been in business since 1865. In 1924, the company offered eight styles of hair-chain mountings. Jewelers could purchase, singly or by the dozen, hair vest chain mountings or mountings for the flat woven fobs. The company did not offer hair braiding or repairs.[57] No other companies have been located who offered either the mountings or braiding, or even repairs of hair jewelry after 1924.

Making one's own hairwork continued into the twentieth century, but the craft had lost much of its appeal. In 1911, E. E. Crofut published an instructional manual. Arguing that the "demand for watch chains made of ladies' hair is constantly increasing" and that "many persons would have hair chains braided as presents for their friends and relatives, if they only knew how. Others would follow it for money making, and as good wages can be demanded for this kind of work as for any other kind of skilled labor."[58] Further job advice was found under the heading "Braiding Hair Chains for Profit." Crofut suggested accepting no less than $2 for each hair chain braided and calculated that that would work out to be about $1 an hour, "good wages for any skilled labor." "Of course at first it may take you

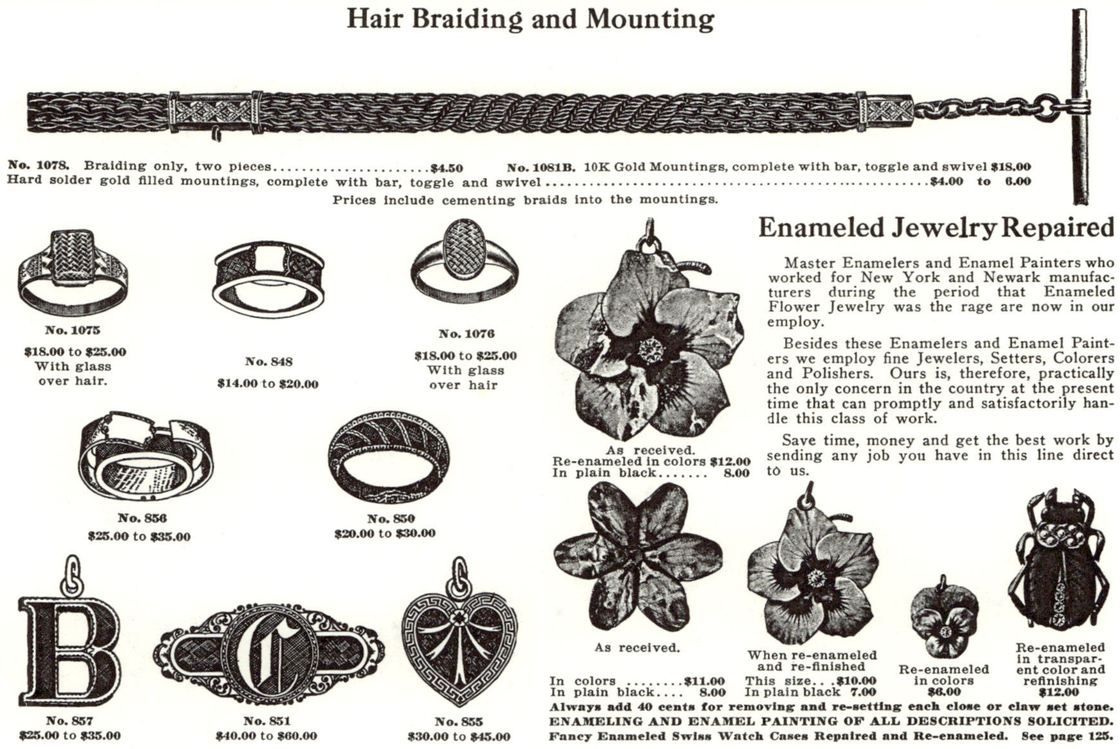

Figure 24. An offer to braid hair for a watch chain, and the mountings to go with it. Interested customers could also consider a hair ring or pendant (displayed on the left). Its partner on the page was also on the wane; as the wholesaler notes about enameled jewelry, it was once "the rage." Enamel workers, like the hair workers, outlasted their products' popularity. W[endell] & Co. *Book of Designs* (1920–1921). Courtesy, National Museum of American History Library.

three, four or maybe five hours to make one chain but the more you make the faster you can make them."[59]

Ironically, in the 1880s and 1890s, unmounted hair chains braided to order cost between $2 to $3.[60] In 1891, Sears offered hair chains braided to order for a mere $1.35.[61] The wages for braiding ornamental hairwork had actually fallen by 1911, making it all the more unlikely that the craft would experience a resurgence of popularity as an occupation. There was no way for a hair worker, who could make hairwork only so fast given the physical limitations of hand manufacture, could compete with the prices offered by wholesalers. Wholesalers could pay extraordinarily little to individual hair workers and consolidate their savings, then charge far less than an actual hair worker could. If machines were in fact introduced in this scheme (and there is no actual evidence that they were) the downward economic pressures would be impossible to resist for artisans.

One indication of the decline of the sentimentality attached to hair was in a short story from 1901.[62] The author, Jennette Lee, described the ritual haircuts received by four young children living on a farm. One of the children, Tommy, undergoes his shearing. "Tommy's mouth opened and shut rapidly, but no sound issued. The crop of thick, dark curls fell silently and encircled him." As Tommy's hair fell, "there was a scramble for the soft locks. Nelson produced a piece of string, which was broken into short lengths and distributed, a piece for each tuft. As the shearing went on, the stock of string ran short. But a tuft from each head was carefully gathered up." But this was not a sentimental gesture on the part of the children, nor were they preserving their hair for their mother's careful keeping. Instead, Lee noted, "Later these would be labelled and preserved in collections—a process that insured their disappearance within six weeks." In other words, the tufts of hair were collected as the children would have assembled rocks or leaves. It mimicked the sentimental traditions of hair keepsakes without the core of emotional significance. It was a commentary on the shallowness of sentimentality itself.

Contrast this approach to that of Emily Dickinson in the 1840s. Dickinson wrote to a friend, Emily Ford, "I said when the barber came I would save you a little lock, and fulfilling my promise, I send you one to-day. I shall never give you anything again that will be half so full of sunshine as this wee lock of hair, but I wish no hue more sombre might ever fall to you. . . . Dear Emily [Ford], this is all—it will serve to make you remember me when locks are crisp and gray."[63] Dickinson, writing in the 1840s, reflected the sentimentality of her time period. Hair was fundamentally emotional, able to impart one's desires to the recipient, and to preserve that emotional state through time. For the children in Lee's 1901 story, hair was still something to be momentarily treasured, but then forgotten. Their mother had no hand in preserving their hair and, in the end, the tufts of hair were scattered as their other toys were.

In 1901, Amelia Gere Mason asked in an article, "Is Sentiment Declining?" It was, she concluded, for "there is no sentiment in business, and business is a controlling factor in the world of to-day. In nothing does sentiment contribute to visible success."[64] In 1902, a newspaper article observed that hair jewelry was "founded upon fashion. It has survived upon sentiment."[65] Thus, hairwork's decline in popularity was well under way. Fashion and sentiment are shallow words for the emotional resonance that hair jewelry held from the 1770s to the early 1900s in American culture. Sentiment, as emotion that was not primary but reiterated and relived, was always wedded to fashion, with its concern for the superficial. But for most nineteenth-century middle-class Americans, hairwork was far more than merely sentimental fashion. It was their life encapsulated within the neat borders of a frame holding a wreath or a chain of hair attached to a metal clasp. The hair of their mothers, fathers, brothers, sisters, children, and dearest friends was woven into an object of sentiment, of fashion, and of emotion. The laborious production of hairwork, where every strand was literally produced by someone's body and then every strand was carefully woven with the others to form a singular object, represented the very difficult work of the living itself. And what endured, even after hairwork fell out of favor and was criticized for its overly effusive appearance and its supposedly affected meaning, was that life itself had been lived. Hairwork satisfied what its owners hoped it would—the physical body and the ephemeral emotions of an individual were given continuing life.

Epilogue

Hairwork ceased to be available as a commercial product in 1925, when jewelry companies no longer offered hair-jewelry repair or work. Hair wreath making also largely ended at this point, although the craft of making hair flowers did not. And certainly, the practice of saving hair has never died. Many families today are taken aback as elderly female family members die, and they find a long hank of hair tied with a tag attached, often reading "my own hair, bobbed, 1923." Their great (or even great-great aunt), having died in her nineties, had as a young woman saved her hair, whether to have a source of hair for artificial hairpieces or as a memorial to her youth. But with hair jewelry so out of favor and unlikely to become fashionable again, and with no professionals making it anymore, most of the long hanks were either thrown away or carefully saved and never used.

Hairwork has not been acknowledged as a valuable artifact of the past or as an important part of America's cultural heritage, partly because the feminine associations of hairwork—the very connotations that lent it such prominence in the nineteenth century—made hairwork easy to ignore. Hairwork represented individual stories of everyday people, and that narrow focus did not position hairwork as historically important either. In addition, hairwork, divorced from its context of nineteenth-century sentiment and personal associations, seemed creepy and morbid, and thus hard for those who were not part of that culture to understand.

Hairwork was never actually forgotten, although certainly it was very soon overlooked or misunderstood. As early as 1924, writers reflected on the "bygone" craft of human hairwork. Josephine Fitch, writing in *Antiques* magazine that year, marveled that "the thought of having the tresses of a deceased relative decoratively dangling at one's ear made stronger appeal to the sentimental notions of the past century than to the sanitary code of the present."[1] That same year, hair watch chains were offered for the final time by a national jewelry wholesaler. Six years later, John Hill Morgan wrote in *Antiques* about how mourning miniatures, including hairwork, "were only one indication, among many other symptoms, of the false standards and mock sentimentality of an age."[2] Morgan focused on eighteenth-century miniatures, but he referred to his own nineteenth-century example of a braided watch chain. He argued that the "fashion seems to have gone out with the mourning brooches of our grandmothers."[3] In her 1931 compendium of American handicrafts, Ella Shannon Bowles wrote of "hair-wreaths, mementoes both of the living and the dead! Ornamental hair-work, as it was designated, seems to have been one of the chief handicrafts of our grandmothers."[4] At least Bowles's interest in women's work leavened her condemnation of hairwork itself.

Antique collectors and amateur historians rarely mentioned hairwork either as a collectible or as historical evidence. But beginning in the late 1950s, there was a revived interest in the craft and the artifacts. In 1959, Ila A. Wright was interviewed about her life in Idaho as a Mormon woman, and she discussed at great length hairwork, both jewelry and wreaths, and how to make it. She described weaving the tubular chain around a shoelace that was left inside the finished tube, and then the process of having it mounted by a jeweler. She concluded by remarking that "it had great sentimental value because usually the wife's hair was used to make the husband's watch chain." In addition, hair watch chains had a special position in Mormon culture, according to Ila, since "young girls had hair watch chains made from their own hair to send as presents to the fiancés when they were on missions for the Latter-Day Saints Church."[5]

In the 1960s and 1970s, most discussions of hairwork focused on its secondary role as memento mori, argued it was popular only in the 1850s and 1860s, and acknowledged its commercial as well as handicraft origins.[6] Lillian Baker Carlisle's 1972 essay begins, "In the 1850s and 1860s, hair jewelry was the darling of fashion." Using *Godey's Lady's Magazine* as her source, Carlisle discussed how women could mail order jewelry from the magazine or use its 1859 instructions to make the jewelry at home.[7] In an essay in the collector's magazine, *The Antiques Journal* in 1971, Carlisle predicted the imminent revival of many nineteenth-century crafts, but she doubted hairwork would be one of those. After all, she pointed out, "It would not now be possible to acquire the long hair necessary to make up one of these wreaths. If you are among the fortunate owning a hair wreath, guard it well," she advised.[8]

Perhaps Carlisle was correct. In 1975, the Stellers, jewelry store owners in Wisconsin, issued a pamphlet of hairwork jewelry they could make for customers. "A most personal gift from your own hair," they promised customers. The styles offered were relatively simple and, while some were modeled on those popular in the nineteenth century, such as flat woven bracelets ("for him or her"), the family also introduced more contemporary styles, such as watch bands and a bracelet described as "small & smart." Prices started as $39.95 to a complete watch set in 14-carat gold for $195.00.[9] It made sense, with the popularity of long hair on women, and a revived interest in crafts in general, that hairwork could be revived. But the Stellers do not appear to have been successful in their efforts.

It was the World Wide Web and the Internet that helped. In the early 1990s, as the Web allowed far greater access to the antiques and to entrepreneurial craftspeople, custom-made hairwork became, if not popular, at least available. There had always been devoted collectors of eighteenth- and nineteenth-century hairwork. Without their efforts, many surviving hairwork examples would have disappeared from the historical, artifactual record. Leila Cohoon is one of the most notable of these; Mrs. Cohoon not only collected hairwork throughout the 1960s, 1970s, 1980s, to the present, she started her own (and the world's only) Hair Museum in Independence, Missouri, to house and exhibit her large collection. Another collector, C. Jeanenne Bell, not only collected hair jewelry when it was unpopular as an antique, she has written a thorough and engaging encyclopedia of hairwork to encourage present and future collectors.[10] Other major collectors are Carmelita Johnson, Ruth Gordon, Leila Cohoon, and Anna Sparr. Prices for hairwork have steadily risen since the 1990s, and hairwork jewelry and wreaths now garner between $200.00 and $800.00 on eBay.com, one of the major purveyors of hairwork today.

For mid–twentieth-century collectors such as Bell and Cohoon and historians of nineteenth-century domestic life, the persistent mischaracterizations of hairwork are frustrating. A typical example of how hairwork was presented from the 1950s through the 1970s is found in a short story by Pauline C. Smith published in *Alfred Hitchcock's Mystery Magazine* in 1968. A young girl was lured to her death by a "mountain woman," Aunt Abbie, who has killed her for her red hair, perfect for her ongoing hair wreath project. The victim was terrified not by her impending death (of which she has no warning) but by the sight of the hair wreath itself. " 'You mean that's hair?' The girl clung to the arms of the chair because here was substance, here reality. 'Human hair? All of it?' " The "mountain woman" pointed out that she had only one flower left to complete the wreath: a rose. Drugging her victim, shearing her hair, and then tossing the body over a nearby gorge, Aunt Abbie is seen in her parlor by her niece, placidly completing the red hair rose of her wreath. Aunt Abbie, surrounded with the fruits of "her talent for keeping the record," finished her final stitch of hair.[11] Hairwork, severed from its context of sentimentality and of acceptable commercialism, was the stuff of horror stories. For the victim, the hair in the wreath was ephemeral and ghastly, whereas the chair's arm she grasps was "substance . . . reality." By the 1960s, hairwork had lost almost all its ability to metaphorically represent emotional relationships or act as a neutral material object, so overwhelming was its connotation of death and morbidity. In fact, hairwork makes its now-macabre appearance in mysteries and horror novels from the 1960s on, lending its air of antiquated creepiness to whatever plot turns the author created.[12]

In the 1850s, Harry Egy wrote in Emma Miller's hair album:

This lock of hair once did grow.
Upon a persons head you know,
But now is placed within this book
For those to see that may chance to look.

Think of this when this you see,
And bear in mind, Miss Emily,
Though oer my grave the grass grows green,
A friend to you I've always been.[13]

Harry and Emma understood the value of hairwork. Hair grew from the self, could be severed and cut short just as the body that originated it, and, yet, through that hair the self could continue long after the body's death. In fact, hair could be kept alive with an investment of sentiment and memory and act as a regenerative agent. Grass will grow and friendships will endure as long as one remembers to remember "when this you see."

In 2000, I sat in the reading room of the Virginia Historical Society, and carefully pulled a bulky letter from its envelope. I unfolded the paper and began to read. It was the words of Mrs. Mary Elizabeth (Wise) Garnett, writing to her husband in 1867. Their rambunctious three-year-old daughter, Annie, had cut off a large piece of her golden blond hair. Mrs. Garnett attached the hair to a card, and inscribed the card with Annie's comments about the proceedings.

"Look here Mama what I cut off"
"Oh Annie I am so sorry you cut your hair" "Mama is you going to sew it on"
"Mama is you going to put it in the paper to dream"

And, with that, Mrs. Garnett dated the card and sent it to her husband.[14]

Annie's mother succeeded in doing what so many wished to accomplish: she transfixed a moment in time. Annie's hair, cut from her head, attached to a card, accompanied with Annie's own words, was "in the paper to dream." It was Annie saved there, but it was also her mother's experience, her father's experience; it was their life together that was preserved. The hair, real, tactile, true, embodied the moment in time. But as Annie understood, even at age three, something had been done to her hair—her hair had been transformed from a part of herself to something that now would "dream." And, oddly enough, it did. One hundred and forty years later, Annie's hair tells its own story—a story about Annie but also about her generation, her race, her social position, and the ways her culture understood and translated the deepest and most intimate experiences of individual lives.

When nineteenth-century Americans said to one another, "when this lock of hair you do see, think of me," they were addressing the dynamic, transformative aspects of their sentimental culture. Hairwork was a practice of white, middle-class Americans that attempted to marry stability to class and race identities, wed sentiment to commerce, and unite sincerity and action. While all these unions were constantly subject to degradation and dissolution, the middle-class Americans that created, owned, and were memorialized in hairwork succeeded in one goal: they did indeed render themselves and their loved ones into lasting, evocative monuments of self. "When this lock of hair you do see," we can indeed do little else but "think of me," for what we see is what they were—individuals transformed through the market, through sentimentalism, and through the act of making the nontangible physical.

Notes

Prologue

1. There are many contemporary artists who explore the discomfort of audiences regarding human hair; I will not be listing contemporary artists working with hair. *Frontiers: A Journal of Women's Studies* 17, no. 2 (1996) published a special issue that provides a useful overview of the uses of hair in memory, art, narrative, and identity. See also Alison Ferris, *Hair*, exhibition catalogue, John Michael Kohler Arts Center, Sheboygan, Wisc. December 6, 1992–February 14, 1993 (Sheboygan, Wis.: John Michael Kohler Arts Center, 1992).

2. Emma Egy Miller album, ca. 1860s. Watkins Community Museum, Lawrence, Kansas. The verse continues: "Emma may our friendship ever prove/ United both with truth and love./ Thus may we soar to realms on high/ Heaven born friendship never dies."

3. See Nancy Tomes, *The Gospel of Germs: Men, Women, and the Microbe in American Life* (Cambridge, Mass.: Harvard University Press, 1998), 165. See Mary Douglas, *Purity and Danger: An Analysis of Concepts of Pollution and Taboo* (New York: Praeger, 1966).

4. Studies about the relationship between debates over slavery and the development of the consumer market are Jane Tompkins, *Sensational Designs: The Culture Work of American Fiction, 1790–1860* (New York: Oxford University Press, 1985); Gillian Brown, *Domestic Individualism: Imagining Self in Nineteenth-Century America* (Berkeley: University of California Press, 1990); Shirley Samuels, ed., *The Culture of Sentiment: Race, Gender, and Sentimentality in Nineteenth-Century America* (New York: Oxford University Press, 1992); Lori Merish, *Sentimental Materialism: Gender, Commodity Culture, and Nineteenth-Century American Literature* (Durham, N.C.: Duke University Press, 2002). The literature on the relationship between the roles of women and consumerism is extensive. See especially Victoria de Grazia with Ellen Furlough, eds., *The Sex of Things: Gender and Consumption in Historical Perspective* (Berkeley: University of California Press, 1996); Wendy Gamber, *The Female Economy: The Millinery and Dressmaking Trades, 1860–1920* (Urbana: University of Illinois Press, 1997); Karen Halttunen, *Confidence Men and Painted Women: A Study of Middle-Class Culture in America, 1830–1870* (New Haven, Conn.: Yale University Press, 1982); Anne Rose, *Voices of the Marketplace: American Thought and Culture, 1830–1860* (New York: Twayne, 1995). For discussions of class identity and consumerism in the nineteenth century, see Elaine S. Abelson, *When Ladies Go A-Thieving: Middle-Class Shoplifters in the Victorian Department Store* (New York: Oxford University Press, 1992); Susan Porter Benson,

Counter Cultures: Saleswomen, Managers, and Customers in American Department Stores, 1890–1940 (Urbana: University of Illinois Press, 1988); Stuart Blumin, *The Emergence of the Middle Class: Social Experience in the American City, 1760–1900* (Cambridge: Cambridge University Press, 1989); Halttunen, *Confidence Men and Painted Women*; Catherine E. Kelly, *In the New England Fashion: Reshaping Women's Lives in the Nineteenth Century* (Ithaca, N.Y.: Cornell University Press, 1999);

5. The distinction between sensibility and sentimentality are outlined in the following: Mary Louise Kete, "Sentimental Literature," in *Oxford Encyclopedia of American Literature,* vol. 3, ed. Jay Parini (New York: Oxford University Press, 2004), 545–554; Alison Scott, "Sensibility," in *Encyclopedia of the Romantic Era, 1760–1850,* vol. 2, ed. Christopher John Murray (New York: Fitzroy Dearborn, 2004), 1039–1040; Janet Todd, *Sensibility: An Introduction* (London: Methuen, 1986); and Raymond Williams, "Sensibility," in *Keywords: A Vocabulary of Culture and Society* (London: Fontana/Croom Helm, 1976), 235–239.

6. Amelia Gere Mason, "Is Sentiment Declining?" *Century Illustrated Magazine* 61, no. 4 (YEAR), 627. See Mary Chapman and Glenn Hendler, eds., *Sentimental Men: Masculinity and the Politics of Affect in American Culture* (Berkeley: University of California Press, 1999) for essays examining the polarities, and consonances, between the masculine world of business and the feminized realm of sentiment.

7. Henry James, *Washington Square* (New York: Modern Library/Random House, 1997).

8. Lori Merish, "'The Hand of Refined Taste' in the Frontier Landscape: Caroline Kirkland's *A New Home, Who'll Follow?* and the Feminization of American Consumerism," *American Quarterly* 45, no. 4 (December 1993), 491; see also chapter 2, "Gender, Domesticity, and Consumption in the 1830s: Caroline Kirkland, Catharine Sedgwick, and the Feminization of American Consumerism," in Merish, *Sentimental Materialism,* 88–134.

9. The phrase "moral market culture" comes directly from Elizabeth White Nelson, *Market Sentiments: Middle-Class Market Culture in Nineteenth-Century America* (Washington, D.C.: Smithsonian Books, 2004), 9. The original sentence reads "Sentimentalism [is] a useful language for describing and defining the terms of a moral market culture." See also Amy Dru Stanley, "Home Life and the Morality of the Market," in *The Market Revolution in America: Social, Political, and Religious Expressions, 1800–1880,* ed. Melvyn Stokes and Stephen Conway (Charlottesville: University Press of Virginia, 1996), 74–98.

10. Nancy Dunlap Bercaw, "Solid Objects/Mutable Meanings: Fancywork and the Construction of Bourgeois Culture, 1840–1880," *Winterthur Portfolio* 26, no. 4 (Winter 1991), 233.

11. Nelson, *Market Sentiments,* 7.

12. For other studies focused on the relationship between production and consumption, see Ann Bermingham and John Brewer, *The Consumption of Culture, 1600–1800: Image, Object, Text* (London: Routledge, 1995); Regina Lee Blaszczyk, *Imagining Consumers: Design and Innovation from Wedgwood to Corning* (Baltimore: Johns Hopkins University Press, 2000; Colin Campbell, *The Romantic Ethic and the Spirit of Modern Consumerism* (Oxford: Basil Blackwell, 1987); Neil McKendrick,

John Brewer, and J. H. Plumb, *The Birth of Consumer Society: The Commercialization of Eighteenth-Century England* (Bloomington: Indiana University Press, 1982); Daniel Miller, *Material Culture and Mass Consumption* (London: Basil Blackwell, 1987); and Nelson, *Market Sentiments.*

13. Herbert G. Gutman, *The Black Family in Slavery and Freedom, 1750–1925* (New York: Pantheon Books, 1976), chapter 1, "Send Me Some of My Children's Hair," 3–44. See also Shane White and Graham White, "Slave Hair and African American Culture in the Eighteenth and Nineteenth Centuries," *Journal of Southern History* 61, no. 1 (February 1995), 45–76.

14. See Wendy Cooper, *Hair: Sex Society Symbolism* (New York: Stein and Day, 1971); Gananath Obeyeskere, *Medusa's Hair: An Essay on Personal Symbols and Religious Experience* (Chicago: University of Chicago Press, 1984); Anthony Synott, "Shame and Glory: A Sociology of Hair," *British Journal of Sociology* 38, no. 3 (September 1987), 381–413.

15. Laura Peers, "Strands Which Refuse to Be Braided: Hair Samples from Beatrice Blackwood's Ojibwe Collection at the Pitt Rivers Museum," *Journal of Material Culture* 8, no. 1 (2003), 75–96.

16. The literature on the cultural significance of hair in African American culture is exceptionally wide-ranging. For issues pertaining to this discussion, see Ayana D. Byrd and Lori L. Tharps, *Hair Story: Untangling the Roots of Black Hair in America* (New York: St. Martin's Press, 2001); Juliette Harris and Pamela Johnson, eds., *Tenderheaded: A Comb-Bending Collection of Hair Stories* (New York: Pocket Books, 2001).

17. Malcolm X, with the assistance of Alex Haley, *The Autobiography of Malcolm X* (New York: Grove Press, 1966).

Chapter 1. That Curious Art

1. Throughout this book, I use the term "professional" to designate hairwork that is the product of a person who was trained in hairwork and who created hairwork for payment of wages. In the eighteenth century, this would include persons advertising their willingness to do so. In the nineteenth century, these same types of individuals are included, as well as "piece workers," that is, those employed to make hairwork on contraact and who fulfilled mail orders. "Amateur" designates any persons making hairwork at home, for their own pleasure, and with no intention of selling their work. "Amateur" also includes those individuals who make hairwork within their own home, possibly but not necessarily for money, but for a "clientele" that was informal and not determined by a wage structure.

2. Locket-Mourning, number 81.0133, Winterthur Museum and Country Estate, Winterthur, Delaware. Donor, Mr. Roland E. Jester. Curatorial comments suggest the possibility of an English origin. Winterthur designates this as a mourning piece for a number of reasons, including the presence of the urn, a symbol of death, and the initials, date, and age of the deceased.

3. This is an educated guess. The examples of eighteenth-century hairwork

jewelry I have viewed all appear to be by "professionals." This designation denotes that these pieces were made to be bought and is not a qualitative judgment. Hair embroidery may very well have been created for sale as well, but, given that so many middle-class girls went to "ladies' schools" that taught fancy embroidery, it is likely these examples could be amateur creations.

4. David Jaffee's "The Age of Democratic Portraiture: Artisan-Entrepreneurs and the Rise of Consumer Goods," in *Meet Your Neighbors: New England Portraits, Painters, and Society, 1790–1850* (Sturbridge: Old Sturbridge Village and University of Massachusetts Press, 1992), 35–46, specifically addresses the role of artisan portraitists in this emergent consumer culture. Richard L. Bushman, "Shopping and Advertising in Colonial America," in *Of Consuming Interests: The Style of Life in the Eighteenth Century*, ed. Cary Carson, Ronald Hoffman, and Peter J. Albert (Charlottesville: U.S. Capitol Historical Society by University Press of Virginia, 1994), 235, notes that "shops went from being places for obtaining supplies to places for realizing aspirations . . . shops shaped the desires of consumers not for goods alone but for a new social identity."

T. H. Breen, "Narrative of Commercial Life: Consumption, Ideology, and Community on the Eve of the American Revolution," *William and Mary Quarterly*, 3rd ser., 50, no. 3 (July 1993): 471–501, argues that consumerist identity was central to the revolutionary ideology of colonial America and that support for the effort was fueled in part by the colonists' participation in a consumer market threatened by a punitive English Parliament. Other historians have argued that Breen's arguments conflate politics and commodities. See Jean-Christophe Agnew, "Coming Up for Air: Consumer Culture in Historical Perspective," in *Consumption and the World of Goods*, ed. John Brewer and Roy Porter (New York: Routledge, 1993), 19–39.

5. Charles Olton, *Artisans for Independence: Philadelphia Mechanics and the American Revolution* (Syracuse, N.Y.: Syracuse University Press, 1975), 4, categorizes miniaturist, hair worker, and artist under "Fine Arts Crafts" within artisan trades. A notable exception to this statement is Samuel Folwell, whose career will be discussed later in this chapter.

6. James Askew, advertisement, *Charleston Evening Gazette*, no. 75 (October 5, 1785), Decorative Arts and Photograph Collection, Winterthur Museum and Country Estate Library (hereafter referred to as Prime File). Hamilton Stevenson, advertisement, *Royal South Carolina Gazette* (Charleston), no. 141 (June 6, 1782), Prime File. I retain the punctuation in the original advertisements throughout this discussion. I am uncertain what Askew means by "railed" hairwork. Palette work, that is, hair worked into elaborate designs glued on a backing of ivory, did not use a "rail." Given Askew's time period, this kind of flat glued work is most likely what he is referring to, as it was the dominant hairwork style. Francis Rabineau, advertisement, *Wood's Newark Gazette and New-Jersey Advertiser*, no. 256 (April 6, 1796), Prime File.

7. Jeremiah Andrews, advertisement, *Maryland Journal* (Baltimore), page 1, col. 2 (April 13, 1779), Prime File. For a similar listing, see Jeremiah Boone, Dickenson and Robbson, advertisement, *Federal Gazette* (Philadelphia), no. 2294 (March 1, 1796), Prime File; Daniel Carrell, advertisement, *South Carolina Gazette* (Decem-

ber 18, 1794), Prime File; Claudius Chat, advertisement, *Pennsylvania Packet (Dunlac's and Claypoole's American Daily Advertiser)*, no. 5124 (September 12, 1795), Prime File; William Dawson, advertisement, *Pennsylvania Packet (Dunlac's American Daily Advertiser)*, no. 4447 (April 28, 1798), Prime File.

8. M. Sauvage, advertisement, *Charleston City Gazette and Advertiser*, no. 3765 (September 6, 1799), Prime File. I am assuming that Sauvage offered only hairwork and not the jewelry mountings.

9. Edward Greene Malbone, advertisement, *Columbian Centinel* (Boston), no. 2021 (June 29, 1796), Prime File.

10. Edward Greene Malbone, account book and register of portraits, 1794–1807. Collection no. 331, Downs Collection of Manuscripts and Ephemera, Winterthur Museum and Country Estate Library (hereafter, Downs Manuscript Collection).

11. Hamilton Stevenson, advertisement, *Royal South Carolina Gazette*, no. 141 (June 6, 1782), Prime File.

12. Richard L. Bushman, in his essay, "Shopping and Advertising in Colonial America," notes that in the eighteenth century, specialty shops proliferated—especially those of luxury goods (237). See also Karin Calvert, "The Function of Fashion in Eighteenth-Century America," in Carson et al., *Of Consuming Interests*, 252–283. See Dale T. Johnson, *American Portrait Miniatures in the Manney Collection* (New York: Metropolitan Museum of Art, 1991); Susan Strickler, *American Portrait Miniatures: The Worcester Art Museum Collection* (Worcester, Mass.: Worcester Art Museum, 1989); Anne Hollingsworth Wharton, *Heirlooms in Miniature* (Philadelphia, Pa.: J. B. Lippincott Company, 1898), for detailed information on the mechanics of painting miniatures. Robin Jaffee Frank, *Love and Loss: American Portrait and Mourning Miniatures* (New Haven, Conn.: Yale University Press and Yale University Art Gallery, 2000), is a thorough study of the art and the cultural meaning of miniatures.

Edward Norgate, *Miniatura or the Art of Limning*, edited, introduced, and annotated by Jeffrey M. Muller and Jim Murrell (New Haven, Conn.: Yale University Press, 1997), is a seventeenth-century guidebook. Charles William Day, *The Art of Miniature Painting* (London: Winsor and Newton, 1905), is a later guide.

Bruce Laurie, "'Spavined Ministers, Lying Toothpullers, and Buggering Priests': Third-Partyism and the Search for Security in the Antebellum North," in *American Artisans: Crafting Social Identity, 1750–1850*, ed. Howard B. Rock, Paul A. Gilje, and Robert Asker (Baltimore: Johns Hopkins University Press, 1995), 100.

13. John B. Dumoutet, advertisement, *Aurora*, no. 2786 (February 28, 1800), and no. 2779 (February 19, 1800), Prime File. William Coleman, advertisement. *The Maryland Gazette: or the Baltimore General Advertiser*, page 3, col. 3 (June 6, 1783), Prime File. A catalog of designs, probably similar to the "patterns" Coleman and other contemporaries offered, is in the Winterthur Museum and Country Estate Library, Rare Books and Periodicals Collection. See TT880A343, Rare Book Room, "Album of Hair Designs for Hair Jewelry," no author, no date [circa 1800]. All the designs are for palette-worked devices. Davida Tenenbaum Deutsch, "Jewelry for Mourning, Love, and Fancy, 1770–1830," *Antiques* 51 (April 1999), 566–575, suggests this album is English (Pl. X, caption).

Cooke and Company, advertisement, *Maryland Gazette: or the Baltimore General Advertiser*, page 1, col. 2 (September 10, 1784), Prime File.

According to Bruce Laurie's useful definition in *Working People of Philadelphia, 1800–1850* (Philadelphia, Pa.: Temple University Press, 1980), the term *manufactory* "identifies plants with more than twenty-five workers (employed either outside or inside the premises) but without power sources. Or, phrased another way, manufactories are nonmechanized factories" (20). Laurie is defining early nineteenth-century industry. I do not know if Cooke and Company's business actually encompassed twenty-five workers, but it is very likely they had no form of mechanical power, nor would they until the mid-to-late-nineteenth century. See Jonathan Prude, "Capitalism, Industrialization, and the Factory in Post-Revolutionary America," *Journal of the Early Republic* 16:2 (Summer 1996), 237–255, for another discussion of the emergence of the factory from the artisan shops.

Daniel Carrell, advertisement, *South Carolina Gazette* (Charleston), (December 18, 1794), Prime File.

14. John Walters, advertisement, *Pennsylvania Packet* (Philadelphia) (July 20, 1784), Prime File. M. Sauvage, advertisement, *Charleston City Gazette and Advertiser*, no. 3765 (September 6, 1799), Prime File. Joseph Cooke, advertisement, *Pennsylvania Packet* (Philadelphia), no. 5087 (July 31, 1795), Prime File.

15. Raphaelle Peale, advertisement, *Pennsylvania Packet* (Philadelphia), no. 7479 (December 8, 1800), Prime File.

16. Edward Greene Malbone, account book and register of paintings, 1794–1807. Entries, November 11, 1801, and December 10, 1801. Downs Manuscript Collection. See Jennifer J. Hammond, "The William Dunkling [*sic*] Mourning Pendant: Reflection of Early 19th-Century America," October 10, 1995, Winterthur Museum and Country Estate, unpublished paper, for additional information on the pricing structure and miniature art production.

17. Daniel Carrell, advertisement, *South Carolina Gazette* (December 18, 1794), Prime File.

18. Peter Leret, advertisement, *Maryland Gazette, or, The Baltimore Advertiser*, page 3, col. 3 (April 24, 1787), Prime File.

19. Samuel Folwell, advertisement, *Pennsylvania Packet* (Philadelphia), no. 3987 (November 7, 1791), Prime File, and *Pennsylvania Packet* (Philadelphia), no. 4481 (April 8, 1792), Prime File. Cooke and Company, advertisement, *Maryland Gazette, or the Baltimore General Advertiser*, page 1, col. 2 (September 10, 1784), Prime File.

20. The *Oxford English Dictionary* provides definitions of the word *device* that vary from the "action of devising, contriving; the faculty of devising, inventive faculty"; that of "will, pleasure, inclination, fancy, desire"; to "an emblematic figure or design." See *Oxford English Dictionary* (Oxford: Clarendon Press, 1933).

21. Rivington & Brown, advertisement, *Maryland Gazette, or The Baltimore General Advertiser*, page 2, col. 3 (August 5, 1761), Prime File. Philip Tidyman, advertisement, *South Carolina Gazette* (Charleston), no. 1935 (January 21, 1772), Prime File. John Miot, advertisement, *South Carolina and American General Gazette* (Charleston), no. 836 (September 16, 1774), Prime File. G. Smithson, advertisement. *South Carolina Gazette* (Charleston), no. 2036 (April 3, 1775), Prime File. James

Askew, advertisement, *Charleston Evening Gazette*, no. 75 (October 5, 1795), Prime File.

22. Hamilton Stevenson, advertisement, *Royal South Carolina Gazette* (Charleston), no. 141 (June 6, 1782), Prime File. See also George Aiken, advertisement, *Maryland Gazette, (or the Baltimore Advertiser)*, page 3, col. 3 (March 2, 1787), Prime File. Francis Rabineau, advertisement, *Woods Newark Gazette and New-Jersey Advertiser*, no. 256 (April 6, 1796), Prime File. Desaignes, advertisement, *General Advertiser* (Philadelphia), no. 394 (January 3, 1792), Prime File. Desaignes, it should be noted, listed himself only as a miniature painter of artist, not as a hair worker. Josiah Flagg, advertisement, *Maryland Journal and Baltimore Advertiser*, page 3, col. 1 (August 31, 1784), Prime File. Joseph Cooke, advertisement, *Pennsylvania Packet* (Philadelphia), no. 5087 (July 31, 1795), Prime File. M. Sauvage, advertisement, *Charleston City Gazette and Advertiser*, no. 3765 (September 6, 1799), Prime File. John Walters, advertisement, *Pennsylvania Packet* (Philadelphia), (July 20, 1784), Prime File.

23. Brooks and Warrock, advertisement, *Norfolk Herald*, no. 117, Vol. 2 (May 26, 1796), Prime File.

24. Samuel Folwell, advertisement, *Pennsylvania Packet* (Philadelphia), no. 2293 (June 10, 1786), Prime File. Betty Ring, *Girlhood Embroidery: American Samplers and Pictorial Needlework, 1650–1850* (New York: Alfred A. Knopf, 1993), 378–387, provides a detailed account of Folwell's career. Davida Tenenbaum Deutsch provides two detailed essays regarding Samuel Folwell. See "Samuel Folwell of Philadelphia: An Artist for the Needlework," *Antiques* 119 (February 1981), 420–423, and "Collector's Notes," *Antiques* 128 (September 1985).

25. Samuel Folwell, advertisement, *Pennsylvania Packet* (Philadelphia), no. 2852 (March 26, 1788), Prime File.

26. J[eremiah] Boone, J[oseph] Anthony, and J[oseph] Cooke, advertisement, *Pennsylvania Packet* (Philadelphia), no. 2855 (March 29, 1788), Prime File.

27. Samuel Folwell, advertisement, *Pennsylvania Packet* (Philadelphia), no. 2857 (April 1, 1788), Prime File.

28. Folwell is calling Cooke an uneducated fool who cannot recognize "art" when he sees it. The reference is the mythological figure of Midas, who was a fool himself. Midas was asked to judge a musical contest between Apollo and Pan. Pan played little ditties on his pipes, while Apollo played the music of the gods on his lyre. Unfortunately, Midas could not hear the music of the gods, and expressed his preference for Pan's lowly pipe music. At that, Apollo changed Midas's ears into those of an ass. See Edith Hamilton, *Mythology: Timeless Tales of Gods and Heroes*, 48th printing (New York: New American Library, 1969), 278–279.

29. Joseph Cooke, advertisement, *Pennsylvania Packet* (Philadelphia), no. 2859 (April 3, 1788), Prime File.

30. Laurie, "'Spavined Ministers, Lying Toothpullers, and Buggering Priests,'" asserts that the apprenticeship system survived longer depending on one's urban or rural location.

31. Daniel Carrell, advertisement, *South Carolina Gazette* (Charleston), (December 18, 1794), Prime File. Claudius Chat, advertisement, *Gazette of the United*

States, no. 578 (July 15, 1794), Prime File. Claudius Chat, advertisement, *Pennsylvania Packet* (Philadelphia). no. 5124 (September 12, 1795), Prime File.

32. See Bruce Laurie, *Artisans into Workers: Labor in Nineteenth-Century America* (New York: Hill and Wang, 1989), 36. For a full-length study of the apprenticeship system in American industry, see W. J. Rorabaugh, *The Craft Apprentice: From Franklin to the Machine Age in America* (New York: Oxford University Press, 1986). For a study of women's apprenticeship in a traditionally female-dominated craft industry, see Wendy Gamber, *The Female Economy: The Millinery and Dressmaking Trades, 1860–1930* (Urbana: University of Illinois Press, 1997).

33. Billy G. Smith, *The "Lower Sort": Philadelphia Laboring People, 1750–1800* (Ithaca, N.Y.: Cornell University Press, 1990), 67.

34. Cooke and Company, advertisement. *Maryland Gazette: or the Baltimore General Advertiser*, Page 1, Col. 2 (September 10, 1784), Prime File.

35. Stuart W. Bruchey, ed., *Small Business in American Life* (New York: Columbia University Press, 1980), 6.

36. J[eremiah] Boone, J[oseph] Anthony, and J[oseph] Cooke, advertisement, *Pennsylvania Packet* (Philadelphia), no. 2855 (March 29, 1788), Prime File.

37. Alfred F. Young, "Revolutionary Mechanics," in *Working for Democracy: American Workers from the Revolution to the Present*, ed. Paul Buhle and Alan Dawley (Urbana: University of Illinois Press, 1985), 9. Young does not provide a source for this characterization.

38. Samuel Folwell, advertisement, *Pennsylvania Packet* (Philadelphia), no. 2857 (April 1, 1788), Prime File.

39. See Steven Rosswurm, *Arms, Country, and Class: The Philadelphia Militia and "Lower Sort" during the American Revolution, 1775–1783* (New Brunswick, N.J.: Rutgers University Press, 1987); Ronald Schultz, "The Small-Producer Tradition and the Moral Origins of Artisan Radicalism in Philadelphia, 1720–1810," *Past and Present* 127 (May 1990), 84–116; Sean Wilentz, *Chants Democratic: New York City and the Rise of the American Working Class, 1788–1850* (New York: Oxford University Press, 1984).

40. Artisans were not simply overrun by change; they were complicit in encouraging changes in their professions. See Susan E. Hirsch, "From Artisan to Manufacturer: Industrialization and the Small Producer in Newark, 1830–1860," in Bruchey, ed., *Small Business in American Life*, 80–99, and see Paul A. Gilje, "The Rise of Capitalism in the Early Republic," 159–181, and Richard Stott, "Artisans and Capitalist Development," 257–271, both in *Journal of the Early American Republic* 16:2 (Summer 1996).

41. Samuel Folwell, *Charleston City Gazette and Advertiser*, no. 1779 (May 17, 1791), Prime File. Four minutes would have been extremely fast.

42. Ring, *Girlhood Embroidery*, 378.

43. Samuel Folwell, advertisement, *Pennsylvania Packet* (Philadelphia), no. 4481 (April 8, 1792), Prime File.

44. Diary (1834–1858), Jane Chancellor Payne. MSS51P2934:1. Virginia Historical Society, Richmond, Virginia.

45. Raphaelle Peale, advertisement, *Pennsylvania Packet* (Philadelphia), no. 7479 (December 3, 1800), Prime File.

46. Strickler, *American Portrait Miniatures,* gives a thorough account of the construction of the miniature cases. See also Carol Aiken, "The Emergence of the Portrait Miniature in New England," in *Painting and Portrait Making in the American Northeast,* ed. Peter Benes (Dublin Seminar for New England Folklife Annual Proceedings 1994), (Boston: Boston University, 1995), 30–45; Robin Bolton-Smith, *Portrait Miniatures in the National Museum of American Art* (Chicago: University of Chicago Press, 1984); Wharton, *Heirlooms in Miniature*; Johnson, *American Portrait Miniatures in the Manney Collection*; Arthur Mayne, *British Profile Miniaturists* (Boston: Boston Book and Art, 1970); R. W. Norton Art Gallery, *Portrait Miniatures in Early American History, 1750–1840,* April 18–June 13, 1976, exhibition, Shreveport, La); Desmond Shawe-Taylor, *The Georgians: Eighteenth-Century Portraiture and Society* (London: Barrie and Jenkins, 1990).

47. Bolton-Smith, *Portrait Miniatures in the National Museum of American Art,* 1.

48. Jean H. Baker, *Mary Todd Lincoln: A Biography* (New York: W. W. Norton and Company, 1987), note 1, letter from Robert Smith Todd to Elizabeth Humphreys, January 13, 1826, in the Illinois State Historical Society, Springfield, Illinois. Ellen K. Rothman, *Hands and Hearts: A History of Courtship in America* (New York: Basic Books, 1984), has commented on men's "almost ritualized incantations of sincerity" issued during courtship, as did Robert Todd (43).

49. Robert A. Sobieszek and Oddette M. Appel, *The Spirit of Fact: The Daguerreotypes of Southworth and Hawes, 1843–1862* (Boston: David R. Godine and the International Museum of Photography, 1976), xx.

50. T. H. Breen, "'The Meaning of Likeness': Portrait-Painting in an Eighteenth-Century Consumer Society," in *The Portrait in Eighteenth-Century America,* ed. Ellen G. Miles (Newark: University of Delaware, 1993), 39. Breen does not recognize sentimentality as one of those possible "cultural meanings," instead focusing on how details in eighteenth-century portraits, such as draperies and lace, revealed to the viewer the depicted individual's middle-class status. See also Margaretta M. Lovell, "Reading Eighteenth-Century American Family Portraits," *Winterthur Portfolio* 22, no. 4 (Winter 1987), 244–264.

51. Cooke and Company, advertisement, *Maryland Gazette: or the Baltimore General Advertiser,* (September 10, 1784), and Josiah Flagg, advertisement, *Maryland Journal and Baltimore Advertiser,* (August 31, 1784), Prime File. James Askew, advertisement, *Charleston Evening Gazette,* no. 75 (October 5, 1785), Prime File.

52. For discussion of the relationship between a developing consumer market and middle-class culture in the eighteenth-century, see Breen, "The Meaning of Likeness"; T. H. Breen, "'Baubles of Britain': The American and Consumer Revolutions of the Eighteenth Century," *Past and Present* 199 (1988): 73–104; Breen, "Narrative of Commercial Life"; Grant McCracken, *Culture and Consumption: New Approaches to the Symbolic Character of Consumer Goods and Activities* (Bloomington: Indiana University Press, 1990); Neil McKendrick, John Brewer, and J. H. Plumb, *The Birth of a Consumer Society: The Commercialization of Eighteenth-Century England* (Bloomington: Indiana University Press, 1982); and Victoria de Grazia with Ellen Furlough, eds., *The Sex of Things: Gender and Consumption in Historical Perspective* (Berkeley: University of California Press, 1996).

53. The cultural constructions of the idea of "fancy" are discussed in Sumter Turner Priddy, *Fancy: Acceptance of an Attitude, Emergence of a Style* (master's thesis, University of Delaware, 1981).

54. T. H. Breen, in "The Meaning of Likeness," notes that "Americans expected portrait painters to produce a 'likeness,'" but that was an "extremely elusive term" (48). The slipperiness of the term is because of the sometimes conflicting expectations, Breen argues, of proper interpretation of character as well as an immediately recognizable likeness.

55. Peter Leret, advertisement, *Maryland Gazette: or the Baltimore General Advertiser*, page 3, col. 3 (April 24, 1787). For similar phrasing, see also in the Prime File, advertisements for Cooke and Company (1784), William Donovan (1784), George Aiken (1787), Dan. Carrell (1792), and Samuel Folwell (1792). Oliphant and Henderson, advertisement, *South Carolina and American General Gazette*, no. 433 (February 27, 1767); Prime File, advertisement.

In addition, the hair could be finely chopped, mixed with glue, and applied to the ivory miniature, and then augmented with "couleurs," or paints. Thus, almost any desired design could be created.

56. For general histories of the practices of mourning in the eighteenth- and nineteenth-centuries, see John Morley, *Death, Heaven and the Victorians* (Philadelphia, Pa.: Temple University Press, 1980); Martha V. Pike and Janice Gray Armstrong, *A Time to Mourn: Expressions of Grief in Nineteenth Century America* (Stony Brook, N.Y.: Museums at Stony Brook, 1980); Anita Schorsch, *Mourning Becomes America: Mourning Art in the New Nation* (Philadelphia, Pa.: Main Street Press, 1976).

57. Mourning Locket, number 74.0166, Winterthur Museum and Country Estate. Dated 1807. See also Jennifer J. Hammond, "The William Dunkling [sic] Mourning Pendant: Reflection of Early 19th-Century America," Winterthur Museum and Country Estate, October 10, 1995, which examines mourning jewelry in particular.

58. Anita Schorsch, "A Key to the Kingdom: The Iconography of a Mourning Picture," *Winterthur Portfolio* 14, no. 1 (Spring 1979), 41–71, examines the imagic roots of the type of mourning scene we see on the Dunklin miniature. Schorsch focuses on the work of Samuel Folwell, who created paintings on silk, miniature and full-size portraits, and, as we have seen, hairwork.

59. Dated 1808 by Aldridge (or Oldridge), the Bell portrait was painted by an artist named either Eldridge or Oldridge in Virginia who was active in 1808. See pages 39–40, Abby Aldrich Rockefeller Folk Art Center, *American Folk Portraits: Paintings and Drawings from the Abby Aldrich Rockefeller Folk Art Center* (New York: Graphic Society, 1981). The issues related to the wearing of jewelry, especially the intimacy and expression of power it represents, will not be discussed here. See Marcia Pointon, "Intriguing Jewellery: Royal Bodies and Luxurious Consumption," *Textual Practice* 11, no. 3 (1997): 493–516, and "Valuing the Visual and Visualizing the Valuable: Jewellery and Its Ambiguities," *Cultural Values* 3, no. 1 (1999): 1–27.

60. Robin Jaffee Frank, *Love and Loss: American Portrait and Mourning miniatures* (New Haven, Conn.: Yale University Art Gallery, 2000), discusses the Sarah

Bell portrait, 31. The language of the caption of the image of Sarah Bell reflects Jaffee Smith's arguments.

61. Bolton-Smith, *Portrait Miniatures in the National Museum of American Art*, 9.

62. *Ladies' National Magazine* [becomes *Peterson's Magazine* in 1848] (November 1844), 179.

63. There are, of course, many working definitions of *fashion*. Valerie Steele, in *Fashion and Eroticism: Ideals of Feminine Beauty from the Victorian Era to the Jazz Age* (New York: Oxford University Press, 1985), defines fashion as "a distinct subcategory of dress . . . that is characterized by a sequence of relatively rapid changes in style. The expressions "in fashion" and "outmoded" indicate the association of fashion with a regular pattern of change" (8–9). Hairwork, and especially hair jewelry, was popular for over a hundred years, but the styles of jewelry changed rapidly, paralleling changes in clothing styles and more traditional forms of jewelry.

For an explicit discussion of the fashionable qualities of sentimentality, see Karen Halttunen, *Confidence Men and Painted Women: A Study of Middle-Class Culture in America, 1830–1870* (New Haven, Conn.: Yale University Press, 1982), esp. 80. To be regarded as unfashionable in nineteenth-century, middle-class culture could mean one was literally left out in the rain. In H. Hastings Weld's short story "The Mourning Ring," *Godey's Lady's Magazine* 26 (June 1843), 277–285, our heroine is left standing in the rain "ankle deep in mud and water? Why? She was not fashionable—not even in last year's fashion" 277.

64. Especially useful in this discussion is Karen Halttunen's chapter, "Sentimental Culture and the Problem of Fashion" (56–91), in *Confidence Men and Painted Women.*

65. Halttunen, *Confidence Men and Painted Women*, 65. Halttunen is not discussing hairwork here.

66. Mary's grandmother outlines exactly how a hair ring or another piece of hair jewelry might change hands. The grandmother complains, "It was such good oldfashioned gold that the jeweller gave you twelve for it . . . You might have had the hair saved—your own poor father's, and his father's—but there. It is swept into the street long before this, without they saved it to put into a new ring, for it was beautiful hair" (H. Hastings Weld, "The Mourning Ring," *Godey's Lady's Magazine* 26 [June 1843], 280). See Melanie Tebbutt, *Making Ends Meet: Pawnbroking and Working-Class Credit* (New York: St. Martin's Press, 1983), about the tradition of pawning.

67. (Mrs.) D. Ellen Goodman, "The Two Shreds of Hair," *Ladies' National Magazine* [became *Peterson's Magazine* January 1848] 14 (June 1848), 209–210.

68. Mrs. Alfred H. Reip, "The Hair Neck-Lace," *The Ladies' Companion and Literary Expositor: A Monthly Magazine Embracing Every Department of Literature* (October 1843): 284–291.

69. According to the rules of fiction, Lucy's fear was well-founded. In 1853, one magazine noted, "The question is sometimes asked, 'What will cure love?' We answer, scissors." "The Hair," *International Magazine of Literature, Art, and Science* 1, no. 4 (July 22, 1850), 103.

70. Todd Steven Gernes, "Recasting the Culture of Ephemera: Young Women's Literary Culture in Nineteenth-Century America" (Ph.D. diss., Brown University, 1987), chapter 2, 57–109, discusses at length the role of the autograph and friendship albums in nineteenth-century women's culture. Also, Anya Jabour, "Albums of Affection: Female Friendship and Coming of Age in Antebellum Virginia," *Virginia Magazine of History and Biography* 107, no. 2 (Spring 1999), 125–158, has a detailed analysis of albums and argues that many of these represent young women's coming of age. Tamara Plakins Thornton, in *Handwriting in America: A Cultural History* (New Haven, Conn.: Yale University Press, 1996), 114, discusses autograph albums. Thornton argues that, until the 1860s, album contributors did not even sign their full names (she bases this conclusion on a study of seventy-seven albums, dating 1820 to 1850, at the American Antiquarian Society, Worcester, Massachusetts).

71. This is not always true, of course. In 1862, Rachel Bowman recorded in her diary that she had started making a scrap album with her fiancé, Samuel. Diary entry, March 31, 1862, in Mohr, *The Cormany Diaries*, 163.

72. "Remember Me" (no author given). *The Souvenir*, Wednesday, July 18, 1827 (Philadelphia, Pa.), no pagination.

73. Mrs. Clarissa Packard, *Recollections of a Housekeeper* (New York: Harper and Brothers, 1834), F2.

74. "Remember Me," *Souvenir*, Wednesday, July 18, 1827, no pagination.

75. Mary Edes, Autograph Album, no. 649, dated 1828, Washington County Historical Society, Fort Calhoun, Nebraska. Donor, Mrs. Louise Stegner.

76. Edes, Autograph Album.

77. Accession no. 9506, Putney Housewife album, dated June 14, 1839 (inside cover). Waukesha County Museum and Historical Society, Waukesha, Wisconsin. The beginning line of this 1839 verse, "How dear to my heart are the scenes of my childhood," also begins James Whitcomb Riley's poem, "The Old-Fashioned Bible." See *The Complete Poetical Works of James Whitcomb Riley* (Bloomington: Indiana University Press, 1993), 229. Riley lived from 1844 to 1939. (Riley's poem was satirized by Samuel Woodworth in "The Old Oaken Bucket," and Woodworth's poem was satirized by an anonymous poet in "The Old Oaken Bucket (As Censored by the Board of Health)." This third version begins, "With what anguish of mind I remember my childhood." See Hazel Felleman, *The Best Loved Poems of the American People* (New York: Doubleday and Company, 1936), 385, 386. Riley's poem was something of a cultural phenomenon, spawning not only a parody but numerous affiliated products, including trade cards, giveaway chromolithographs, and store promotional brochures. The verse was popular among autograph album owners. See, for instance, Hattie Lyon's autograph album, Warshaw Collection, Box 1 Autograph Albums, Folder 1. Lyon's book opens with a glued image of a well and four lines from Riley's poem.

Chapter 2. An Article of Commerce

1. See Janet Todd, *Sensibility: An Introduction* (London: Methuen, 1986); and Mary Louise Kete, "Sentimental Literature," in *Oxford Encyclopedia of American*

Literature, ed. Jay Parini, vol. 3 (New York: Oxford University Press, 2004), 545–554. There is an extensive literature on nineteenth-century sentimentality. In terms of issue of self-control over the ideal middle-class body and emotions, there are histories of etiquette such as Karen Halttunen's *Confidence Men and Painted Women: A Study of Middle-Class Culture in America* (New Haven, Conn.: Yale University Press, 1982), and John Kasson's *Rudeness and Civility: Manners in Nineteenth-Century Urban America* (New York: Hill and Wang, 1990). For an emphasis on the issues of bodily control and self-control, see C. Dallett Hemphill, *Bowing to Necessities: A History of Manners in America, 1620–1860* (New York: Oxford University Press, 1999), and Tamara Plakins Thornton, *Handwriting in America: A Cultural History* (New Haven, Conn.: Yale University Press, 1996). The ideal of emotional self-control is described in Peter N. Stearns, *Battleground of Desire: The Struggle for Self-Control in Modern America* (New York: New York University Press, 1999).

2. Mark Campbell, advertisement in Isaac Guyer, *History of Chicago* (Chicago: Goodman and Cushing, 1862), 60.

3. "Fashions for November," *Peterson's Magazine* 24 (October 1853): 260. The set of open-weave globes described here are the popular "beads" which characterized one of the most common styles of hairwork jewelry in the mid-nineteenth century.

4. *Peterson's Magazine*, 24 (November, 1853): 260.

5. "Fashions for April," *Peterson's Magazine* 33 (April 1858): 328.

6. "Editor's Table," *Peterson's Magazine* 35 (June 1859): 462.

7. Mark Campbell, advertisement in Guyer, *History of Chicago*, 61.

8. See Philip Scranton, "Manufacturing Diversity: Production Systems, Markets, and an American Consumer Society, 1870–1930," *Technology and Culture* 35, no. 3 (July 1994): 476–505; "The Politics of Production: Technology, Markets, and the Two Cultures of American Industry," *Science in Context* 8, no. 2 (1995): 369–395; "Diversity in Diversity: Flexible Production and American Industrialization, 1880–1930," *Business History Review* 65 (Spring 1991): 27–90.

9. "Household Decorative Art: Working in Hair," Peter Cassell, *Cassell's Household Guide: Being a Complete Encyclopedia of Domestic and Social Economy, and Forming a Guide to Every Department of Practical Life* (London: Peter Cassell and Galpin, 1869–1871 [?]), 337.

10. "The Art of Ornamental Hair-Work," *Godey's Book and Magazine* 58 (February 1859): 121. The title of this journal varied throughout the nineteenth century, from *Godey's Magazine and Lady's Book* (July 1848–June 1854), *Godey's Lady's Book* (July 1854–December 1882, October 1892–August 1898), and *Godey's Book and Magazine* (January 1883–September 1892). The title in use at the time of the referenced publication will appear; the title *Godey's Lady's Magazine and Book* is used in the bibliography.

11. "Household Decorative Art: Working in Hair," *Cassell's Household Guide*, 337.

12. Mrs. C. S. Jones and Henry T. Williams, *Ladies' Fancy Work: Hints and Helps to Home Taste and Recreations* (New York: Henry T. Williams Publisher, 1876), 4. The language suggests a tablet made for the hair-working market; I have not located such a product listing in catalogues.

13. Gold-beaters' skin is, according to *Funk and Wagnalls Standard Dictionary, International Edition* (1970), "the outer coat of the cecum of the ox [that is, the intestinal cavity], prepared for the use of the gold beater." Gold-beating is to hammer gold flat. Gold leaf is paper-thin sheets of gold that can be applied by rubbing onto the surface of an object.

14. Henry T. Williams and Mrs. C. S. Jones, *Ladies' Fancy Work: Hints and Helps to Home Taste and Recreations* (New York: Henry T. Williams Publisher, 1876) 51; "Household Decorative Art—Working in Hair," *Cassell's Household Guide*, 337.

15. Ruel Pardee Tolman, "Human Hair as a Pigment," *Antiques* 8, no. 6 (December 1925) 353, and "A Document on Hair Painting," *Antiques* 17, no. 3 (March 1930), 231. Tolman concludes in "Human Hair as a Pigment" that it is correct to say that this technique is hair painting. He found that one could, using finely ground hair and glue, produce a paint that would adhere to an ivory or a glass backing. He concludes such a technique was "attributable solely to its capabilities of appeal to a somewhat lachrymose sentiment . . . . The American public has, indeed, always cherished a fondness for sweets made syrupy with tears" (353).

16. National Artistic Hair Work Company, *Catalogue of Designs for Artistic Hair Scenery and Ornaments Executed by National Artistic Hair Works of Chicago* (Chicago: National Artistic Hair Work Company, 1886). The researcher is Tolman, "Human Hair as a Pigment."

17. Alexanna Speight, *The Lock of Hair, Its History, Ancient and Modern, Natural and Artistic, with the Art of Working in Hair* (London: A. Goubaud, 1872), no pagination.

18. "The Art of Ornamental Hair-Work," 121.

19. "The Art of Ornamental Hair-Work," 121.

20. Mark Campbell, *Self-Instructor in the Art of Hair Work, Dressing Hair, Making Curls, Switches, Braids, and Hair Jewelry of Every Description* (New York: M. Campbell, 1875), 30.

21. "Weaving or Plaiting Hair Ornaments—No. 1," *Peterson's Magazine* 38 (September 1860): 224.

22. "The Art of Ornamental Hair-Work," 219, recommended the bath. "Weaving or Plaiting Hair Ornaments—No. III," *Peterson's Magazine* 38 (November 1860): 395–396, is an example of the open-work braid. See Campbell, *Self-Instructor in the Art of Hair Work, Dressing Hair, Making Curls, Switches, Braids, and Hair Jewelry of Every Description* (New York: Mark Campbell, 1875), for examples of "plain open braid," and "open fine braid" (110, 111).

23. Receipt, January 22, 1859, C. Linherr, Artist in Hair, and Jeweller, New York, to Miss Colgate. Hair, Box 2; Folder, Lewinson, L., Warshaw Collection. There are two separate Linherrs. See trade cards, T. A. Linherr, Artist in Hair Jewelry, New York. Hair, box 2; Folder, Lewinson. C. Jeanenne Bell notes in her *Collector's Encyclopedia of Hairwork Jewelry: Identifications and Values* (Paducah, Ky.: Collector Books, 1998), that in 1853 at the Crystal Palace exhibition in New York a "Limherr and Company" displayed a tea set (23). In fact, C. Linherr exhibited "hair bracelets, breast-pins, rings and watch-chains" at the 1853 New York Exhibition (see *Official Catalogue of the New York Exhibition of the Industry of All Nations* [New York: G. P. Putnam, 1853], 79).

24. Madame K. Schmitt, advertisement. Hair, Box 2; Folder, Sanderson, Charles, Warshaw Collection.

25. Trade card, Robert Link, "Hair Braiding Establishment." Hair, Box 2; Folder, Logan, Mrs. M., Warshaw Collection.

26. Vincent Brandly, advertisement, *Le Bon Ton* (New York), June 1857, p. 111.

27. Samuel Parrott, Receipt Book, 1860–1869. Document 248, Downs Manuscript Collection. See records from July 28, 1863; October 6, 1863; February 2, 1864; March 19, 1864; April 2, 1864; April 4, 1867; and August 6, 1867.

28. *Godey's* was begun in 1830 by Louis A. Godey as *The Lady's Book* and the title varied after that. The magazine is accepted as one of the most influential women's periodicals of the 1830s to 1870s. Ros Margaret Ballaster, Elizabeth Frazer, and Sandra Hebron, *Women's Worlds: Ideology, Femininity, and the Woman's Magazine* (New York: MacMillan, 1991), view women's periodicals in the eighteenth and nineteenth centuries as the site of struggles over the meaning of femininity. Karen Halttunen, *Confidence Men and Painted Women in America, 1830–1870* (New Haven: Yale University Press, 1982), *A Study of Middle-Class Culture in America, 1830–1870* (New Haven: Yale University Press, 1982), argues *Godey's* promulgated 1830s–1850s sentimental culture and was the leader in attacking "fashion" as hypocritical at the same time that it presented fashion as desirable (see 65–68 especially). Isabelle Lehuu, "Sentimental Figures: Reading *Godey's Lady's Book* in Antebellum America," in *The Culture of Sentiment: Race, Gender, and Sentimentality in Nineteenth-Century America*, ed. Shirley Samuels (New York: Oxford University Press, 1992), 73–91, views *Godey's* as central in the construction of a feminine ideal; see also chapter 5, "The 'Lady's Book' and the Female Vernacular in Print Culture," in her book, *Carnival on the Page: Popular Print Media in Antebellum America* (Chapel Hill: University of North Carolina Press, 2000). Barbara Welter, "The Cult of True Womanhood," in *Dimity Convictions: The American Woman in the Nineteenth Century* (Athens: Ohio University Press, 1976), uses *Godey's* to explore the ideology of the "true woman." Other historians, notably Nelson, have taken issue with Welter's use of the magazine. Elizabeth White Nelson, *Market Sentiments: Middle-Class Market Culture in Nineteenth-Century America* (Washington, D.C.: Smithsonian Books, 2004), views *Godey's* marketing strategy as dependent on the production of a sentimental ethos (see chapter 5, "The 'Lady's Book' and the Female Vernacular in Print Culture," 102–125). Gail Caskey Winkler, "Influence of *Godey's Lady's Book* on the American Woman and Her Home: Contributions to a National Culture (1830–1877)," (Ph.D. diss., University of Wisconsin—Madison, 1988), examines the actual influence of the magazine on women's decorating activities.

Despite this lengthy entry, there is, unfortunately, no cultural history, full-length study, or even in-depth analysis of *Godey's Lady's Book and Magazine*. Finally, Bertha Stearns, "Philadelphia Magazines for Ladies: 1830–1860," *Pennsylvania Magazine of History and Biography* 69 (July 1945), 207–219, reminds historians that *Godey's* had predecessors and challengers, namely in the form of regional and local periodicals. See also Cynthia L. White, *Women's Magazines, 1693–1968* (London: Michael Joseph, 1970).

29. "The Art of Ornamental Hair-Work," *Godey's Lady's Book* 41 (December 1850): 377.

30. Marion Edmonds Roe, "How to Dress Well on a Small Allowance," in *How Six Girls Made Money: Occupations for Women* (Mount Morris, Ill.: Brethren's Publishing Company, 1887), 87.

31. *Godey's* and other mail-order retailers depended on the postal system to conduct their business. In 1863, letter rates were as low as three cents per half-ounce, and by 1869 the Transcontinental Railroad provided seven-day mail service. The Rural Free Delivery was not in place until 1896, and therefore played no role in the mail-order business of hairwork until that decade.

32. "Description of Fashion-Plate for July," *Godey's Lady's Book* 49 (July 1854): 93.

33. "Philadelphia Agency," *Godey's Book and Magazine* 49 (November 1854): 470.

34. "Philadelphia Agency," *Godey's Book and Magazine* 54 (April 1857): 380.

35. "Philadelphia Agency," *Godey's Book and Magazine* 55 (October 1857): 380.

36. "Notices," *Godey's Book and Magazine*, 64 (February 1862): 204. The title advertised is Madame Levina B. Urbino, Professor Henry Day et al. *Art Recreations: Being a Complete Guide to Pencil Drawing, Oil Painting . . . Wax Work, Shell Work* (Boston: J. E. Tilton and Company, 1869). "A List of Articles We Can Supply," *Godey's Book and Magazine* 65 (October 1862): 411, mentions Matilda Marian Pullan's *The Lady's Manual of Fancy-Work: A Complete Instructor in Every Variety of Ornamental Needle-Work* (New York: Dick & Fitzgerald, 1859), 298.

37. "Philadelphia Agency," *Godey's Book and Magazine* 56 (February 1858): 212.

38. "Hair-Manufactures," *English Cyclopaedia*, ed. Charles King (London: Bradbury and Evans, 1860), 607–608.

39. Virginia Penny, *How Women Can Make Money* (Springfield, Mass.: D. E. Fisk and Company, 1870, 281; reprint, New York: Arno and the New York Times, 1971).

40. Louisa May Alcott, *Little Women* (1868; New York: Puffin Books, 1952), chapter 15, "A Telegram," 205–216. The 1952 edition has an evocative illustration of the shearing, with Jo depicted as a surly and determined young woman with hair cascading down to her shoulders (illustration by Shirley Hughes, p. 213).

41. Mrs. S. W. Holbrook, advertisement, *Fitchburg (Massachusetts) Sentinel*, Saturday, March 9, 1872.

42. Penny, *How Women Can Make Money*, 281.

43. Francis J. Bailey, trade cards (2). Hair, Box 1; Folder, Babcock, Dr. Geo. W. Warshaw Collection.

44. "The Trade in Locks," *Every Saturday* 8, no. 184 (July 10, 1869): 40–44. See also the same story, *London Society* 15 (May 1869): 547–552.

45. Thomas Gardner, advertisement (no date). Hair, Box 1; Folder, Gammon, D.S. Warshaw Collection.

46. Thomas Gardner, advertisement (no date). Hair, Box 1; Folder, Gammon, D.S. Warshaw Collection.

47. Halttunen, *Confidence Men and Painted Women*, 179.

48. Daniel Miller, "A Theory of Christmas," in *Unwrapping Christmas*, ed. Daniel Miller (Oxford: Clarendon Press, 1993), 17, argues that mass consumption

increasingly relied on "the negation of the abstract nature of the commodity through rituals of appropriation," such as gift giving. See also James G. Carrier, "Alienating Objects: The Emergence of Alienation in Retail Trade," *Man: The Journal of the Royal Anthropological Institute* 29, no. 2 (June 1994): 359–380.

49. Russell Belk, "The Perfect Gift," in *Gift Giving: A Research Anthology*, ed. Cele Otnes and Richard F. Beltramini (Bowling Green, Ohio: Bowling Green State University Popular Press, 1992), 59. The term "bad commodities" is used by James Carrier, *Gifts and Commodities: Exchange and Western Capitalism since 1700* (London: Routledge Press, 1995), 13–43.

50. James Carrier has not ignored the productionist arguments (that to make something makes that object a gift), but he is more concerned with the transactional elements. See Carrier, *Gifts and Commodities*, and Carrier, "Alienating Objects." For a discussion of how advertising can affect the transactions of commodities as gifts, see James Carrier, "The Symbolism of Possession in Commodity Advertising," *Man: The Journal of the Royal Anthropological Institute* 25, no. 4 (December 1990): 693–706.

51. William Waits, *The Modern Christmas in America: A Cultural History of Gift Giving* (New York: New York University Press, 1993), 16 and 19. See also Penne L. Restad, *Christmas in America* (New York: Oxford University Press, 1995), 129, where Restad relies on Waits's argument.

52. Waits, *The Modern Christmas in America*, 20–21.

53. I can find no demographic or statistical study that supports this claim. Restad notes that in one study, a store manager observed that "people are making smaller presents to more persons. . . . Where a man would come in years ago and say, 'Give me twenty-five yards of $4 silk,' and sent it to his favorite maiden aunt for a present, he'll buy twenty $5 presents for all his sisters and cousins as well as his aunts." Restad, *Christmas in America,* note 5, 200, citing Phillip Synder, *December 25th, The Joys of Christmas Past* (New York: Dodd, Mead, 1985), 79.

54. Alice B. Neal, "Gift-Making," *Godey's Book and Magazine* 55 (November 1857): 421–427. All further references to this story will not be cited in the text.

55. The reference to the village blacksmith is an allusion to Henry Wadsworth Longfellow's popular parlor poem, "The Village Blacksmith," in *Ballads and Other Poems* (Cambridge: John Owen, 1842).

56. Susan Porter Benson, *Counter Cultures: Saleswomen, Managers, and Customers in American Department Stores, 1890–1940* (Urbana: University of Illinois Press, 1988), discusses male-manager–female-customer relations later in the century, in chapter 3, "'An Adamless Eden': Managing Department-Store Customers," 75–123. She notes that often "the male managers treated the female customers with a contemptuous indulgence that spoke both of paternalism and of the sexual conflict" inherent in a world of shopping built around anticipating female desires (94).

57. "The Framing and Hanging of Pictures," *Ladies' Floral Cabinet* (November 1884): 363.

58. Solon J. Buck, ed. *William Watts Folwell: The Autobiography and Letters of a Pioneer of Culture* (Minneapolis: University of Minnesota Press, 1933), 77. William Watts Folwell served as the first president of the University of Minnesota. His autobiography sternly notes that after having written his book, Folwell burned all "pri-

vate" notes pertaining to the relationship between himself and his wife but not his diary. Luckily, his wife, Sarah Heywood Folwell, did not destroy hers.

59. Letter from Sarah Heywood to William Watts Folwell. July 13, 1860. Box 6, Folder 1. Folwell Manuscript Room, Minnesota Historical Society Library, St. Paul, Minnesota. An ambrotype is known as "amphipositives" in France, and "collodian positives" in England. A negative plate, treated with collodion (a viscous solutions of nitrocellulose in alcohol and ether), was underexposed and, when the glass negative was displayed on a dark background, the image appeared. The process was created in 1851 by J.-R. Le Moyne. See Jean-Claude Lemagny and André Rouillé, *A History of Photography: Social and Cultural Perspectives* (Cambridge: Cambridge University Press, 1987); Naomi Rosenblum, *A World of Photography*, 2nd ed. rev. (New York: Abbeville Press, 1989).

In 1853, J. H. Croucher published his book, *Plain Directions for Obtaining Photographic Pictures*, and the word *ambrotype* was coined in 1854 to describe these wet-plate glass negative images. Beaumont Newhall, in his *The History of Photography from 1839 to the Present*, 2nd ed. (New York: Museum of Modern Art, distributed by New York Graphic Society Books, Little, Brown and Company, 1982), notes that by 1863 the *American Journal of Photography* declared ambrotypes were becoming obsolete in the face of new and improved photographic techniques, including the tintype (invented in 1856).

60. Letter from Sarah Heywood to William Watts Folwell. July 16, 1860. Box 6, Folder 1. Folwell Papers, Manuscript Room, Minnesota Historical Society Library, St. Paul, Minnesota. The ambrotypes Sarah refers to are in the Folwell Papers, N7.1 r 19–20, Photo Box.

61. Letter from Sarah Heywood to William Watts Folwell, August 10, 1860. Box 6, Folder 1. Folwell Papers, Manuscript Room, Minnesota Historical Society Library, St. Paul, Minnesota.

62. Walter Benn Michaels, *The Gold Standard and the Logic of Naturalism* (Berkeley: University of California Press, 1987), chapter 7, "Action and Accident: Photography and Writing," 217–244.

63. Rachel Bowman, diary entry, February 8, 1860, in *The Cormany Diaries: A Northern Family in the Civil War*, ed. James C. Mohr (Pittsburgh, Pa.: University of Pittsburgh Press, 1982), 71–72.

64. Samuel Cormany, diary entry, February 6, 1860 in Mohr, *The Cormany Diaries*, 65.

65. Rachel Bowman, diary entry, February 7, 1860, in Mohr, *The Cormany Diaries*, 71.

66. Michaels, *The Gold Standard*, quoting John Berger, 237. See John Berger and Jean Mohr, *Another Way of Telling* (New York: Pantheon, 1982).

67. Accession file notes, artifact no. 7010.111, watch fob. Minnesota Historical Society, St. Paul, Minnesota.

68. Ann Douglas, *The Feminization of American Culture* (New York: Anchor Books, 1977), 205. For general histories of death practices in America, see Martha V. Pike and Janice Gray Armstrong, *A Time to Mourn: Expressions of Grief in Nineteenth Century America* (Stony Brook, N.Y.: Museums at Stony Brook, 1980); Charles O. Jackson, ed., *Passing: The Vision of Death in America* (Westport, Conn.:

Greenwood Press, 1977); James Stevens Curl, *A Celebration of Death: An Introduction to Some of the Buildings, Monuments, and Settings of Funerary Architecture in the West European Tradition* (New York: Scribner, 1980); James J. Farrell, *Inventing the American Way of Death, 1830–1920* (Philadelphia: Temple University Press, 1980); Jessica Mitford, *The American Way of Death Revisited*, rev. ed. (New York: Alfred A. Knopf, 1998); Lou Taylor, *Mourning Dress: A Costume and Social History* (London: Allen and Unwin, 1983). For mourning jewelry, see chapter 2 of Taylor's *Mourning Dress*, 219–224; Margaret Hunter, "Mourning Jewellery: A Collector's Account," *Costume* 27 (1993), 9–22. For general overviews of mourning objects, including hairwork, see Martha Pike, "In Memory Of: Artifacts Relating to Mourning in Nineteenth Century America," in *American Material Culture: The Shape of Things Around Us*, Edith Mayo, ed. (Bowling Green, Ohio: Bowling Green State University Popular Press, 1984), 48–65, and *Women in Mourning*, exhibition catalogue of the Museum of the Confederacy, Richmond, Virginia, November 14, 1984–January 6, 1986.

69. Mrs. Lydia H. Sigourney, "The Lock of Hair," *The Lady's Almanac for 1860* (Boston: Shepard, Clark, and Brown, 1860), no pagination.

70. "The Last Good Night," in Frances E. Percival, ed., *The Angel Visitor, or The Voices of the Heart* (Boston: L. P. Crown and Company, 1857), 192.

71. Mrs. Harriet E. Francis, "A Mother's Trial," *Godey's Book and Magazine* (October 1862): 276.

72. Thomas Hood, "Mother and Child," in *Golden Thoughts on Mother, Home and Heaven*, ed. Theodore L. Cuyler (New York: E. B. Treat, 1882), 64.

73. "A Home Picture," in *The Angel Visitor*, 217.

74. Ibid.

75. *Lady's Almanac for 1860*, no pagination.

76. Epitaph card with hair, no. 86 x 1.16, Mobley Collection, Folder, Mourning Cards and Funeral Notices. Downs Manuscript Collection, Winterthur Museum and Country Estate Library.

77. Timothy Shay Arthur, *Our Homes; Their Cares and Duties, Joys and Sorrows* (New York: John W. Lowell Co., 1888), 204.

78. Mrs. Mattie D. Britts, "My Treasures," *Peterson's Magazine* 42 (October 1862): 290.

79. Memorial poem and lock of hair, no date. Winterthur Museum and Estate, Winterthur, Delaware.

80. E. C. Shriner, advertisement, Fancy Work, Philadelphia, PN. Undertakers, Box 1, Folder Receipts,Warshaw Collection.

81. W. R. Seymour and Company, advertisement, Wax Flower Memorials. Philadelphia, Pennsylvania. Museum no. 86x1.125-Col. 6, Mobley Collection, Winterthur Museum and Country Estate Manuscripts Room, Winterthur Library. Neither the Shriner advertisement nor the Seymour advertisements are dated. The Shriner advertisement is circa 1860s or even slightly earlier, based on the fibrous paper and typeface, while the Seymour memorial wreaths, with their elaborate appearance, would be appropriate in parlors of the last quarter of the nineteenth century.

82. Donna Bassin, "Maternal Subjectivity in the Culture of Nostalgia: Mourn-

ing and Memory," in *Representations of Motherhood*, ed. Donna Bassin, Margaret Honey, and Meryle Mahrer Kaplan (New Haven, Conn.: Yale University Press, 1994), 168, 162. Bassin borrows the term "mourning play" from H. Loewald, *Sublimation: Inquiries into Theoretical Analysis* (New Haven, Conn.: Yale University Press, 1988). Caveats to the use of Bassin: I am transposing her late twentieth-century analysis onto a nineteenth-century phenomenon; she takes a Freudian approach to mourning; and she views nostalgia (or, prolonged mourning) as a case of arrested psychological development of the infant-mother relationship. Nancy Bercaw, "Solid Objects/Mutable Meanings: Fancywork and the Construction of Bourgeois Culture, 1840–1880," *Winterthur Portfolio* 26, no. 4 (Winter 1991): 231–247, suggests that mourning hairwork was "full of defiance and play" (244).

Chapter 3. The Gem That Binds

1. *The Young Lady's Companion: or, Sketches of Life, Manners, and Morals at the present day*. Edited by a Lady. (Philadelphia: H. C. Peck and Theodore Bliss, 1851), 37. Vincent J. Bertolini, "Fireside Chastity: The Erotics of Sentimental Bachelorhood in the 1850s," *American Literature* 68, no. 4 (December 1996): 707–738, deconstructs the tropic images of "the scene of the solitary lounging bachelor dreaming before the glowing embers" (707). These images were the literary manifestation of what Bertolini calls the "highly problematized social identity" of the bachelor, as the "bachelor's sociosexual identity is undefined and unregulated" (709).

2. Beverly Gordon, "Victorian Fancywork in the American Home: Fantasy and Accommodation," in *Making the American Home: Middle-Class Women and Domestic Material Culture, 1840–1940*, ed. Marilyn Ferris Motz and Pat Browne (Bowling Green, Ohio: Bowling Green State University Popular Press, 1988), argues this point, and includes the infamous lobster-claw figurines, figure 2, 54.

3. Gail Caskey Winkler, "Influence of Godey's *Lady's Book* on the American Woman and Her Home: Contributions to a National Culture (1830–1877)" (Ph.D. diss., University of Wisconsin–Madison, 1988, chapter 6, 283–373), discusses the issues of frugality, economy and fancywork. Winkler argues that fancywork was a way to make commercial objects more personable, and that much fancywork could be the result of genuine economic necessity combined with creative expression (286).

4. Mrs. Hannah Robertson, *The Young Ladies School of Arts, Containing a Great Variety of Practical Receipts* (York: New Printing-Office, 1777), 4th ed., viii. In her study of the role of fancywork in women's education in the nineteenth century, Patricia T. Herr includes an early 1800s letter from a Sister Pentry to her friend Mrs. Driliker: "Last week our Children had the Examination. . . . They were examin'd in Spelling, reading and writing, German and English—arithmetic grammar geography Music Sewing Knitting Tambour and embroidery or Satin Stitch." Letter from Sister Pentry to Mrs. Driliker, Linden Hall Archives, Lititz, Pennsylvania, Box 16. Quoted in Patricia T. Herr, *The Ornamental Branches: Needlework and Arts from the*

Lititz Moravian Girls School Between 1800 and 1865 (Lancaster County: Heritage Center Museum of Lancaster County, Pennsylvania, 1996), 18.

5. Annie S. Frost, *The Ladies' Guide to Needlework, Embroidery, etc.: Being a Complete Guide to All Kinds of Ladies' Fancy work* (New York: Henry T. Williams, 1877), 3.

6. George E. Blakelee, *Blakelee's Industrial Cyclopedia: A Ready Reference and a Reservoir of Useful Information. A Simple, Practical Home Guide for Men, Women, and Children* (New York: Useful Information Exchange, 1887), n.p.

7. "Duty. A Tale," *The Young Lady's Companion: or, Sketches of Life, Manners, and Morals at the Present Day, Edited by a Lady* (Philadelphia: H. C. Peck and Theodore Bliss, 1851), 97–110.

8. "Duty. A Tale," *The Young Lady's Companion,* 110. For a similar fictionalized account see Julia McNair Wright, *The Complete Home: An Encyclopedia of Domestic Life and Affairs . . .* (Philadelphia: J. C. McCurdy and Company, 1879), where "Aunt Sophronia" lectures her two nieces on "what is the first thing needful in starting a home." Aunt Sophronia answers that a common religion was necessary, and her niece Helen declares, "'I should have thought you would have said *love* came first." (20).

9. See Mary Jaene Edmonds, *Samplers and Samplermakers: An American Schoolgirl Art, 1700–1850* (New York: Rizzoli for the Los Angeles County Museum of Art, 1991); Betty Ring, *Let Virtue Be a Guide to Thee: Needlework in the Education of Rhode Island Women, 1730–1830* (Providence, R.I.: Rhode Island Historical Society, 1983); Ring, "Needlework Pictures from Abby Wright's School in South Hadley, Massachusetts," *Antiques* 131 (September 1986): 482–493; Susan Burrows Swan, *Plain and Fancy: American Women and Their Needlework, 1700–1850* (New York: Holt, Rinehart and Winston, 1977).

10. Nancy Bercaw, "Solid Objects/Mutable Meanings: Fancywork and the Construction of Bourgeois Culture, 1840–1880," *Winterthur Portfolio* 26, no. 4 (Winter 1991): 231–247, argues that through making nature-themed fancywork, "women often softened or denied harsh realities by transforming the world around them" (243). Gordon, "Victorian Fancywork in the American Home," 48–68, explicitly frames fancywork as a transformative escape mechanism for women.

11. These are some of the most popular nineteenth-century women's fancywork. Berlin work is embroidery using Berlin wools, and relied on mass-produced patterns. Tatting is a form of lace-making using a shuttle and cotton or silk thread. Embroidery is the ornamental stitching of patterns on cloth. See Molly J. Proctor, *Victorian Canvas Work: Berlin Wool Work* (London: B. T. Batsford, 1972), and Margaret Vincent, *The Ladies' Work Table: Domestic Needlework in Nineteenth-Century America*, exhibition catalogue (Allentown, Pa.: Allentown Art Museum, 1988), 32–34, for discussions of the craft, including its commercial roots. For complete definitions of these and other nineteenth-century needlework terms, see Sophia Frances Anne Caulfield and Blanche C. Saward, *Encyclopedia of Victorian Needlework [Dictionary of Needlework]*, 2 vols. (London: A. W. Cowan, 1887; reprint, Mineola, N.Y.: Dover Publications, 1972), and Therese de Dillmont, *The Complete Encyclopedia of Needlework* (Philadelphia, Pa.: Running Press, 1978); see also Margaret Vincent, *The*

Ladies' Work Table. Gail Caskey Winkler, "Influence of Godey's *Lady's Book* on the American Woman and Her Home," 299–301, surveys its American presence.

12. Laurel Thatcher Ulrich, *Good Wives: Image and Reality in the Lives of Women in Northern New England, 1650–1750* (New York: Vintage Books, 1982), and *A Midwife's Tale: The Life of Martha Ballard, Based on Her Diary, 1785–1812* (New York: Alfred A. Knopf, 1990), and *The Age of Homespun: Objects and Stories in the Creation of an American Myth* (New York: Vintage Books, 2001); Joan Jensen, *Loosening the Bonds: Mid-Atlantic Farm Women, 1750–1850* (New Haven, Conn.: Yale University Press, 1986). Jensen discusses how women became increasingly involved in visible "commodity production" in the first half of the nineteenth century through their butter-making activities. For the concept of "Republican motherhood," see Linda Kerber, *Women of the Republic: Intellect and Ideology in Revolutionary America* (Chapel Hill: University of North Carolina Press, 1980). For discussion of the development of the "separate sphere" ideology in relationship to this issue of visible versus invisible production, see Nancy F. Cott, *The Bonds of Womanhood: "Woman's Sphere" in New England, 1780–1835* (New Haven, Conn.: Yale University Press, 1977), and Jeanne Boydston, *Home and Work: Housework, Wages, and the Ideology of Labor in the Early Republic* (New York: Oxford University Press, 1990).

13. Theodore Cuyler, ed. *Golden Thoughts on Mother, Home and Heaven* (New York: E. B. Treat, 1882), 8.

14. See Harvey Green, *The Light of the Home: An Intimate View of the Lives of Women in Victorian America* (New York: Pantheon Books, 1983), 34–38, for an overview of the move from Enlightenment to late 1900s and the parallels between women's child nurturance and gardening, both activities that the "entwining" imagery in both fictional accounts and material creations such as hair jewelry personify. See Ruth H. Bloch, "American Feminine Ideals in Transition: The Rise of the Moral Mother, 1785–1815," *Feminist Studies* 4, no. 21 (June 1978): 100–126, for a discussion of the shift in ideals of motherhood from the eighteenth to the nineteenth centuries.

15. Mary J. Muckle, "Mother, Home, and Heaven," in Cuyler, *Mother, Home and Heaven*, 35.

16. For example, Reverend Daniel Wise, in his *The Young Lady's Counsellor; or, Outlines and Illustrations of the Sphere, the Duties, and the Dangers of Young Women* (New York: Carlton and Phillips, 1852), relates the example of Mary Washington, mother of George. Walking behind her esteemed son during a celebration of the American revolutionary victory, Wise notes that Mary "had trained him in his boyhood. . . . Her early influence over her glorious son was well understood, and silently acknowledged, in that gay assembly . . . she shared the richest enjoyments of [the war's] success; but she did it through her heroic son" (98–99). Thus, a woman's duty to her children, and especially her son's, was to form their character and to never seek explicit acknowledgment or reward of their own labors.

17. This is an ideal of maternal love, not its reality. Gillian Brown, *Domestic Individualism: Imagining Self in Nineteenth-Century America* (Berkeley: University of California Press, 1990), discusses Harriet Beecher Stowe's images of this maternal heaven. E. Anthony Rotundo, *American Manhood: Transformations in Masculinity from the Revolution to the Modern Era* (New York: Basic Books, 1993), 29–30, notes

this as well, although Rotundo does not explore the significance of such transcendent language. The term "mother love" is used by Jan Lewis, "Mother's Love: The Construction of an Emotion in Nineteenth-Century America," in *Social History and Issues in Human Consciousness: Some Interdisciplinary Connections*, ed. Andrew E. Barnes and Peter N. Stearns (New York: New York University Press, 1989), 209–229.

18. This is taken directly from Jan Lewis, "Mother's Love." She notes that maternal love was eternal "in another sense, as well, for it was reincarnated in her children, who carried it with them always, as a talisman and an almost corporeal part of themselves" (215).

19. Doris Green, "Hair Jewelry," *Antiques Journal* 18, no. 6 (June 1963): 16–17, mentions this 1812 example. Unfortunately, she does not provide any provenance information. The instructions she pictures are almost exactly those published by *Peterson's Magazine*, *Godey's Lady's Book and Magazine*, and Mark Campbell's various guides, all of the 1850s and 1860s.

20. Directions for making hairwork at home appear in *Godey's Book and Magazine*, in a series beginning in volume 58 (February 1859): 123, and in *Peterson's Magazine* beginning in volume 28 (September 1860): 222–224. Innumerable domestic craft and fancywork manuals were published for middle-class women in the nineteenth century. Those that mention hair fancywork include Mark Campbell, *Self-Instructor in the Art of Hair Work, Dressing Hair, Making Curls, Switches, Braids, and Hair Jewelry of Every Description/Compiled from Original Designs and the Latest Parisian Patterns by Mark Campbell* (New York: Mark Campbell, 1867); Peter Cassell, *Cassell's Household Guide: Being a Complete Encyclopedia of Domestic and Social Economy, and Forming a Guide to Every Department of Practical Life*, vol. 4 (London: Peter Cassell and Galpin, 1869–71[?]), 337–338, 356–357; E. E. Crofut, *The Art of Hair Chain Braiding* (Malta, Mont.: E. E. Crofut, 1911); Mrs. C. S. Jones and Henry T. Williams, *Ladies' Fancy Work: Hints and Helps to Home Taste and Recreations* (New York: Henry T. Williams Publisher, 1876); Mrs. Matilda Marian Pullan, *The Lady's Manual of Fancy-Work: A Complete Instructor in Every Variety of Ornamental Needle-Work* (New York: Dick & Fitzgerald, 1859); Madame Levina B. Urbino, Professor Henry Day, et al. *Art Recreations: Being a Complete Guide to Pencil Drawing, Oil Painting . . . Wax Work, Shell Work* (Boston: J. E. Tilton and Company, 1869).

21. Mark Campbell, advertisement in Isaac Guyer, *History of Chicago* (Chicago: Goodman and Cushing, 1862), 61.

22. Mark Campbell, advertisement, Guyer, *History of Chicago*, 61.

23. Cassell, "Household Decorative Art: Working in Hair," *Cassell's Household Guide*, 337.

24. National Artistic Hair Work Company. *Catalogue of Designs for Artistic Hair Scenery and Ornaments Executed by National Artistic Hair Works of Chicago* (Chicago: National Artistic Hair Work Company, 1886).

25. "The Art of Ornamental Hair Work," *Godey's Lady's Book* 41 (December 1850), 377.

26. Urbino et al., *Art Recreations*, 294.

27. Henry Bucklin Scammell, "Hair Work," in *Scammell's Universal Treasure-House of Useful Knowledge: An Encyclopaedia of Valuable Receipts in the Principal Arts of Life* (Philadelphia, Pa.: Scammell and Company, 1885), 1487.

28. Pullan, *The Lady's Manual of Fancy-Work*, 298. The advertisement for hairwork orders appears at the end of her instructional manual. Matilda Pullan was a prolific writer of fancywork instructions. See Elizabeth White Nelson, *Market Sentiments: Middle-Class Market Culture in Nineteenth-Century America* (Washington, D.C.: Smithsonian Books, 2004), 146–148, for a biographical sketch of Pullan.

29. National Artistic Hair Work Company, *Catalogue of Designs*, 3–4.

30. Jones and Williams, *Ladies' Fancy Work*, 4. Urbino et al., *Art Recreations*, 294.

31. "The Art of Ornamental Hair-Work," *Godey's Lady's Book* 41 (December 1850), 377.

32. Campbell, *Self-Instructor in the Art of Hair Work* (Chicago: Mark Campbell, 1859), preface.

33. "The Art of Ornamental Hair-Work," *Godey's Lady's Book* 41 (December 1850): 377.

34. "The Art of Ornamental Hair-Work," *Godey's Lady's Book* 58 (March 1859); 219; "The Art of Ornamental Hair-Work," *Godey's Lady's Book* 41 (December 1850), 377.

35. Campbell, *Self-Instructor* (1859), 137.

36. C[hristopher] R. Edwards, advertisement under "Hair Worker." *The Syracuse Directory* (Syracuse, N.Y.: William H. Boyd, 1857).

37. Both the letter and the pin are in the private collection of Jan Odegaard, Wisconsin Historical Society, Madison, Wisconsin.

38. Museum no. 1945.1326, Wisconsin Historical Society, Madison, Wisconsin. Donor, Miss Mary S. Foster. Necklace created circa 1850.

Mark Campbell provides several different styles of "open braids," (see pages 94–121) with directions on using two different colors of hair to produce a "diamond," "spiral," "check," or even "scotch plaid" design (*Self-Instructor* [1875]), pages 108, 109, 111, 112, respectively).

39. Museum no. 8030.33 (watch chain) and no. 8030.31 (brooch), Minnesota Historical Society, St. Paul, Minnesota. Donor, Nellie Cardoza. Additional information is on a card reading, "The jewelry made of hair and gold were made of her and her sister's hair—when they were quite young," letter from Dr. Robert Rosenthal. Nellie Cardoza was born in 1855. The date of 1860s is derived from Nellie's birth date and Rosenthal's commentary.

40. Locating information about the colors and patterns of cloth used in women's clothing (as opposed to the "newest styles" reported in women's periodicals) is very difficult. See Betty J. Mills, in her book *Calico Chronicle: Texas Women and Their Fashions, 1830–1910* (Lubbock: Texas Tech Press, 1985), for a chart of each decade's most popular fabrics, colors, designs, trim, and so on. She reports that the 1850s, 1860s, and 1870s all relied on plaids, and the colors of browns, tans, and creams were popular as well. Joan L. Severa, *Dressed for the Photographer: Ordinary Americans and Fashion, 1840–1900* (Kent, Ohio: Kent State University Press, 1995), and *My Likeness Taken: Daguerrian Portraits in America* (Kent, Ohio: Kent State University Press, 2006), agrees with this. In the 1870s, Severa notes, colors remain in the browns and deep colors, and "cotton dresses, now even for dressy occasions,

sometimes consisted of three patterns of fabric with shared colors, often using plain, plaid, and stripes as various parts of the dress. Most often the skirts were of the dark, plain shade and the overskirt and bodice of a lighter mix, with either or both used in trimming all three pieces." (*Dressed for the Photographer*, 303). By the 1880s, color preferences have shifted to deep burgundies, greens and coppers, and fabrics used with silks, velvets, and wools. Thus, dual-colored hair jewelry would work well in the 1860s and 1870s against the tans and browns with simple cottons and wools dominant, but the 1880s would demand a different style of hair jewelry.

41. Museum no. 1951.1909, Wisconsin Historical Society. Donor, Dr. and Mrs. C. A. Harper. Dated 1896. The brooch was donated, according to the Wisconsin Historical Society records, in 1951. Thus, its original owner was most likely Mrs. C. A. Harper's parent.

42. Lynn A. Bonfield and Mary C. Morrison, *Roxana's Children: The Biography of a Nineteenth-Century Vermont Family* (Amherst: University of Massachusetts Press, 1995), preface.

43. Letter, Sarah Rivers to husband. Bruce Family Papers 1836–1906, MSS1 B 8306d 5–14, Section 3. Virginia Historical Society, Richmond, Virginia.

44. Emma Egy Miller album, Watkins Community Museum, Lawrence, Kansas. George Garber's verse is a fine example of the "rote verse," for which there were manuals of instruction. See *Madam Worth's Kensington and Fancy Work Manual* (Wallingford, Conn.: R. L. Spencer, 1886), "The Album Writer's Assistant," advertisement, "The Album Writer's Assistant" advertisement notes that many "have found it impossible at the moment to draw from the well of their own thoughts the sentiment they desire to express. . . . A few moments' research of the pages of this manual will always disclose some attractive expression in prose or poetry, expressive of almost every human feeling and sentiment . . . with this book at hand you can readily oblife [oblige] all your friends that request you to inscribe your expression of friendship." R. L. Spencer Company, advertisement, in *Madam Worth's Kensington and Fancy Work Manual.*

45. Commonplace Book, 1865–1867. Boswell, Virginia Catherine (Persinger). In Persinger Family Papers, 1865–1932. MSS1 P4314a1. Virginia Historical Society, Richmond, Virginia.

46. Letter, Overton Bernard to Martha Jane (Thomas) Bernard. Bernard Family Papers, 1821–1903. Folder, Martha Jane (Thomas) Bernard, Sec. 1. MSS1 B4568b24–29. Virginia Historical Society, Richmond, Virginia.

47. Letter, Sarah Rivers to husband. Bruce Family Papers 1836–1906, MSS1 B 8306d 5–14, Section 3. Virginia Historical Society, Richmond, Virginia.

48. Winkler, "Influence of Godey's *Lady's Book* on the American Woman and Her Home," discusses the decoration and functions of the parlor space (311–325). Winkler also notes that the sitting room, being a less formal space, may have been a more likely display area for a woman's fancywork (325–333).

49. Jones and Williams, *Ladies' Fancy Work*, 52.

50. I make the assertion that hair wreaths were used primarily to decorate parlor walls with some reservations. The privacy of bedrooms would argue against displaying hair wreaths in that space, given that wreaths were intended to be displayed in public. Carolyn Brucken, in her "Victorian Privacy: An Analysis of Bed-

rooms in American Middle-Class Homes from 1850–1880" (Master's thesis, University of Delaware, 1991), suggests that while the bedroom was considered a private, often unadorned space, the guest or spare bedroom "was routinely opened to the public," as it frequently functioned as a transitional space for visitors, who would be allowed to use the bedroom to "freshen up" and compose themselves (61). It is possible, then, that hair wreaths might be used to decorate the spare bedroom space.

51. The best overview of the development and changes in American parlors is Katherine C. Grier, *Culture and Comfort: Parlor Making and Middle-Class Identity, 1850–1930*, rev. 2nd ed. (Washington, D.C.: Smithsonian Institution Press, 1997). I recommend for precise chronological information Grier's *Culture and Comfort: People, Parlors, and Upholstery, 1850–1930* (Rochester, N.Y.: Strong Museum, 1989). See also Foy and Marling, *The Arts and the American Home,* for various essays regarding later parlor developments. See also William Seale, *The Tasteful Interlude: American Interiors through the Camera's Eye, 1860–1917*, rev. 2nd ed. (Nashville, Tenn.: American Association of State and Local History, 1981). For how parlors structured behavior within its walls, see Karen Halttunen, *Confidence Men and Painted Women: A Study of Middle-Class Culture in America, 1830–1870* (New Haven, Conn.: Yale University Press, 1982), and John F. Kasson, *Rudeness and Civility: Manners in Nineteenth-Century Urban America* (New York: Hill and Wang, 1990), 173–181.

52. Elizabeth Alice White, "Sentimental Enterprise: Sentiment and Profit in American Market Culture, 1830–1880" (Ph.D. diss., Yale University Press, 1995), mentions fancywork shops, 172, 174. White relies on fictional accounts, recommendations for women to make money, and at least two advertisements. The date of 1830s reflects White's conclusion.

Virginia Penny, *How Women Can Make Money* (Springfield, Mass.: D. E. Fisk, and Company, 1870; reprint, New York: Arno and the New York Times, 1971), includes as possible occupations for women "keepers of fancy stores." Penny is not clear what was to be sold in such stores.

53. Timothy Shay Arthur, "Taking Boarders," *Godey's Magazine and Lady's Book* 42 (March 1851): 163. Complete story appears in 42 (January 1851): 13–20; 42 (February 1851), 81–87; and 42 (March 1851): 160–167.

54. "Stamens," *Godey's Lady's Book* 63 (November 1861), cited by Lilian Baker Carlisle, "Hair Today, Shorn Tomorrow (sorry!)," *Yankee* (January 1974): 97. Hair wire spools, Henry Bristow, Price List, *Trade Catalogue: Ornaments, Novelties, Paper Flowers* (Washington, D.C., 1886), 30, Printed Books and Periodical Collection, Winterthur Library, Winterthur, Delaware (hereafter, Winterthur Library). Flower-making supplies, Waterman and Hunt, *Price List for Tools and Materials for Wax Flowers and Fruitmaking* (Boston: circa 1885), Winterthur Library. See Nelson, *Market Sentiments*, 136, for a brief mention of an entrepreneurial flower-making instruction manual. Ladies' Art Company (St. Louis, Missouri), *Illustrated Catalogue and Price List*, circa 1897, 14–15, Winterthur Library.

55. In addition to Urbino et al., *Art Recreations*, see Scammell, "Hair Work," *Scammell's Universal Treasure-House*, 1487. The Dodge County (Minnesota) Historical Society has a note "Instructions for Making a Hair Wreath" (1984), from Mrs.

Mabel Krause, Fenton, Iowa, born 1900. Krause's instructions use a knitting needle, wire, and hair in a different technique. I have found no nineteenth-century origin for this technique.

56. Jones and Williams, *Ladies' Fancy Work*, 55. Urbino et al., *Art Recreations*, 295.

57. See "Making Feather Flowers," *Peterson's Magazine* 40 (October 1861): 315; and "Feather-Work," *Peterson's Magazine* 52 (July 1867): 76. "Star-Flower in Filigree Point," *Harper's Bazaar* (August 14, 1880): 516, 520; "Crochet Leaf for Newspaper Rack," *Harper's Bazaar* (October 18, 1886): 672; "The Work Table: An Entire New Style of Crochet Embellishment—Flower-Work," *Godey's Magazine and Lady's Book* 39 (September 1849): 218. To gain a sense of the close link made between fancywork and "natural" forms, see Anne Hulbert, *Victorian Crafts Revived* (New York: Hastings House, 1978); she offers directions on making nineteenth-century crafts ranging from shellwork, silhouettes, pressed flowers, and so on, and Ella Shannon Bowles, *Homespun Handicrafts* (Philadelphia: J. B. Lippincott Company, 1931). Both provide comprehensive overviews of the range of fancywork crafts.

58. The series "Worsted Flowers" ran in March 1862 and April 1862, *Godey's Lady's Magazine*. See also Molly J. Proctor, "Wool Work Flowers," in *Victorian Canvas Work*, 129–131, for a comprehensive overview of the craft.

59. Wreath, no. 12764. Waukesha County Museum and Historical Society, Waukesha, Wisconsin. Donor, L. V. Imig in behalf of Mother Imig (Louise). Donor's note: "wreath and frame were handmade by mother of donor, Mrs. Louise Imig, about 1872."

60. Wreath, no. 81519U02. Domestic Life Division, National Museum of American History. On the back of the frame is written, "Wreath made of hair in the / Theyer and McMaster families / Flowers (large) of dark brown hair / are of my grandfather; Dr. John A. Theyer / Lighter reddish brown hair at bottom / is of our great grandfather, Judge Robert McMaster."

61. Wreath is in the private collection of Leila Cohoon, The Hair Museum, Independence, Missouri.

62. All quotes from typescript letter, dated Jan. 1, 1894, Folder, Hair Wreath (4 of 4), Mrs. Stickney's statement, Manuscripts Room, Chicago Historical Society. The wreath cannot be traced. A similar "wreath" is at the Smithsonian Institution, at the National Museum of American History. This panel was displayed at the U.S. Patent Office and presents, according to its original card, "Hair of the Presidents of the United States with other persons of distinctions." The panel was created by John Varden. Accession no. 13152, catalog no. 16157A, Division of Political History.

63. One ongoing problem with dating such things as the frames of hair wreaths is that often a wreath may have been reframed to maintain an up-to-date appearance in the parlor. See Kenneth L. Ames, introductory essay of *The Arts and the American Home, 1890–1930*, ed. Jessica H. Foy and Karal Ann Marling (Knoxville, University of Tennessee Press, 1994), xv–xxiv, for a discussion of this problem.

64. Wreath, no. 9828. Minnesota Historical Society, St. Paul, Minnesota. Donor, Mrs. H. McLean. Wreath, no. 61. Goodhue County Historical Society, Goodhue, Minnesota. No donor.

65. Hair picture, no. 8347/HH05D, Minnesota Historical Society, St. Paul, Minnesota. Donor, Mrs. C. G. Schulz. Dated 1890.

66. Hair wreath, no. 94.41.1., Blue Earth County Historical Society, Blue Earth, Minnesota. Donor, Lou Ella Schroeder. Donor's note: "Hannah's hair was used for this wreath. She was born January 1882 and died February 1894 from scarlet fever. Siblings of Hannah were Sarah, Peder, and Alfred."

67. Rachel Bowman Cormany, August 17, 1863, Mohr, *The Cormany Diaries*, 377. Rachel Bowman Cormany periodically resorts to making money through her sewing skills. As the editor notes, Rachel did so throughout the period of her diary, as an unmarried student, then as teacher, as a newly-married homesteader, and, here, as a soldier's wife.

68. Rachel Bowman Cormany, August 18, 1863, Mohr, *The Cormany Diaries*, 378.

Chapter 4. Made to Order

1. Wendy Gamber's *The Female Economy: The Millinery and Dressmaking Trades, 1860–1930* (Urbana: University of Illinois Press, 1997), is an excellent study of similar industries. The parallels between the millinery and dressmaking trade and the hair-working trade are in their custom-work production, the personal and emotional relationships between customers and producers, and the roles each industry held in the development of the twentieth-century market of fashion and personal goods.

2. Mark Campbell, *The Art of Hair Work* (New York: Mark Campbell, 1867). See Duhme and Company, advertisement, *Jewelers' Circular and Horological Review* (December 1881), 54, and Enos Richardson and Company, advertisement, *Jewelers' Circular and Horological Review* (September 1882), 50, for similar gender-segregated labor-force images.

3. Emil Wilhelm Moutoux was born in Frankenburg, Hesse, in 1839, and his brother Ernst Louis was born in Friedrichsdorf, Taunus. Moutoux Genealogy, compiled by Ruth Wales, 1982. National Museum of American History, Costume Collection, Foote Files, "Memorial or Mourning Jewelry."

4. For a general overview of African American businesses in the United States, see Juliet E. K. Walker, *The History of Black Business in America: Capitalism, Race, Entrepreneurship* (New York: Macmillan Library Reference Series [Twayne's Evolution of Modern Business Series], 1998). Walker specifically cites black women hairdressers, 130.

5. *Halpin's Eighth Annual Edition Chicago City Directory 1865–1866* (Chicago: T. M. Halpin, 1865). On page 56, Ohswaldt is listed as "col'd." In the same directory, Ohswaldt advertised himself as offering "Premium Wigs & Hair Jewelry." Ohswaldt appears in several listings in the years 1861 to 1865. Jared Gray is listed as "col'd" in 1868 under the listing of "wig makers." *Bailey and Edwards' Chicago Directory 1868* (Chicago: Edwards and Co. Publishers, 1868), 1357. Gray is listed as a hair jeweler in 1862 in *Halpin's and Bailey's Chicago City Directory* (Chicago: Halpin and Bailey,

Publishers, 1862), under the category "hair jewelry." Gray appears to have focused on wigs instead of jewelry, however. In following years, he is usually listed as a hairdresser and wig maker. George Stewart is listed in 1855 as a hairdresser. In 1859, George Stewart is listed as "col'd" under the category of "Hair (Ornamental, Manufacturers)" in *Boyd's Philadelphia City Business Directory* comp. Wm. H. Boyd (Philadelphia, Pa.: Joseph Monier, 1859). This category could also include wig makers. In 1861 Elizabeth Stewart, living five houses down the street from George, is listed as a hair jeweler and as "(c)olored" wig maker. *McElroy's Philadelphia City Directory for 1861* (Philadelphia: Edward C. & J. Biddle and Company, 1861), 1169.

6. Juliet E. K. Walker states that "for both free black men and women, merchandising required capital and credit, which few antebellum blacks had, a condition that limited their participation in the business community as shopkeepers." *The History of Black Business in America*, 148.

7. Marion Edmonds Roe, *How Six Girls Made Money; or, Occupations for Women* (Mount Morris, Ill.: The Brethren's Publishing Company, 1887), 19. Susan Ingalls Lewis, "Female Entrepreneurs in Albany 1840–1885," *Business and Economic History* 2nd ser., 21 (1992), 65–73, mentions one hair-working establishment, that of Mr. and Mrs. Theodore Yaumans, 69. See also Wendy Gamber, "Gendered Concerns: Thoughts on the History of Business and the History of Women," *Business and Economic History*, 23 (1994): 129–140, and *The Female Economy*, and Angel Kwolek-Folland's *Incorporating Women: A History of Women and Business in the United States* (New York: Twayne Publishers, 1998).

8. Katherine Schmitt was awarded a prize by the Franklin Institute. She also was a partner in a hairwork shop with F. Steubenrauch. She was listed in various Philadelphia city directories until 1900. After 1900, she is not listed. Schmitt would have been eighty-two years old in that year, according to her reported age in the 1860 census (Bureau of the Census, *Eighth Census of the United States*, Pennsylvania Free Schedule, City of Philadelphia, Ward Eight, M653, Roll 1158, p. 336).

Friedrich Steubenrauch advertised in the *Daily Gazette and Comet* (Baton Rouge, Louisiana) on January 3, 1860, page 3, col. 5, "that he is fully prepared to execute any order in his line, such as Bracelets, Necklaces . . . &c., &c., . . ." and assured readers that he would never attempt, as others were, of "substituting work imported from the North and Europe, and passing it off as if executed with the Hair furnished by customers." His business was at 27 Chartres Street, New Orleans, Louisiana (newspaper listing courtesy Vicki Betts, University of Texas at Tyler).

9. *McElroy's Philadelphia Directory, for 1855* (Philadelphia: Edward C. and John Biddle, 1855), listed under "Hair Plaiting" and "Jewelers."

10. Figures according to 1870 and 1874 to 1880 R. G. Dun and Company reports. For a discussion of the increasing prominence of the credit agency, see James H. Madison, "The Evolution of Commercial Credit Reporting Agencies in Nineteenth-Century America," *Business History Review* 48, no. 2 (Summer 1974): 164–178. Madison comments at length on the agencies' information-gathering techniques, see 171–173. See also James D. Norris, *R. G. Dun and Company, 1841–1900: The Development of Credit-Reporting in the Nineteenth Century* (Westport, Conn.: Greenwood Press, 1978).

11. *1860 Eighth Census of the United States*, Philadelphia Free Schedule, City of

Philadelphia, Ward 8, microfilm location M653, Roll 1158, p. 336. *Non-Population Census Schedules for Pennsylvania, 1870–1880: Industry and Manufacturing*, District 28, Ward 10, 1870. Microfilm location M1796, Roll 3, p. 5. In adopting the title "Madame," Mrs. Schmitt followed a time-honored method of female entrepreneurs to attain an elevated class status and the aura of fashionable authority. See Gamber, *The Female Economy*, 107, for a discussion of women milliners and dressmakers who did the same.

12. "In bus. some years . . ." New York, vol. 395, p. 100, June 28, 1869, R. G. Dun and Company Collection, Baker Library, Harvard Business School. "Not now living . . ." New York, vol. 395, p. 100, January 21/1871, R. G. Dun and Company Collection, Baker Library, Harvard Business School. "Active business . . ." New York, vol. 395, p. 100, January 4, 1872 and December 5, 1872, R. G. Dun and Company Collection, Baker Library, Harvard Business School.

13. *Catalogue of the Thirteenth Exhibition of American Manufactures, held in Philadelphia, 1842* (Philadelphia: William S. Young, 1842), 24, from *Franklin Institute and the Making of Industrial America*, microfiche 237. This is the same Dressler that did subcontracted hairwork for Samuel Parrott (see Chapter 2). Dressler was very poorly rated by R. G. Dun and Company in 1849. The credit agent noted his shop was twenty feet square, "his stk [stock] looks old + he is in a part of the city where he cant do much, not like to trust him." Philadelphia, Pa., vol. 1, p. 131, March 29, 1848, R. G. Dun and Company Collection, Baker Library, Harvard Business School.

14. See *Reports of the First Exhibition of the Middlesex Mechanic Association* (Lowell, Massachusetts) (Lowell, Mass.: S. J. Varney, 1852), 61, 67; *A Record of the First Exhibition of the Metropolitan Mechanics' Institute* (Washington, D.C.) (Washington, D.C.: H. Polkinhorn, 1853), 33, 38, 39; *Catalogue of the Third Annual Exposition of the New England Manufacturers' and Mechanics' Institute* (Boston: Tolman and White, 1883), 58, 257.

15. Madame K. Schmitt, advertisement, *Gopsill's Philadelphia City Directory for 1877* (Philadelphia: James Gopsill, 1877), 1280; Schmitt claims to have received "First Premium at the Centennial. Two Premiums of Franklin Institute for 1854 & 1874." In 1875, Schmitt placed a half-page illustrated advertisement highlighting her Franklin Institute medals. Madame K. Schmitt, advertisement, *Gopsill's Philadelphia City Directory for 1875* (Philadelphia: James Gopsill, 1875), front materials, no pagination. Indeed, Mrs. Schmitt had earned the medals. *Report on the Twenty-Fourth Exhibition of American Manufactures* (Philadelphia: Barnard and Jones, 1855), lists Schmitt and "Stubensaule" under "Hair Plaiting," 32. In the *Report of the Twenty-Seventh Exhibition of American Manufactures* (Philadelphia: Barnard and Jones, 1874), Mrs. Schmitt again has won commendation. United States Centennial Commission, *Reports and Awards: International Exhibition, 1876, vol. 5, Groups 8–9*, ed. Francis A. Walker (Washington, D.C.: Government Printing Office, 1880), Group X, Citation #33, Mrs. K. Schmitt, 98. Madame K. Schmitt, advertisement, *Gopsill's Philadelphia City Directory for 1881* (Philadelphia: James Gopsill, 1880), 1447.

16. Patent record no. 31,735 (March 19, 1861), John S. Palmer.

17. Patent record no. 56,618 (July 24, 1866), Lorenzo Sauter.

18. "Specimens of Hair Work" in "Report on the New York Crystal Palace

Exhibition," *Gleason's Pictorial Drawing-Room Companion*, August 13, 1853, 233. Zim Collection, Series 1, Box 60.

19. Receipt, January 22, 1859, C. Linherr, in Hair, Box 2, Folder, Lewison, L., Warshaw Collection, National Museum of American History. There are two Linherrs, Christian and John A. While they joined forces for the 1853 exhibition, they usually conducted business separately. For price comparisons, see the price list for Mark Campbell's breastpins, which range from $4.00 to $16.00 in 1875. And in 1859, *Godey's Book and Magazine* offered hairwork breastpins through its mail-order service that ranged in price from $4.00 to $12.00 (8: October 1859), 375.

20. Dates derived from the partnership of Stubenrauch and Schmitt, whose business was located at 928 Chestnut Street, Philadelphia, Pennsylvania, the address on the box label, from 1863 to 1867. After 1867, the partners split up, but as late as 1870 the company of Stubenrauch and Schmitt were rated by R. G. Dun and Company. For similar examples, see the A. Bernhard and Company Catalog of 1870, no. 395, reprinted in C. Jeanenne Bell's *Collector's Encyclopedia of Hairwork Jewelry* (Paducah, Ky.: Schroeder Publishing Company, 1998), 239; Mark Campbell's *Self-Instructor* (1875), style no. 52 and no. 53.

21. The fob and box are in the National Museum of American History's jewelry collections, no. 323595.1 and no. 323595.2. The 1871 advertisement appears in *Gopsill's Philadelphia City Directory for 1871* (Philadelphia: James Gopsill, 1871).

22. Mrs. A. S. Rollo, trade card, no date. Hair, Box 2, Warshaw Collection. See also N. G. Pearsons, trade card, no date. Hair, Box 2, Folder, Pearsons, N. G., Warshaw Collection. Here, Pearsons terms her- or himself as a dealer of "Human Hair Goods" and pictures a row of hair jewelry and lists a variety of artificial hairpieces also available.

23. Misses M. A. Shaw and A. M. Shafer, trade card, no date. Hair, Box 2, Folder, Shaw, L., Warshaw Collection.

24. For broader studies, see Wendy Cooper, *Hair: Sex Society Symbolism* (New York: Stein and Day, 1971), chapter 6, "The Hair Industry," 151–181, and J. Stevens Cox, *An Illustrated Dictionary of Hairdressing and Wigmaking* (Philadelphia: George S. MacManus Company, 1966). Both Cooper and Cox discuss the development of modern hairdressing and both note the popularity of hair jewelry in the nineteenth century.

Surprisingly little has been done on the historical development of the hair industry and hairdressing in America, with the exception of the attention paid to the African American beauty industry and African American beauty salons, especially (and rightly so) the career of Madame C. J. Walker. See A'Lelia Bundles, *On Her Own Ground: The Life and Times of Madam C. J. Walker* (New York: Scribner, 2001). For a profile of Martha Harper, another pioneer of the American hairdressing industry, see Jane R. Plitt, *Martha Matilda Harper and the American Dream: How One Woman Changed the Face of Modern Business* (New York: Syracuse University Press, 2000). Don Herzog, "The Trouble with Hairdressers," *Representations* 53 (Winter 1996): 21–43, discusses the political role of male hairdressers in pre- and post-Revolutionary France.

25. Stanley C. Hollander, "The Effects of Industrialization of Small Retailing

in the United States in the Twentieth Century," in *Small Business in American Life*, ed. Stuart W. Bruchey, (New York: Columbia University Press, 1980), 212–239.

26. The information on the rise and subsequent decline of jobbers is derived from Timothy B. Spears, *100 Years on the Road: The Traveling Salesman in American Culture* (New Haven, Conn.: Yale University Press, 1995). See also Lewis Atherton, *The Pioneer Merchant in Mid-America* (New York: Da Capo Press, 1969) and Glenn Porter and Harold C. Livesay, *Merchants and Manufacturers: Studies in the Changing Structure of Nineteenth-Century Marketing* (Baltimore: Johns Hopkins University Press, 1971).

27. "O. Schwencke, advertisement," *Jewelers' Circular and Horological Review*, June 1877 and February 1878. "Business Notes," *Jewelers' Circular and Horological Review*, November 1879.

28. New York, vol. 426, p.100A19, July 28, 1877, and February 11, 1879, R. G. Dun and Company Collection, Baker Library, Harvard Business School. John Linherr resurrected his business under his wife's name in 1880, and shifted from hair jewelry to "jewelry." This business apparently thrived, although both John and his wife refused to actually talk with the R. G. Dun and Company agents who were sent to their store every six months. John appears to have acted as an agent for their store. In another change, Mrs. M. A. Linherr, John's wife, simply did not apply for credit any longer, and borrowed from friends instead. The business was still continuing in 1893, when the R. G. Dun and Company ceased rating them. (New York, vol. 426, sub100/A80 and sub100/A12, R. G. Dun and Company Collection, Baker Library, Harvard Business School, "Mrs. J. Gray".)

29. See Philip Scranton, "Manufacturing Diversity: Production Systems, Markets, and an American Consumer Society, 1870–1930," *Technology and Culture* 35, no. 3 (July 1994): 476–505; "The Politics of Production: Technology, Markets, and the Two Cultures of American Industry," *Science in Context* 8, no. 2 (1995): 369–395; "Diversity in Diversity: Flexible Production and American Industrialization, 1880–1930," *Business History Review* 65 (Spring 1991): 27–90.

30. To give a sense of the small numbers of hair workers I am discussing, in 1884 the following jewelers advertised themselves as hair workers to the trade in *Jewelers' Mercantile Agency Limited Directory for the Jobbing Trade Only:* A. Bernhard, Charles Menge [*sic*] (who also advertised in the 1880s in *Jewelers' Circular and Horological Review*), William Moutoux, Lorenzo Sauter, and O. Schwencke, all of New York City. In addition to these jewelers, the following hair workers advertised in various trade publications from 1870 to 1889: Charles Francke and Co., New York, in *The Watchmaker and Jeweler: Devoted to the Interests of Watchmakers, Jewelers, Silversmiths*, etc. 2, no. 1 (September 1870): 32; William M. Fisher of Providence, Rhode Island, in *Jewelers' Circular and Horological Review*, March 1881; Max and Albert Friedenthal of New York City, in *Jewelers' Circular and Horological Review*, in March 1880 and continuing until 1882; Fanning and Potter (who specified they worked "for the jobbing trade only") of Providence, Rhode Island, in *Manufacturing Jeweller* 1, no. 2 (November 1884): 79, and also in 1886 and 1888 issues; and C. E. Hayward in *Manufacturing Jeweller* 2, no. 5 (February 1886): 249.

31. New York, vol. 329, p. 1454, March 27, 1875 "Charles F. Menge" [*sic*], R. G. Dun and Company Collection, Baker Library, Harvard Business School.

32. New York, vol. 329, p. 1454, October 12, 1885, "Charles F. Menge" [*sic*], R. G. Dun and Company Collection, Baker Library, Harvard Business School.

33. "Lorenz[o] Sauter: Manufacturer of Fine Jewelry," advertisement, *The Watchmaker and Jeweler: Devoted to the Interests of Watchmakers, Jewelers, Silversmiths, etc.* 4, no. 3 (December 1871): 122. See also Sauter advertisements, 3, no. 5 (June 1872); 3, no. 8 (April 1872).

34. New York, vol. 409, p. 301, April 16, 1880, R. G. Dun and Company Collection, Baker Library, Harvard Business School.

35. Isaac Guyer, *History of Chicago* (Chicago: Goodman and Cushing, 1862), 60–61. Guyer published "mugbooks," a commercial promotional tool. See David E. Kyvig and Myron A. Marty, *Nearby History: Exploring the Past Around You*, 2nd ed. (New York: Rowman and Littlefield, 2000), 67–69, for a brief discussion of these.

36. Mark Campbell, Circular, "Ladies' Guide to M. Campbell's *Self-Instructor.* Art of Hair Work" (Chicago: Mark Campbell, 1867). His instructional guide, *Self-Instructor in the Art of Hair Work, Dressing Hair, Making Curls, Switches, Braids, and Hair Jewelry of Every Description / Compiled from Original Designs and the Latest Parisian Patterns by Mark Campbell* (New York: Mark Campbell, 1867), provided detailed instructions for the home creation of hairwork.

37. Illinois, vol. 33, p. 39, April 18, 1868, R. G. Dun and Company Collection, Baker Library, Harvard Business School.

38. Illinois, vol. 33, p. 39, June 3, 1871, R. G. Dun and Company Collection, Baker Library, Harvard Business School. This is the last recorded entry for Campbell. Mark Campbell applied for several patents for hair implements in the 1890s. See Patent Record no. 463,328 (November 17, 1891) for "Crimping and Curling Iron"; Patent Record no. 466,057 (December 29, 1861) for "Curling-Iron"; Patent Record no. 11,237 (reissued April 26, 1892) for "Curling Iron"; Patent Record no. 489,217 (January 3, 1893) for "Crimping Iron."

39. In 1859, a listing for "Gray, J. and Co. (Jay Gray and Jacob Harper)" at 77 Clark Street appears in the Chicago City Directory, under the headings of "Hair Dressers" and "Hair Ornaments and Jewelery." J. Gray continued to list his business at 77 Clark Street each year in the Chicago City Directories. By 1865–66, the listing is "Jared Gray" at 77 Clark Street. Directories, *Halpin's Eight Annual Edition Chicago City Directory* (Chicago: T. M. Halpin, respective years).

40. "He denies it . . ." Illinois, vol. 35, p. 66, December 15, 1869, R. G. Dun and Company Collection, Baker Library, Harvard Business School. "No credit in this city . . ." Illinois, vol. 35, p. 66, May 18, 1870, R. G. Dun and Company Collection, Baker Library, Harvard Business School.

41. Losses in fire, see Illinois (Chicago), vol. 37, p. 162, R. G. Dun and Company Collection, Baker Library, Harvard Business School, "Gray and Barrows," dated October 8, 1871. Here the agent notes that the partnership of Gray and Barrows was "burnt out" during the fire, and the business destroyed. They received no insurance settlement, and outstanding debts precluded any new credit extension. It is unclear what Barrows did, but Gray reopened his business under his wife's name. But in 1876 an agent reported that Gray still had outstanding debts of $11,567.48 and had no assets (Illinois [Chicago], vol. 37, p. 162, R. G. Dun and Company Collection, Baker Library, Harvard Business School, "Gray and Burrows," dated March

14, 1876). "lost everything . . ." Illinois, vol. 37, p. 258, June 1872, R. G. Dun and Company Collection, Baker Library, Harvard Business School, "Mrs. J. Gray."

42. See Edward J. Balleisen, *Navigating Failure: Bankruptcy and Commercial Society in Antebellum America* (Chapel Hill: University of North Carolina Press, 2001), esp. 78–79. This "hiding behind the wife's skirts," as one contemporary cartoon termed it (see 79) was a common practice. Some agents chose to continue to file reports under the husband's name, while others began a new listing under the wife's name.

43. "Human Hair: The Magnitude and Importance of the Trade: J. Gray, Chicago," *Republican Daily Journal* (Lawrence, Kansas), July 4, 1873.

44. Illinois, vol. 37, p. 258, March 6, 1875, R. G. Dun and Company Collection, Baker Library, Harvard Business School, "Mrs. J. Gray."

45. Clapp and Company, *Catalogue* (New York: Clapp and Company, 1888), 117; J. H. Purdy and Company, *Twentieth Century Catalogue of Supplies for Watchmakers, Jewelers and Kindred Trades* (Chicago: J. H. Purdy and Company, 1899), 747; S. H. Clement Company, *Wholesale Jewelers' Pamphlet* (Chicago: S. H. Clement, 1889); A. C. Becken Company, *Fourteenth Annual Illustrated Catalogue and Price List* (Chicago: A. C. Becken, 1905), 768.

46. Montgomery Ward and Company, *1894–95 Catalogue and Buyers Guide, No. 56* (republished by DBI Books, Northfield, Ill.: 1977), 153.

47. *Ehrich's Fashion Quarterly* 6 (Spring 1880): 107. Dry Goods, Box 9, Folder Ehrich Bros. 1880, Warshaw Collection.

48. Busiest House in America, *Illustrated Catalogue; Jeweler's Wholesale Supply Depot* (Chicago: 1883), 231.

49. Busiest House in America, *Illustrated Catalogue; Jeweler's Wholesale Supply Depot* (Chicago: 1884), 224.

50. Mrs. C. S. Jones and Henry T. Williams, *Ladies' Fancy Work: Hints and Helps to Home Taste and Recreations* (New York: Henry T. Williams, 1876), 4.

51. National Artistic Hair Work Company, *Catalogue of Designs for Artistic Hair Scenery and Ornaments* (Chicago: 1886), 4.

52. See Miles Orvell, *The Real Thing: Imitation and Authenticity in American Culture, 1880–1940* (Chapel Hill: University of North Carolina Press, 1989).

53. Philippe Perrot, *Fashioning the Bourgeoisie: A History of Clothing in the Nineteenth Century*, trans. by Richard Bienvenu (Princeton, N.J.: Princeton University Press, 1994), 71–72, states that "such newly discovered chemical processes and products as pinchbeck, electroplating, paste jewelry, and imitation leather" provided imitations of formerly expensive materials.

Chapter 5. Fancies of the Heart

1. Some women made hair wreaths but purchased hair jewelry. See, for example, the wreath made by Martha Doege Schultz, and the purchased jewelry. Wreath, no. 68.158.5, Minnesota Historical Society, St. Paul, Minnesota. Donor comments: "made when young [maker born 1850]." Donor, Gertrude and Esther Schultz. Watch fob, no. 68.158.2, and ring, no. 68.158.5, also owned by M. D. Schultz.

2. "Be Gentle to Thy Husband," *Lady's Almanac for 1860* (Boston: Shepard, Clark, and Brown, 1860), 9.

3. James C. Mohr, ed., *The Cormany Diaries: A Northern Family in the Civil War*, (Pittsburgh, Pa.: University of Pittsburgh Press, 1982), Samuel Cormany, October 8, 1860, 89. See Angel Kwolek-Folland, "The Elegant Dugout: Domesticity and Moveable Culture in the United States, 1870–1900," *American Studies* 25 (Fall 1984): 21–37, and "The Useful What-Not and the Ideal of 'Domestic Decoration'," *Helicon Nine* 8 (1983): 72–83, for discussions of this phenomena.

4. Henry T. Williams published, and sometimes co-wrote, many domestic manuals, including *The Ladies' Complete Manual of Home Duties* (New York: World Manufacturing Company, 1885), with "Daisy Eyebright"; with Mrs. C. S. Jones, *Beautiful Homes, or, Hints in House Furnishing*, vol. 4, Williams Household Series (New York: Henry T. Williams, 1878); and Annie S. Frost, *The Ladies' Guide to Needlework, Embroidery, etc. etc.* (New York: Henry T. Williams, 1877). Williams and Jones, *Beautiful Homes*, 6. See Elizabeth White Nelson, *Market Sentiments: Middle-Class Culture in Nineteenth-Century America* (Washington, D.C.: Smithsonian Books, 2004), 149–150, for a discussion of Williams and Jones's "household elegancies."

5. Julia McNair Wright, *The Complete Home: An Encyclopaedia of Domestic Life and Affairs* (Philadelphia: J. C. McCurdy and Company, 1879), 25.

6. Mary Virginia (Hawes) Terhune, *House and Home; a Complete Housewife's Guide by Marion Harland* [pseudonym] (New York: Union Publishing House, circa 1889), 15.

7. Wright, *The Complete Home*, 151.

8. Julia Darrow Cowles, *Artistic Home Furnishings for People of Moderate Means* (New York: F. M. Lupton Publishers, 1898), 201.

9. Wright, *The Complete Home*, 464.

10. John A. Anderson, "Policy of the Regents," *State Board of Agriculture: The Third Annual Report to the Legislature of Kansas for the Year 1874* (Topeka, Kans.: George W. Martin, State Printing Works, 1875), 259–319. This essay lays out the rationale for creating in the Kansas Agricultural College four distinct courses of study: Farmer, Mechanic, Professional, Woman. These courses of study were not adopted; although, in 1874, the Kansas Normal School was created. See Clifford S. Griffin, *The University of Kansas: A History* (Lawrence: University Press of Kansas, 1974), 111, for a discussion of the Normal School. See pages 280–282 for a discussion of the early 1900s institution of the department of "Household Science," a course of study specifically for women.

11. George A. Peltz, ed. *The Housewife's Library* (Englewood, N.J.: Englewood Publishing Company, 1885), 490.

12. Williams and Jones, *Beautiful Homes*, 5.

13. Wright, *The Complete Home*, 26.

14. "Home After Business Hours," *Godey's Lady's Book* (January 1883), 43. For a discussion of the centrality of the image of the fireside in middle-class nineteenth-century homes, see Kate Roberts, "Fireside Tales to Fireside Chats: The Domestic Hearth," in *The Arts and the American Home, 1890–1930*, ed. Jessica H. Foy and Karal Ann Marling (Knoxville: University of Tennessee Press, 1994), 44–61. For the

"lonely man" view of the fireside as the site of unfulfilled revery, see Vincent J. Bertolini, "Fireside Chastity: The Erotics of Sentimental Bachelorhood in the 1850s," *American Literature* 68, no. 4 (December 1996): 707–738. For a delightful visual representation of the bachelor-at-hearth image so popular in the nineteenth century, see *The Sportsman's Dream* by C. F. Senior, reprinted in Harold L. Peterson, *Americans at Home: From the Colonists to the Late Victorians; a Pictorial Source Book of American Domestic Interiors with an Appendix of Inns and Taverns* (New York: Scribner, 1971), plate 177. As Peterson described this work, "It is a cheery masculine interior, comporting well with Victorian coziness," while, Peterson continues, it wholly misrepresented the gun, fishing tackle, and the fox rug, which "must certainly have been one of the largest in creation!"

15. Effie Woodward Merriman, comp., *Home Decorative Work* (Minneapolis, Minn.: Buckeye Publishing Company, 1891), n.p.

16. Williams and Jones, *Beautiful Homes*, 3.

17. See Colleen McDannell, *The Christian Home in Victorian America, 1840–1900* (Bloomington: Indiana University Press, 1986), 49. McDannell argues that religion itself was used to accomplish this as well: "By linking morality and religion with the purchase and maintenance of a Christian home, the Victorians legitimized acquisition and display of domestic goods."

18. Williams and Jones, *Beautiful Homes*, preface.

19. Williams and Jones, *Beautiful Homes*, 7. Williams and "Daisy Eyebright," *The Ladies' Complete Manual of Home Duties*, 94. In her book *France at the Crystal Palace: Bourgeois Taste and Artisan Manufacture in the Nineteenth Century* (Berkeley: University of California Press, 1992), Whitney Walton argues that for the French immediately after the exhibition in 1851 phrases like "simple" and "elegant" were often used to describe the most ornate objects in the exhibition, and such terms allow the emergent middle class to contrast itself from the prolifigacy of the aristocracy. Thus, no matter an object's ornate appearance, a term such as "simple" was used to designate an object appropriate for the refined, bourgeois taste. While Walton's thesis works well for French middle-class society post-1850s, I would argue that the American tastemakers used the term "simple" to suggest a mythical colonial past of frugality, uprightness, and morality. See David Shi, *The Simple Life: Plain Living and High Thinking in American Culture* (New York: Oxford University Press, 1985), for a detailed discussion of the concept of simple living in American culture, especially its literature. Leo Marx, *The Machine in the Garden: Technology and the Pastoral Ideal in America* (New York: Oxford University Press, 1964), and T. J. Jackson Lears, *No Place of Grace: Antimodernism and the Transformation of American Culture, 1880–1920*, 3rd ed. (Chicago: University of Chicago Press, 1994), both examine the strand of antimodern thought in American culture.

20. Wright, *The Complete Home*, 150.

21. Ibid.

22. Ibid.

23. *Madam Worth's Kensington and Fancy Work Manual* (Wallingford, Conn.: R. L. Spencer, 1886), introductory page (no pagination).

24. Ibid. It should be noted that in this context, "public" has a limited connotation. As Lewis O. Saum noted in *The Popular Mood of Pre-Civil War America*

(Westport, Conn.: Greenwood Press, 1980), "Family, friends, church and immediate community were construed as society" xx. Ms. (Jenny Jone) Croly, ed., *Needlework: A Manual of Stitches and Studies in Embroidery and Drawn Work* (New York: A. L. Burt, 1885), 83.

25. While for married women the parlor was the venue of self-expression, for their daughters, especially young women of the 1880s on, the bedroom could serve as a private/public place of "writing one's self" through display of goods. For girls, bedroom decoration was viewed as a form of self-cultivation, and "the bedroom was significant in legitimizing the privatization of the home as it provided a site for self-cultivation." Carolyn E. Brucken, "Victorian Privacy: An Analysis of Bedrooms in American Middle-Class Homes from 1850–1880" (Master's thesis, University of Delaware, 1991). "The Daughter's Bedroom," *Demorest's Family Magazine* 28, no. 8 (June 1892): 497–499, gives detailed instructions on the decoration of an ideal room. The author of "The Daughter's Bedroom" suggested a divan, books, watercolors on the wall and a washstand curtain; such a room was clearly intended to serve public, quasi-parlor functions for a young, unmarried middle-class daughter. See also Sally McMurry's analysis of young women's bedrooms in *Families and Farmhouses in Nineteenth Century America: Vernacular Design and Social Change* (New York: Oxford University Press, 1988).

26. Croly, *Needlework: A Manual of Stitches and Studies*, 83.

27. "The Useful and the Ornamental in Ladies' Work," *Godey's Book and Magazine* 50 (May 1855), 424.

28. Laura Carter Holloway Langford, *The Hearthstone; or, Life at Home* (Beloit, Wis.: Inter-State Publishing House, 1883), in *Gerritsen Collection of Women's History* (microform series or gerritsen.chadwyck.com), 53–54, f#A1622.3.

29. Williams and "Daisy Eyebright," *The Ladies' Complete Manual of Home Duties*, 144. Charles E. Sargent, *Our Home, or Influences Emanating from the Hearthstone* (Springfield, Mass.: King-Richardson Company, 1900), 33. *Madam Worth's Kensington and Fancy Work Manual*, introduction. Mary Virginia (Hawes) Terhune, *House and Home* in *Gerritsen Collection of Women's History* (microform series or gerritsen.chadwyck.com), p. 15, f#2814.1.

30. Mary P. Ryan, *Cradle of the Middle Class: The Family in Oneida County, New York, 1790–1865* (Cambridge: Cambridge University Press, 1981), 33.

31. See *Transactions of the Kansas State Board of Agriculture*, ed. Alfred Gray (Topeka, Kans.: S. S. Prouty, 1872); *Report of the State Board of Agriculture to the Legislature of Kansas for the Year 1873* (Topeka, Kans.: George W. Martin, State Printing Works, 1874); *State Board of Agriculture: The Third Annual Report to the Legislature of Kansas for the Year 1874* (Topeka, Kans.: George W. Martin, State Printing Works, 1875).

32. Catherine E. Kelly, "'The Consummation of Rural Prosperity and Happiness': New England Agricultural Fairs and the Constructions of Class and Gender, 1810–1860," *American Quarterly* 49, no. 3 (September 1997): 574–602. Kelly discusses the inclusion of fancywork, the criticism with which these products of women's work were met, and the shift from more overtly economic production (that is, woven cloth) to more decorative items.

33. Mrs. J. W. Likins, *Six Years' Experience as a Book Agent in California* (San

Francisco: Women's Union and Job Printing Office, 1874), 52–80. Selection reprinted in *So Much to Be Done: Women Settlers on the Mining and Ranching Frontier*, ed. Ruth B. Moynihan, Susan Armitage, and Christiane Fischer Dischamp (Lincoln: University of Nebraska Press, 1990), 45.

34. *Transactions of the Kansas State Board of Agriculture* (1872), Class K "Textile Fabrics," Lot 47, 182. Also listed is Mrs. E. Wilder of Topeka, Kansas. In 1874, Class J "Fine Arts," held Lot 50 "Jewelry and Silverware," where Mrs. D. A. Smith of Topeka is noted for "best display of hair jewelry and fancy hairwork made in Kansas" (182). Mrs. D. A. Smith may very well have been a businesswoman in hairwork, for another lot, Lot 53 "Needle and Fancy Work," lists a prize for Mrs. Rhoda Hayes, Grasshopper Falls, Kansas, for best hairwork (183). For a complete history of the county fairs in Kansas, see Cathy J. Ambler, "The Look of the Fair: Kansas County Fairscapes, 1854–1994," (Ph.D. diss., University of Kansas, 1996).

Other state fairs featured women's domestic crafts, including hairwork. For instance, Karal Ann Marling, *Blue Ribbon: A Social and Pictorial History of the Minnesota State Fair* (St. Paul: Minnesota Historical Society Press, 1990), 236, has a photograph of the state fair art gallery in the 1880s with hair wreaths displayed.

35. Mrs. Mary T. Gray, "Report of the Superintendent of Fine Arts and the Children's Department," *State Board of Agriculture: The Third Annual Report to the Legislature of Kansas for the Year 1874* (Topeka, Kans.: George W. Martin, 1875), 79–81. Mary Gray is the first female superintendent of this category listed, with those heading the class lots in 1872 and 1873 being male. Although it is extremely unlikely that Mary Gray's call for financial support was a contributing factor, it should be noted that the following year, the State of Kansas temporarily ceased holding a state fair. In the *Fourth Annual Report of the State Board of Agriculture to the Legislature of the State of Kansas (1875)* (Topeka, Kans.: Office of the State Board of Agriculture, 1875), an unknown officer of the State Board stoutly maintains that "state fairs under the auspices of the State, and at the expense of the public treasury, are more than a humbug—they are a gross wrong," 6.

36. John A. Anderson, "Woman's Course," *State Board of Agriculture: The Third Annual Report to the Legislature for the Year 1874* (Topeka, Kans.: Office of the State Board of Agriculture, State Printing Works, 1874), 278.

37. John A. Anderson was a member of the Kansas Board of Regents in 1872 and 1873, and was also pastor of the Junction City Presbyterian Church, and later president of the Agricultural College. In 1876, the Board required by legislation that a "Normal" department be created at the University of Kansas (see *Eleventh Annual Catalogue of the Officers and Students of the University of Kansas, 1875–6* (Lawrence, Kans.: H. A. Cutler Book and Job Printer, 1877). The Normal School was filled with predominantly female students (in 1875–76, its first year, there were 2 men and 33 women). See Griffin's *The University of Kansas.*

38. Mary E. Wilkins Freeman, "A Souvenir," *Harper's New Monthly Magazine* 70, no. 418 (March 1885): 590–596. I thank Susan Strasser, who in turn thanks Ann Romines, for bringing this short story to my attention. All quotes hereafter are from this text.

39. This wreath is designated as the Peffer family wreath. Museum no. 1882, Waukesha County Museum and Historical Society, Waukesha, Wisconsin, Donor,

Alvina Peffer, 1867. A handwritten caption on the wreath reads: "The wreath is made from the hair of the children of Mr. and Mrs. Harry A. Luke, a sister of Mr. Luke made it. The children are: Lewis Luke, Mrs. Emelia Ruppert nee Luke, Mrs. Tim Breheim nee Luke, Mrs. Nettie West nee Luke, Mrs. Alvina Peffer nee Luke, and Harry Luke. All living in the town of New Berlin, Waukesha Co., WIS. A Pioneer family that settled in New Berlin in 1840."

40. See *Obituary Notebook* and *Pioneer Notebook*, Waukesha County Museum and Historical Society, Waukesha, Wisconsin, for the family records of the Luke family. In addition, the wreath probably does not date later than 1883–1885 given to the manufacture style and use of small, vibrant colored glass beads, which do not appear in many wreaths of known dated provenance post-1885. Such a precise listing of the individuals whose hair is used to create the wreath is revealing. Despite her central role as creator of the wreath itself, Luke's sister neglected to include her own hair and name.

41. Wreath, no. 1966.54, Ruth Ketterer Harris Costume and Textile Collection, Helen Louise Allen Textile Collection, University of Wisconsin—Madison. Donated by Milton F. Hulburt, with handwritten caption. The Daniel Webster referred to is the Unionist senator and representative, born in 1782 and dying in 1852. As the *Encyclopedia Americana*, International edition (Danbury, Conn.: Grolier Inc.), noted in 1993, "No descendant bearing the Webster name is now alive," 558.

42. Wreath, no. 3840, Waukesha County Museum and Historical Society, Waukesha, Wisconsin. Donors Mrs. Charles Bartlett, Mrs. Laura Kober, and Mrs. Frank Nevins of Big Bend, Wisconsin.

43. Wreath, no. 7770.32. Minnesota Historical Society, St. Paul, Minnesota. Donor, G. E. Tuttle, from the estate of Mrs. Jessie Hale Tuttle.

44. Hair tree, no. 7479.1, Minnesota Historical Society, St. Paul, Minnesota. Donor, Richard R. Sackett. Dimensions are 7.5 inches tall, and 5.5 inches wide at the widest part.

45. Hair picture, no. 8347/HH05D, Minnesota Historical Society, St. Paul, Minnesota. Donor, Mrs. C. G. Schulz. Dated 1890.

46. Hair wreath, no. 94.41.1., Blue Earth County Historical Society, Blue Earth, Minnesota. Donor, Lou Ella Schroeder. Donor's note: "Hannah's hair was used for this wreath. She was born January 1882 and died February 1894 from scarlet fever. Siblings of Hannah were Sarah, Peder, and Alfred."

47. Adelaide Dickinson, Scrapbook, undated. Museum no. 61.14.6/MC-06/HC-M2-H-0-6. Donor, Scott DeLong, Anoka, Minnesota. Minnesota Historical Society, St. Paul, Minnesota. This arrangement appears in all pages in which a male-female pair are arranged at the top of a page.

48. See also, for instance, the album, accession no. 2941, Sheboygan County Historical Research Center, Sheboygan, Wisconsin, and the Mabel Marvin Hair Scrapbook, dated 1858, no. 9530.109, Minnesota Historical Society, St. Paul, Minnesota.

49. Hair family album, private collection of Leila Cohoon, The Hair Museum, Independence, Missouri.

50. Rachel Bowman, diary entry, March 31, 1862. Several days later, she continues her scrapbook activity, this time by herself. On April 3, 1862, she writes,

"Worked at my scrapbook. finished one. & am so well pleased with it that I have commenced another." Mohr, *The Cormany Diaries*, 163; 164.

51. "Scrap-Books," *Harper's Bazaar* 9, no. 27 (July 1, 1876): 1. This article suggests two kinds of scrap albums: the decorative fancy album for the drawing room, and a plainer, larger album.

52. Patricia P. Buckler and C. Kay Leeper, "An Antebellum Woman's Scrapbook as Autobiographical Composition," *Journal of American Culture* 14, no. 1 (Spring 1991): 1–8, also argue that scrap albums are autobiographical.

53. It may be guessed, though without any definitive proof, that Salome Flanagan was a young woman, probably in her teenage years. Her indulgence in the more sentimentalized elements of mourning, the gift itself, and even the mere fact it is a scrap album, suggest a young woman in her teens as the creator. Gaye Smith, *Sentimental Souvenirs: Victorian Scrap Albums from the Sir Harry Page Collection*, Catalog of exhibition, Holden Gallery, Faculty of Art and Design, Manchester Polytechnic, April 10–May 12, 1987, Manchester, England, notes that "provenance of albums in this exhibition reveals that ownership was often in the hands of teenage girls from well-educated families," 1.

54. Unfortunately, Salome Flanagan does not often provide full names or familial relationship terms, instead simply using a set of initials. This makes it difficult to "read" the text of the captions, as relationships between represented individuals are difficult to ascertain.

55. On mid-Victorian markers, the female (signified by a ruffle at the wrist) and male (signified by a plain, austere cuff) were joined together in a handclasp. The clasped-hand motif has been explained as a cemetery symbol of the Second Great Awakening Protestant revival; see Parker B. Potter, Jr., and Mark P. Leone, eds., *The Recovery of Meaning: Historical Archaeology in the Eastern United States* (Washington, D.C.: Smithsonian Institution Press, 1988), 468, and Louise Ann Wurst, "'A Rope of Sand': Second Great Awakening Symbolism on Gravestones of the Rural Elite in Broome County, New York" (master's thesis, Temple University, 1986), 37. The Flanagan album is from Upper New York, a primary locale of the Great Awakenings. At the same time, cemetery studies have made clear that the clasped hand is as much a product of commercial popularity as it is a folk symbol (see Colleen Nutty, "Cemetery Symbolism of Prairie Pioneers: Gravestone Art and Social Change in Story County, Iowa," *Journal of the Iowa Archeological Society* 31 [1984]:1–135). Finally, see Leonard V. Huber, *Clasped Hands: Symbolism in New Orleans Cemeteries* (Lafayette: University of Southwestern Louisiana, 1982), 1–10. Here, Jessie J. Poesch in her preface notes that the hands and other symbols were folk motifs.

56. Such creative blending of the commercial and noncommercial differs from many scrap albums of the time period. As Gaye Smith noted in *Sentimental Souvenirs*, with the prescriptive literature and instructions, the "scrap kits," and the array of scrapbook tools to buy (lithographs, gum arabic, etc.), "even attempts at handmade souvenir scrapbooks had become mechanical exercises, almost 'painting by numbers' in characters."

Chapter 6. A Man's Precious Talisman

1. Ellen K. Rothman, *Hands and Hearts: A History of Courtship in America* (New York: Basic Books, Inc., 1984), remarks that "it was his relationship with his mother that carried the emotional current in [his] life" (116).

2. See E. Anthony Rotundo, *American Manhood: Transformations in Masculinity from the Revolution to the Modern Era* (New York: Basic Books, 1993), 35–38, 45–46 for a discussion about men and violence, and the role of mother in ameliorating this. As Anthony Rotundo observes, "Life in a middle-class household taught children to associate the female with nurture, interdependence, and restraint, while linking maleness to power, independence, and freedom of action" (176).

3. Rothman, *Hands and Hearts*, 69.

4. Museum no. 1968.0417.0004, Wisconsin Historical Society, Madison, Wisconsin. Dated 1875, no donor information available.

5. Museum no. 602, Waukesha County Museum and Historical Society, Waukesha, Wisconsin. Donor, Florence Hengen. Donor note: "Taken of Jacob Hengen's mother sent to him by his brother in Germany." For a similar style of bookmark, without a verse, see "Bible Book-Mark," *Godey's Book and Magazine* 64(May 1862), 494.

6. For discussion of the historical evidence supporting this perspective, see Mark C. Carnes, *Secret Ritual and Manhood in Victorian America* (New Haven, Conn.: Yale University Press, 1989), 116–119; Rothman, *Hands and Hearts*, 69, 116; Rotundo, *American Manhood*, 25, 92; and Samuel Watson, "Flexible Gender Roles During the Market Revolution: Family, Friendship, Marriage, and Masculinity Among U.S. Army Officers, 1815–1846," *Journal of Social History* 29, no. 1 (1995): 81–107. The quotation, "exalted . . ." is from Rotundo, *American Manhood*, 93. Rotundo notes that while often intensely emotional, brother-sister relationships were also political (see page 95). In his essay, Watson, "Flexible Gender Roles During the Market Revolution," discusses how men were often more tolerant of women's independence when carried out by their sisters (as opposed to, for instance, their prospective wives) (85–91).

7. See Mary Kelley's discussion of the relationship between Catharine Maria Sedgwick and her brother, Robert Sedgwick, December 1821, Catharine Maria Sedgwick Papers, Massachusetts Historical Society, as cited by Mary Kelley, "Introduction," *The Power of Her Sympathy: The Autobiography and Journal of Catharine Maria Sedgwick*, ed. Mary Kelley (Boston: Massachusetts Historical Society, distributed by Northeastern University Press, 1993), 26, note 34. I am also thinking of Carroll Smith-Rosenberg, "The Female World of Love and Ritual: Relations Between Women in Nineteenth-Century America," *Disorderly Conduct: Visions of Gender in Victorian America* (New York: Oxford University Press, 1985), 53–76, in which Smith-Rosenberg carefully outlines the autonomous, intensely emotional, same-sex friendships of young middle-class American women during this same time period.

8. Museum no. 62.140, Minnesota Historical Society, St. Paul, Minnesota. Donor, Clara F. O'Connor. Donor note: "man who owned it, Daniel O'Connor,

was born January 1, 1847, died May 26, 1898. Chain was made of sister hair, Anna O'Connor Bruce, who died 1924. He was born in Lowell, Massachusetts, and lived in Richmond, Virginia and came to St. Paul [Minnesota] 1860 on river steamer 'Mary Kent.'"

9. I never found any hairwork that suggested a male-to-male friendship or romantic connection. While it is certainly possible that some men exchanged hair gifts, there is no evidence of this.

10. Eva Illouz, *Consuming the Romantic Utopia: Love and the Cultural Contradictions of Capitalism* (Berkeley: University of California Press, 1997), 7, characterizes romantic love as utopian both in her title and in her discussion.

11. Both Illouz, *Consuming the Romantic Utopia*, and Karen Lystra, *Searching the Heart: Women, Men, and Romantic Love in Nineteenth-Century America* (New York: Oxford University Press, 1989), discuss romantic love as a avenue toward self-discovery for nineteenth-century Americans.

12. Rothman, *Hands and Hearts*, chapter 3, for a more complete discussion of how men and women used romance to balance conflicting gender distinctions that often seemed to contradict the blending demanded of a "successful" partnership.

13. This sketch of the shift from public to private display of engagements is derived from Rotundo, *American Manhood*, 116–117.

14. Mrs. Bradley, "The Hair Ring," *Home Magazine* (March 1855) vol. 5, issue. 3: 71.

15. For the historical significance of finger rings, see William Jones, *Finger-Ring Lore, Historical, Legendary and Anecdotal* (London: Chatto and Windus, 1898); George Frederick Kunz, *Rings for the Finger, from the Earliest Known Times to the Present* (Philadelphia: J. B. Lippincott Company, 1917); and Rachel Jean Monfredo, "American Finger Rings: Representing Bonds of Relationships" (master's thesis, University of Delaware, 1990).

16. Illouz, *Consuming the Romantic Utopia*, 26. Kathy Peiss, *Cheap Amusements: Working Women and Leisure in Turn-of-the-Century New York* (Philadelphia: Temple University Press, 1986), discusses the courtship practices of working-class women from 1880 to 1920.

17. Blanche Butler Ames, editor. *Chronicles from the Nineteenth Century: Family Letters of Blanche Butler Ames and Adelbert Ames* (Clinton, Mass.: Colonial Press, 1957). Anya Jabour's *Marriage in the Early Republic: Elizabeth and William Wirt and the Companionate Ideal* (Baltimore: Johns Hopkins University Press, 1998) account of a middle-class marriage between the years 1802 to 1834 resembles the relationship between Blanche Butler Ames and Adelbert Ames.

18. Letter from Adelbert Ames to Blanche Butler, April 25, 1870, *Chronicles from the Nineteenth Century*, 117. Similar ready-made paperweights, ready to be adorned with an image on the bottom, are still available. For instance, in 2006, paperweight blanks similar to those purchased by Ames (today, made of plastic or polystyrene) were available at national chains such as Walgreens, a drugstore chain, and Hobby Lobby, a crafts-supply store. Memorial paperweights were popular during the nineteenth century. See Geraldine J. Casper, *Glass Paperweights in the Art Institute of Chicago* (Chicago: Art Institute of Chicago, 1991), 95.

19. Adelbert Ames's status as a Civil War hero and his subsequent public ser-

vice has accorded him persistent recognition by both his family and American culture well into the twentieth century. See Blanche Butler Ames, *Adelbert Ames, 1835–1933; General, Senator, Governor; the Story of His Life and Times* (New York: Argosy-Antiquarian Press, 1964), for an extensive biography of a man written by his daughter. For an equally biased biographical sketch, see "Adelbert Ames," in *The Cyclopaedia of American Biography*, ed. Rossiter Johnson (Boston: Biography Society, 1904; reprint, Detroit: Gale Research Company, 1968), no pagination.

20. See Susan Stewart, *On Longing: Narratives of the Miniature, the Gigantic, the Souvenir, the Collection* (Baltimore: Johns Hopkins University Press, 1984). Colleen McDannell, in *Material Christianity: Religion and Popular Culture in America*, 2nd ed. (New Haven, Conn.: Yale University Press, 1995), 39–43, discusses souvenirs and relics. She examines the public and private dimensions of *memento mori* of the dead. Illustration 17 is of an example of hairwork. McDannell relies on Stewart for much of her interpretation.

21. Letter from Blanche Butler to Adelbert Ames, May 18, 1870, *Chronicles from the Nineteenth Century*, 129.

22. There were nineteenth-century beliefs that different hair colors had specific, historical significance. See "Red Hair," *Bentley's Miscellany* 29 (1851), 532–537, and "A Chapter on Human Hair," *Peterson's Ladies National Magazine* 24 (1853): 33–34. Echoing Blanche's self-scorn, the *Peterson's Ladies National Magazine*'s writer comments that red hair's "biological" components suggest that "to call red hair brimstone is, it thus appears, no exaggeration," since, according to the author, red hair is caused by an overabundance of carbon. In her novel, *Rose in Bloom* (Boston: Roberts Brothers, 1876; New York: Virago Press, 1990), Louisa May Alcott alludes to the "unromantic" qualities of red hair.

23. Susan Stewart, *On Longing*, suggests lockets "create an additional secret recess of the body" and, as such, "are always vulnerable to exposure," 127.

24. Letter from Adelbert Ames to Blanche Butler, May 27, 1870, *Chronicles from the Nineteenth Century*, 143.

25. For an example of a watch chain made of hair with a locket attached, see hair watch chain, no. 4528, Waukesha County Museum and Historical Society, Waukesha, Wisconsin.

26. Letter from Adelbert Ames to Blanche Butler, May 28, 1870, *Chronicles from the Nineteenth Century*, 148.

27. Susan Stewart, *On Longing*, maintains that "a locket is always threatened by loss, for its magic is dependent upon possession," 127.

28. I echo here Susan Stewart's thesis in her book, *On Longing*.

29. Letter from Adelbert Ames to Blanche Butler Ames, October 19, 1871, *Chronicles from the Nineteenth Century*, 336. By this date, Adelbert and Blanche have married, have had their first son, Butler, and have been separated several months as Adelbert campaigns in Mississippi.

30. Angel Kwolek-Folland argues, "Middle-class manhood, then, separated masculine endeavors and privileges from those of womanhood and located the basis of masculinity in men's relationship to their means of earning of living" (45), in her *Engendering Business: Men and Women in the Corporate Office, 1870–1930* (Baltimore: Johns Hopkins University Press, 1994).

31. Anne C. Rose, *Voices of the Marketplace: American Thought and Culture, 1830–1860* (New York: Twayne Publishers, 1995), notes that "antebellum Americans looked at men in the marketplace with divided feelings. They respected ambition and welcomed prosperity yet deeply worried that men were morally '*at risk*' in such competitive environments" (74).

32. Diary, Walter Mason Oddie (1808–1865). Winterthur Museum and Country Estate, Manuscript Collection. Folder 1, no. 3421, contains his diary. In Folder 2, no. 3421 is a lock of hair, wrapped in paper, and on the paper is written "Julia's March 1824." Walter Mason Oddie was a landscape artist. See Annette Blaugrund, "The 'Mysterious Mr. O.': Walter Oddie (1808–1865)," *American Art Journal* 12: no. 2 (Spring 1980): 60–77.

33. I should note here that I am conflating two pieces of evidence. The Winterthur collection separates Oddie's diary and the hair wrapped in the marked piece of paper. While Oddie does not note in his diary entry that he is indeed looking at the hair as he writes, the tokenism of the hair, and its well-worn folds of paper, suggest that he often did take out his wife's hair and look at it. The sentiment of the diary entry strongly suggests that he re-evoked emotion in himself through the practice of holding the hair as well as putting his thoughts on paper.

34. Ann Fabian, "Unseemly Sentiments: The Cultural Problem of Gambling," in *The Culture of Sentiment: Race, Gender, and Sentimentality in Nineteenth-Century America*, ed. Shirley Samuels (New York: Oxford University Press, 1992), 143–156. Fabian presents the habitual gambler Jonathan Green, who presented gambling, stealing, and dealing within the redemptive terms of sentiment, and provides a unique example of masculine sentimentality.

35. Vincent J. Bertolini, "Fireside Chastity: The Erotics of Sentimental Bachelorhood in the 1850s," *American Literature* 68, no. 4 (December 1996): 707–738. Bertolini characterizes such texts of "bachelor sentimentalism" as "female-authored sentimentalism," thus expressive of an ideological desire rather than actual male practice (710).

36. "The Blond Hair," *The Ladies' Magazine of Literature, Fashion and Fine Arts* (April 1844): 173–178.

37. Alice B. Neal, "Gift-Making," *Godey's Book and Magazine* 55 (November 1857): 423.

38. Neal, "Gift-Making," 426.

39. Alice Carey, *Clovernook, or Recollections of Our Neighborhood in the West*, 2nd ser., (New York: Redfield, 1854), 47. The young man's reversed collar is likely a collar that has been turned over, hiding the soiled front surface, or he was wearing his collar backward, imparting an ecclesiastical flavor to his costume.

40. Actually, the fashionable exterior and romantic interior could be considered, at least ideally, as the same thing. See Phyllis G. Tortora and Keith Eubank, *Survey of Historic Costume: A History of Western Dress*, 2nd ed. (New York: Fairchild Publications, 1994), chapter 12, "The Romantic Period: 1820–1850," 275–294.

41. Carey, *Clovernook*, 47.

42. Photograph, Harry Pinkney, Kansas Collection, Spencer Research Library, University of Kansas, Lawrence, Kansas, no. RH PH 18 K:94. The date is tentative. See Joan L. Severa, *Dressed for the Photographer: Ordinary Americans and Fashion,*

1840–1900 (Kent, Ohio: Kent State University Press, 1995), 208–210, for a summary of men's styles of the 1870s, and 387–388 for the 1880s. I chose an 1880s date for the following reasons: Severa suggests that by the 1880s, the oversized sack coat was shortened, took on a narrow fit, and shoulders set high. "Lapels were extremely narrow and small, as the coat was made to be closed high at the throat." For an example of nearly identical suit, dated 1871, see Margot Lister, *Costume: An Illustrated Survey from Ancient Times to the Twentieth Century* (Boston: Plays, Inc., 1968), figure XIV.38, p. 325. And Pinkney's split, high white collar likewise was in fashion. Severa notes that men wore "collars . . . of the stiff, standing style." Pinkney has combined his split high collar with a scarf, or tie. Most often, a man would have worn such a tie with a turn-down collar (the sort with little standout "wings," rather than the straight collar Pinkney wears). For examples of the waist-seamed coat style Pinkney wears, see *Bloomingdale's Illustrated 1886 Catalog (Fashions, Dry Goods, and Housewares)* (New York: Dover Publications, in association with the Henry Ford Museum and Greenfield Village, 1988), 105.

43. Severa, *Dressed for the Photographer*, 314. Severa notes that since the 1860s and well into the 1880s, one stylish touch was to wear one's sack jacket (a loosely cut, ready-made suit coat) "buttoned at the top button only, falling open to show the vest and watch chain." While most costume histories use the term "sack suit" to describe this loosely cut style, Marybelle S. Bigelow, *Fashion in History: Apparel in the Western World* (Minneapolis, Minn.: Burgess Publishing Co., 1970), notes that in the 1860s, "the *ditto* suit was introduced, consisting of matching pants, coat, and vest" (194).

44. Grant McCracken, "The Voice of Gender in the World of Goods: Beau Brummell and the Cunning of Present Gender Symbolism," in *The Material Culture of Gender / The Gender of Material Culture*, ed. Katherine Martinez and Kenneth L. Ames (Hanover, N.H.: University Press of New England, 1997), argues that George Bryan (Beau) Brummell's style of extremely disciplined clothing "made a fetish of self-possession." See also David Kuchta, "The Making of the Self-Made Man: Class, Clothing, and English Masculinity, 1688–1832," in Victoria de Grazia with Ellen Furlough, ed., *The Sex of Things: Gender and Consumption in Historical Perspective* (Berkeley, University of California Press, 1996), 54–78. As Kuchta explains, the self-disciplined model of dress increasingly represented the emerging ideal of masculinity in the nineteenth century. For an opposing view, which argues that men did not settle down into somber black suits, see Christopher Breward, *The Culture of Fashion: A New History of Fashionable Dress* (New York: Penguin Press, 1995), 170–179.

By the 1820s, ready-made suits began to be made for men; by the 1850s, ready-made clothing was fully in place in America; and by the 1870s and 1880s, when Mr. Pinkney shouldered his own lightly padded, wool, waist-seamed, high-buttoned coat, such "business" wear was readily available to most men. The date 1820 for ready-made suits in England is from Hollander, *Sex and Suits* (New York: Knopf, 1994),103–111. Phillipe Perott, *Fashioning the Bourgeoisie: A History of Clothing in the Nineteenth Century*, trans. Richard Bienvenu (Princeton, N.J.: Princeton University Press, 1994), argues that ready-to-wear suits become widespread by the 1840s "because of improved cutting and sewing techniques and an increasingly rational division of labor" (53). Michael Zakim, "Customizing the Industrial Revolution: The

Reinvention of Tailoring in the Nineteenth Century," *Winterthur Portfolio* 33, no. 1 (Spring 1998): 41–58, gives the date of 1850 for the United States, as measured as a sector of economic activity. See Robert Schorman, *Selling Style: Clothing and Social Change at the Turn of the Century* (Philadelphia: University of Pennsylvania Press, 2003), for an overview.

45. Eric Burton, *Dictionary of Clocks and Watches* (London: Arco Publications, 1962), 74. Also see Theodore Patrick Camerer Cuss, *The Story of Watches* (London: MacGibbon and Kai Ltd.; New York: Philosophical Library, 1952), 126. Pocket watches were first made in Europe in the 1600s and were either carried in a pocket or kept on a table or cabinet. See Frederick James Britten, *Old Clocks and Watches and Their Makers* (London: B. T. Batsford; New York: Scribner, 1899), 116.

Further complicating nomenclature matters is the fact that charms attached to the chains and bars were also known as "fobs." For the purposes of this discussion, an attached token will be known as a "charm," to distinguish it from the flat, short ribbon style I will call a "fob." While less prevalent, short fobs remained stylish throughout the nineteenth century. Indeed, as late as 1902, Sears, Roebuck and Company advertised short ribbon fobs, "of the finest silk web . . . The sale of them is increasing continually." *Sears, Roebuck and Company, Catalogue No. 111* (reprint, New York: Crown Publishers, 1969), 66. It should be noted that on the same page with several examples of ribbon fobs there are mountings for hair watch chains. Sales of ribbon fobs might very well have been increasing for, in 1908, *Catalogue No. 117* (reprint, edited by Joseph J. Schroeder (reprint, Chicago: Follett Publishing, 1969), 300, there were fifteen fobs, as compared to six three years earlier. See Doreen Yarwood, *English Costume from the Second Century B.C. to 1950* (New York: Crown Publishers, 1952), 201; Byrde, *The Male Image*, 81, for illustrations of this trouser style.

46. While knee breeches became unfashionable among urban middle- and upper-class men, English farmers and gentry were the holdouts. See Diana de Marly, *Fashion for Men: An Illustrated History* (New York: Holmes and Meier, 1985), 101–102. Penelope Bryde, *The Male Image: Men's Fashions in Britain, 1300–1970* (London: B. T. Batsford, 1979), offers an illustration of the older fob style with tight breeches, 81, and the new watch chain style discreetly hanging to the side of the vest, 84.

"Albert chains" have a bar to be drawn through a buttonhole of the vest. (Bryde, *The Male Image*, 223, dates this term to 1849, when Prince Albert was presented with a watch attachment of this style.) "Fob chains," the older term most specifically referring to the short, flat, ribbon, by mid-nineteenth century denotes a chain with fobs (tokens or charms) attached. "Vest chain" describes a longer, 2/3 length chain (that is, one that can be stretched across two-thirds of a man's torso). Finally, in this discussion, "fob" denotes the flat, short ribbon used to secure a pocket watch to the waistband of a man's trousers. "Watch chain" will refer to the longer chain that attaches a watch to the man's vest (therefore also referring to vest chains). This usage reflects how C. Jeanenne Bell, *Collector's Encyclopedia of Hairwork Jewelry, Identification and Values* (Paducah, Ky.: Collector Books, 1998), categorizes such jewelry. The confusing dual usage of the term "fob" is prevalent not only in fashion histories but also in catalogues of the time. *Funk and Wagnalls* defines a fob as "a watch pocket in the waistband of trousers; a chain or ribbon hanging from it; also, an ornament on a watch chain or ribbon." The chains were often adorned with "fobs," small charms that themselves were decorated with hair.

47. In "Time, Work-Discipline, and Industrial Capitalism," *Past and Present* 38 (December 1967): 56–97, E. P. Thompson argues that with the introduction of wage labor, "time is now currency: it is not passed but spent" (61).

48. As the penultimate development in this link between time and value, by the end of the nineteenth century, scientific management theory promised to make time pay all its worth. See Kwolek-Folland, *Engendering Business*, 73–76; and Martha Banta, *Taylored Lives: Narrative Productions in the Age of Taylor, Veblen, and Ford* (Chicago: University of Chicago Press, 1993).

49. Thompson, "Time, Work-Discipline, and Industrial Capitalism," asks, "If the transition to mature industrial society entailed a severe restructuring of working habits—new disciplines, new incentives, and a new human nature upon which these incentives could bite effectively—how far is this related to changes in the inward notation of time?" (57). Michael O'Malley, *Keeping Watch: A History of American Time* (Washington, D.C.: Smithsonian Institution Press, 1996), uses the word "control" in a dual sense: capitalism's attempt to further its control over workers, and workers' intensified integration of the discipline of self-control. See Michel Foucault, *Discipline and Punish: The Birth of the Prison*, trans. Alan Sheridan (New York: Vintage Books, 1977), for an extended discussion of this process of self-inculcation of control.

50. Stuart Sherman, *Telling Time: Clocks, Diaries, and English Diurnal Form, 1660–1785* (Chicago: University of Chicago Press, 1996), 177.

51. Mrs. Mary Virginia (Hawes) Terhune, *From My Youth Up* (New York: G.W. Carleton and Company, 1874), 297.

52. Michael O'Malley, *Keeping Watch*, 172. Willis I. Milham, *Time and Timekeepers, Including the History, Construction, Care and Accuracy of Clocks and Watches* (New York: Macmillan, 1923), argues that the first cheap pocket watch was attempted in 1875. This watch, if it had been successful, would have been priced at fifty cents. See Donald R. Hoke, *Ingenious Yankees: The Rise of the American System of Manufactures in the Private Sector* (New York: Columbia University Press, 1990), chapter 5, "The Development of Watch Manufacturing at the Waltham Watch Company, Waltham, Massachusetts, 1849–1910," 179–256. See also Milham, *Time and Timekeepers*, 407, for a more detailed account. The $3.00 to $5.00 price was not an insubstantial amount in 1880 dollars. If one calculates the cost in 2005 dollars, a watch cost $59.40 to $99.01. Cost was calculated using the Inflation Calculator, found at www.westegg.com/inflation, in 2006, using 1880 and 2005.

53. G. M. Hansen, *Novelties, Notions, and Jewelry Catalogue*, no date (circa 1870s). Warshaw Collection, Novelties Box, Folder 1. Edwin Creer, advertisement. In *Board-Work; or the Art of Wig-Making* (London: R. Hovendon and Sons, 1887).

54. Busiest House in America, *Illustrated Catalogue; Jeweler's Wholesale Supply Depot* (Chicago: 1888), 318, 319. J. H. Purdy and Company, *Twentieth Century Catalogue for Watchmakers, Jewelers and Kindred Trades* (Chicago: 1899), 600, 612, 613, 620, 621, 639. Winterthur Museum and Country Estate, Library. Montgomery Ward and Company, *Catalogue No. 56* (Fall-Winter, 1894–1895). Reprint edition, ed. Jo-

seph J. Schroeder, Jr. (Northfield, Ill.: DBI Books, 1977), 153; Sears, Roebuck and Company, *Catalogue No. 111.* Reprint edition, introduction by Cleveland Amory (New York: Crown Publishers, 1969), 66; *Catalogue No. 117*, ed. Joseph J. Schroeder (Chicago: Follett Publishing, 1969), 300; Montgomery Ward, *Catalogue No. 56*, 153.

55. Hair watch chain, no. 3363. Waukesha County Museum and Historical Society, Waukesha, Wisconsin. Donor, A. H. Youmans. Donor's notes "worn by Dr. H. A. Youmans, early physician of Mukwonago, for many years. Made of his wife's hair. Circa '1860s' by her son in the Civil War." It is possible that her son worked as a jeweler during the Civil War, and the implication of war service is misleading. This is the only male amateur hair worker of jewelry I found in my research. Samuel Caster, along with five other individuals, participated in the creation of a hair wreath. See "Family Album" wreath, private collection of Leila Cohoon. Wreath mounted on board pen-inscribed "Family Album" and lists six makers. Otherwise, male hair workers were professional men.

56. Hair watch chain, no. 1991.68.55.1, Wisconsin Historical Society, Madison, Wisconsin. Donors, Werner and Norma Wyss. Donors' notes: "Made by Norma's great grandmother, Rose Etta Barnett Sprague Evans, b. 1850, with her own hair. Made for her second husband John D. Evans, b. 1848 at the Columbian Exposition in Chicago." Rose and John lived in Springwater Town, Waukesha County, Wisconsin. There has been much written about the 1893 fair; see David J. Bertuca, chief compiler, *The World's Columbian Exposition: A Centennial Bibliographic Guide* (Westport, Conn.: Greenwood Press, 1996).

57. Hair watch chain, no. 3343, Waukesha County Museum and Historical Society, Waukesha, Wisconsin. Donor's notes: "made from hair of Mrs. Jane O. Hendley, and worn by her husband, Rev. Charles J. Hendley, for years. After his death, it was worn as a necklace."

58. Hair watch chain, no. 13001, Waukesha County Museum and Historical Society, Waukesha, Wisconsin. Donor, Mrytle E. Hawtin Filbey. Donor's notes: "made of the hair of Elizabeth Mills Hawtin, died 1928 used by her husband, William Henry Hawtin, d. 1919."

59. Williams and "Daisy Eyebright," *Beautiful Homes*, 6. "Home After Business Hours," *Godey's Book and Magazine* 66 (January 1863): 43. Leonore Davidoff and Catherine Hall, *Family Fortunes: Men and Women of the English Middle Class, 1780–1850* (Chicago: University of Chicago Press, 1987), 13. Davidoff and Hall are discussing, of course, the English middle class, but the same holds true for American men of the "white collar" class.

60. Davidoff and Hall, *Family Fortunes.*

61. Rotundo, *American Manhood*, 168–169.

62. Kwolek-Folland, *Engendering Business*, 118, notes, "A man's domestic, private space within a public space [and thereby] strengthened corporate claims of executive "fatherhood."

63. Kwolek-Folland, *Engendering Business*, 132.

64. There are many studies of this phenomenon. See Mary P. Ryan, *Women in Public: Between Banners and Ballots, 1825–1880* (Baltimore: Johns Hopkins University Press, 1990), 24–37; Kwolek-Folland, *Engendering Business*, 131.

Chapter 7. The Only Manufacturer Remaining

1. Busiest House in America, *Illustrated Catalogue; Jeweler's Wholesale Supply Depot* (Chicago: 1888), 319, for hair-chain mounts, and page 388 for garnet pins.

2. Clapp and Company, *Catalogue* (New York: Clapp and Company, 1888).

3. H. F. Leland (Worcester, Mass.), advertisement, *The Delineator* (October 1895): 30.

4. See "Notes," by Ruth Wales, 1982, located in the National Museum of American History, Smithsonian Institution, Costume Division, Moutoux File. I thank Shelley Foote, former museum specialist for her generosity in sharing this research.

5. William Ernst Moutoux notes, National Museum of American History, Smithsonian Institution, Costume Collection Files.

6. New York, vol. 179, September 1873, R. G. Dun and Company Collection, Baker Library, Harvard Business School, "William E. Moutoux."

7. "One Gets Old," *Brooklyn Nachrichten* (1909), submitted to the National Museum of American History, Smithsonian Institution, Costume Collection, by the Moutoux family. According to this story, William Ernst Moutoux left New York City and the hairwork business in 1884.

8. William Ernst Moutoux, advertisement, in *Jewelers' Circular and Horological Review* 10, no. 8 (1879): xx, and 15, no. 4 (1884): xxxvii.

9. Mrs. Matilda Marian Pullan, *The Lady's Manual of Fancy-Work: A Complete Instructor in Every Variety of Ornamental Needle-Work* (New York: Dick & Fitzgerald, 1859), 298.

10. Advertisement, *American Jeweler* 17, no. 7 (July 1897): 283. Moutoux ran the same advertisement in *American Jeweler* 17, no. 2 (February 1897): 79, and 17, no. 1 (January 1897): 30.

11. 1900 Census, 1060, p. 4, "Moutoux, William E."

12. "Hair, Ornamental," *The New York, Boston, Philadelphia and Baltimore Business Directory for General Business Reference* (New York: Commercial Publishing Company, 1900). Bourgard, Banout, Gleason, Pauly, and Wittenauer are listed. Of these, only Wittenauer had been conducting business in hairwork for very long.

13. "Katherine Louise M. Schmitt, hair jewelry," *Gopsill's Philadelphia City Directory for 1900* (Philadelphia: James Gopsill, 1900), 128, and *Gopsill's Philadelphia City Directory for 1901* (Philadelphia: James Gopsill, 1901), no listing.

14. *Our Salesman: Illustrated Price List and Jewelers' Reference Magazine* (Chicago: F. M. Sproehnle & Co., 1891), 69.

15. Ibid., hair-chain mountings, 75, repair list, 350.

16. *The A. C. B. Jewelers' Wholesale Price List for 1898* (Chicago: A. C. Becken Company, 1898), 96, 567.

17. *The Restless and the Sleepless Standard Annual Price List, The Jewelers' Encyclopedia* (Chicago: B. F. Norn's and Afisker 1899), gilt hooks, 645, hair-chain mountings, 102, 184, 185.

18. *Wholesale Dealers, St. Louis, MO*, C. R. Hetter Company listing (St. Louis: 1900), 243.

19. Montgomery Ward and Company, *Fall and Winter 1894–95 Catalogue and Buyers Guide No. 56*. Reprint, ed. Joseph J. Schroeder Jr. (Northfield, Ill.: Gun Digest Books, 1970), 153.

20. Sears does not specifically list human-hair vest chains made to order until 1896. See Sears, Roebuck and Company, *Catalogue No. 103* (1896), 409. For 1902, see Sears, Roebuck and Company, *Catalogue No. 111* (1902; reprint, New York: Crown Company, 1969).

21. Sears, Roebuck and Company, *Catalogue No. 117* (1908; reprint, ed. Joseph Schroeder, Chicago: Follet Publishing Company, 1969), 300.

22. This discussion of the market has relied on Walter Benn Michaels, *The Gold Standard and the Logic of Naturalism* (Berkeley: University of California Press, 1987), chapter two, "Dreiser's *Financier*: The Man of Business as the Man of Letters," 65, in particular.

23. Sears, Roebuck and Company, *Catalogue No. 117* (1908), 300. This is the only mention of machine-made hair jewelry I located that was addressed to customers rather than the trade. It is likely that some hairwork prior to this early twentieth-century offering was machine made. C. Jeanenne Bell, in her *Collector's Encyclopedia of Hairwork Jewelry* (Paducah, Ky.: Collector Books, 1998), plate 809, p. 223, notes that one extremely finely woven watch chain "is possibly a machine-made chain of human hair." Ms. Bell's expertise is appraising hairwork results from decades of antique jewelry trade and she is an expert in the field.

24. Cynthia Duval, *Infinite Riches: Jewelry through the Centuries* (Museum of Fine Arts, St. Petersburg, Florida, February 19–April 30, 1989, exhibition catalogue), notes that machine-made jewelry, popular by the 1850s in the United States, dramatically changed the styles of jewelry (17).

25. For a discussion of the importance of Providence, Rhode Island, in the jewelry trade see Philip Scranton, *Endless Novelty: Specialty Production and American Industrialization, 1865–1925* (Princeton, N.J.: Princeton University Press, 1997), 108–132.

26. W. W. Alden, "Braided Jewelry," Patent Application No. 169,940, patented November 16, 1875.

27. I suggest this as a possibility but with no evidence and, in fact, with evidence to the contrary. For example, in 1886 the W. C. Edge and Sons Company advertised its position as the "sole manufacturers and patentees of the woven fabric gold chain, and chain bracelets" and informed retailers that they were "prepared to furnish the trade with flat woven chain" in any length required. No hair is mentioned. W. C. Edge and Sons Company, advertisement, *Manufacturing Jeweler* 2, no. 4 (January 1886): 154.

28. S. F. Myers Company, Catalogue No. 192 (Fall 1901). National Museum of American History, Warshaw Collection, Box 4 Jewelry, Folder S. F. Myers.

29. A. C. Becken Company, *Fourteenth Annual Illustrated Catalogue and Price List* (Chicago: A. C. Becken, 1905), 111, depicts two "Gentlemen's Real Human Hair Vest Chains," and 768 lists hairwork repair. C. R. Hetter Jewelry Company, *Trade Price List (1907–1908)* offered only six styles of hair-chain mountings and a repair service, 97.

30. Louise F. Shaw, Patent Application No. 96,275, October 26, 1869, microfilm number 96275.

31. Ibid.

32. See, for example, "The Hair Trade: Making Merchandise of the Glory of Woman," *New-York Times* (May 15, 1870), p. 8, col. 1; "A Few Objections to the Use of False Hair," *Manufacturer and Builder* 5, no. 7 (July 1873): 163–164.

33. "Human Hair: Wigs, Waterfalls, Rats, Mice, Curls, Fronts, &c.—How They Are Made and All About Them," *New-York Times* (August 3, 1866), p. 8, col. 5. Hair was tariffed, and at relatively high rates, as this article alleged. In an 1869 report, manufactured human hair was taxed at a rate of $1.0926 per pound (by comparison, gilded porcelain was taxed at a rate of $0.091 dollars per pound). See *Monthly Report of the Deputy Special Commissioner of the Revenue* (September 30, 1869), Bureau of Statistics, Treasury Department. National Museum of American History, Warshaw Collection, Commission Merchants Box 2, Folder unmarked (last in box), 129. In a tariff summary of the years 1842 to 1862, it was noted that hair for "bracelets, chains, ringlets, and curls" was taxed at rates that varied from 24 to 35 percent, and unmanufactured hair (raw hair imported into the United States for domestic artificial-hair production) was tariffed at rates from 8 to 10 percent in the 1840s to the high of 30 percent in 1862. See J. Leander Bishop, *A History of American Manufactures from 1820–1868 . . . Comprising Annals of the Industry of the United States in Machinery, Manufacture, and Useful Arts* (Philadelphia: Edward Young and Company, 1866), 623. For insight on the business of a dry-goods commission agent who often purchased artificial hair from manufacturers, and then resold the goods to dry-goods retailers, see the materials on William E. Hawks, Commission Agent, 1867–1869, in the National Museum of American History, Warshaw Collection.

34. "Human Hair: Wigs, Waterfalls, Rats, Mice, Curls, Fronts, &c.—How They Are Made and all About Them," *New-York Times* (August 3, 1866), p. 8, col. 5.

35. Ibid. Most artificial-hairwork catalogues, that is, wig-supply catalogues, reinforce this national and racial hierarchy. See, for example, Madame Fried, *The Coiffure Beautiful*, illustrated catalogue (New York: no date [1890s to early 1900s]), National Museum of American History, Warshaw Collection, Hair Box 1, Folder, Fried, Madame; E. Burnham, *The Coiffure Catalog No. 37 (Illustrated)* (Chicago: 1908), National Museum of American History, Warshaw Collection, Hair Box 1, Folder, Burgess, BF.

36. "Gathering Human Hair in France," *New-York Times* (August 25, 1882), p. 3, col. 6.

37. See, for example, Edwin Creer, *Board-Work; or the Art of Wig-Making* (London: R. Hovendon and Sons, 1887), 14–15; "Human Hair: Wigs, Waterfalls, Rats, Mice, Curls, Fronts, &c.—How They Are Made and all About Them," *New-York Times* (August 3, 1866), p. 8, col. 5; "Gathering Human Hair in France," *New-York Times* (August 25, 1882), p. 3, col. 6; Charles Geniaux, "The Human Hair Harvest in Brittany," *Wide World Magazine* 4 (January 1900): 430–436; Charles Knight, ed., *The English Cyclopedia* (London: Bradbury and Evans, 1860).

38. Geniaux, "The Human Hair Harvest in Brittany," 430.

39. Ibid.

40. Ibid., 433.

41. Ibid., 435.

42. "Human Hair Market in France," *New York Daily Tribune* (August 12, 1860), p. 4, col. 1.

43. See Julius M. Price, *Same Fashion, Paris-London, 1786–1912* (New York: Scribner, 1913), 146.

44. "Human Hair Supplies: An Impending Crisis in the Market," *New-York Times* (Sunday, December 13, 1874), p. 4, col. 3.

45. George S. Coles, "Hair Manufacture," *A Complete Dictionary of Dry Goods* (Chicago: J. B. Herring Publishing Company, 1894), 125–127.

46. Hair picking was not limited to Europe. The R. G. Dun and Company credit agency rated two brothers who were professional hair pickers in 1876. The brothers, the Dougalls (or McDougalls) were "in business as hair pickers and do not purchase anything on their own . . . The McD's are attentive and industrious men, pay their rent promptly and seem to have a fair share of trade." New York, vol. 247, p. 2333, R. G. Dun and Company Collection, Baker Library, Harvard Business School.

47. "The Chinese Trade in Human Hair," *New-York Times* (June 27, 1877), p. 5, col. 1.

48. For a concise overview of the history of nativism in the United States, see Dale T. Knobel, *"America for the Americans": The Nativist Movement in the United States* (New York: Twayne Publishers, 1996); see also John Higham, *Strangers in the Land: Patterns of American Nativism, 1860–1925*, 2nd edition, (New Brunswick, N.J.: Rutgers University Press, 1988).

49. "Eight cars loaded with human hair . . ." *New York Daily Tribune* (November 24, 1893), p. 6, col. 6.

50. See Najia Aarim-Heriot, *Chinese Immigrants, African Americans, and Racial Anxiety in the United States, 1848–82* (Urbana: University of Illinois Press, 2003), for a general discussion of anti-Chinese sentiment in the United States and a detailed discussion of the passage of the 1882 exclusion law in Congress.

51. Harriet Amelia Smith, diary entry, September 1, 1863, in *To Pike's Peak by Ox-Wagon: The Harriet A. Smith Day-Book*, ed. Fleming Fraker Jr. (Iowa City: State Historical Society of Iowa, 1959), 37.

52. J. Fletcher, advertisement, Broadside, undated. Virgina Historical Society, Ho.3. At least one contemporary craftperson specializes in horsehair jewelry: Suzanne Storms offered "custom horsehair jewelry using hair from YOUR horse/pony" on a Web site (Suzanne Storms, Hairwork Artist, Custom Horsehair Jewelry, www.suzannestorms.com, accessed July 10, 2006). She is one of several horsehair jewelers offering goods on the Web. See also Marjorie Congram, *Horsehair: A Textile Resource* (Martinsville, N.J.: Dockwra Press, 1987).

53. "Hair-Device Workers," *Cornhill Magazine* 52, no. S5 (July 1885): 65. The implication in the quote that hairwork was associated with men rather than women, at least in its earliest years of popularity, is also evident in *Demorest's Magazine*. In 1878, that journal observed, "In the first instance [that is, the eighteenth century], hair jewelry was almost exclusively worn by gentlemen, who wore hair-rings and bracelets as souvenirs of their lady-loves." "Mrs. Demorest's 'What-to-Wear,' *Demorest's Family Magazine*, Fall/Winter 1877–1878, 58. The poem in question, *The*

Corsair, was published by Byron in 1814 and was extremely popular. The elaborate story is about a pirate captain whose wife kills herself in despair over his lengthy absence, and he then abandons his new love, a harem slave he had saved from a life of sexual servitude.

54. "Hair-Device Workers," *Cornhill Magazine* 52, no. S5 (July 1885): 65.

55. Graf Brothers, *Illustrated Catalogue and Price List* (New York, no date). National Museum of American History, Warshaw Collection, Hair, Box 1, Folder, Goody.

56. Wendell & Company, *Book of Designs* (New York: 1920–1921), National Museum of American History, Trade Catalog Collection no. 8894, no pagination.

57. Otto Young and Company, *53rd Annual Illustrated Price List of Jewelers' Merchandise* (Chicago: Otto Young and Company, 1924).

58. E. E. Crofut, *The Art of Hair Chain Braiding* (Malta, Mont.: E. E. Crofut, 1911), 5–6.

59. Crofut, *The Art of Hair Chain Braiding*, 37.

60. *Our Salesman*, illustrated catalog (Chicago: 1891), lists hair chains within this price range. Hair-chain mountings, 75.

61. Sears, Roebuck and Company, *Catalogue No. 111* (1902; reprint, New York: Crown Company, 1969).

62. Jennette Lee, "A Hair-Cut," *Living Age* 12, no. 230 (September 7, 1901): 659–661, excerpted from *A Pillar of Salt* (New York: Houghton Mifflin and Company, 1901). The author, Jennette Barbour Perry Lee [Mrs. Gerald Stanley Lee], was a popular novelist and short story author until the late 1930s in the United States. See Annie Russell Marble, *A Study of the Modern Novel: British and American Since 1900* (New York: D. Appleton and Company, 1928), 352, for a brief biography and selective bibliography of Lee's work.

63. Letter from Emily Elizabeth Dickinson to Emily Ford 1848, in *Letters of Emily Dickinson*, vol. 1, Mabel Todd Loomis, ed. (Boston: Roberts Brothers, 1894), 241.

64. Amelia Gere Mason, "Is Sentiment Declining?" *Century Illustrated Magazine* 61, no. 4 (February 1901): 627.

65. "Hair Jewelry To-Day," *New York Daily Tribune* (August 24, 1902), p. 5, col. 4.

Epilogue

1. Josephine H. Fitch, "Some Victorian Oddities," *Antiques* 6, no. 6 (December 1924): 316–318.

2. John Hill Morgan, "Memento Mori: Mourning Rings, Memorial Miniatures, and Hair Devices," *Antiques* 17 (March 1930): 226. See also Ruel Pardee Tolman, "Human Hair as a Pigment," *Antiques* 8, no. 6 (1925): 353, and "A Document on Hair Painting," *Antiques* 17, no. 3 (March 1930): 231.

3. Morgan, "Memento Mori," 229.

4. Ella Shannon Bowles, *Homespun Handicrafts* (Philadelphia: J. B. Lippincott Company, 1931), 179.

5. "Hair Watch Chains and Flowers," Ila A. Wright interview in *Western Folklore* 18 (1959): 114–117.

6. In addition to those articles specifically discussed here, see Doris M. Green, "Hair Jewelry," *Antiques Journal* 18, no. 6 (1963): 16–17; Richard Corson, *Fashions in Hair: The First Five Thousand Years* (New York: Hastings House, 1965), 472, 480–482; Janis Obst, "Hair Wreaths and Ornaments," *Gopher Historian* (Winter 1966–67): 8–9; Deidre O'Day, *Victorian Jewellery* (London: Charles Lett and Company Limited, 1974), 36–37; Lilian Baker Carlisle, "Hair Today, Shorn Tomorrow (sorry!)," *Yankee* 38, no. 1 (January 1974): 95–97, 108–110, 112–113; Virginia L. Rahm, "Human Hair Ornaments," *Minnesota History* (Summer 1974): 70–74.

7. Lilian Baker Carlisle, "Hair Work Jewelry," in *The Spinning Wheel's Complete Book of Antiques*, ed. Albert Christian Revi (New York: Grosset & Dunlap, 1972), 416–417.

8. Lilian Baker Carlisle, "Hair Work Flowers," *Antiques Journal* 26, no. 9 (September 1971): 35. However, in 1974, Carlisle argued that the longer hair in fashion since the 1950s suggested a revival of the craft (see "Hair Today," 97).

9. "Stellers [sic] Hair Jewelry," pamphlet, Steller's Jewelry, Milwaukee, Wisconsin, research files, Sheboygan County Historical Research Center, Sheboygan, Wisconsin.

10. C. Jeanenne Bell, *Collector's Encyclopedia of Hairwork Jewelry* (Paducah, Ky.: Schroeder Publishing, 1998).

11. Pauline C[oggleshall] Smith, "A Flower for Her Hair," in *Alfred Hitchcock The Best of Mystery* (New York: Galahad Books, 1987), 28–34; original version from *Alfred Hitchcock's Mystery Magazine* (July 1968). One side note to this: Smith has Aunt Abbie embroidering hair onto linen; a more likely craft would be wrapping the hair around wire to form the rose's petals.

12. See, for example, Lilian Jackson Braun, *The Cat Who Turned On and Off* (E. P. Dutton, 1968; reprint, New York: Berkley Publishing Group, 1986); Margaret Maron, *Corpus Christmas* (New York: Doubleday, 1989); Barbara Michaels, *Into the Darkness* (New York: Simon and Schuster, 1990); Corrine Holt Sawyer, *Murder by Owl Light* (New York: D. I. Fine, 1992); Cynthia Harrod-Eagles, *Death to Go* (New York: Scribner, 1994). This is undoubtably a partial list. See also Bailey White, *Sleeping at the Starlite Motel* (New York: Addison-Wesley, 1995), and Kathleen Norris, *Dakota: A Spiritual Geography* (New York: Houghton Mifflin, 1993), who mention hairwork in these memoirs. My thanks to Rosemary Arendt Sheumaker for these citations. Note that all the above-mentioned authors are women, suggesting perhaps that female authors in the late twentieth century are more likely to be cognizant of, and interested in, the presence and meanings of hairwork as feminine records of the past, even if the nineteenth-century connotations have all but disappeared in the rhetoric.

13. Emma Egy Miller Autograph Album, Watkins Community Museum, Lawrence, Kansas. Circa 1850s.

14. Garnett Family Papers, 1764–1944. Mss 1 G 1875 a 114–121, Section 15 (8 items), a 121, Virginia Historical Society, Manuscripts Collection.

Selected Bibliography

Artifact Collections

Blue Earth County Historical Society, Blue Earth, Minnesota
Leila Cohoon, Private Collection and The Hair Museum, Independence, Missouri
Minnesota Historical Society, St. Paul, Minnesota
Preble County Historical Society, Eaton, Ohio
Ruth Ketterer Harris Costume and Textile Collection, Helen Louise Allen Textile Collection, University of Wisconsin—Madison
Sheboygan County Historical Research Center, Sheboygan, Wisconsin
Smithsonian Institution, Washington, D.C.
Costume Collection, National Museum of American History
Domestic Life Division, National Museum of American History
Isadore Warshaw Collection of Business Americana, Archives Center, National Museum of American History
Norcross Greeting Card Collection, Archives Center, National Museum of American History
Virginia Historical Society, Richmond, Virginia
Watkins Community Museum, Lawrence, Kansas
Washington County Historical Society, Fort Calhoun, Nebraska
Waukesha County Museum and Historical Society, Waukesha, Wisconsin
Winterthur Museum and Country Estate, Winterthur, Delaware
Wisconsin Historical Society, Madison, Wisconsin

Manuscript Collections

Archives and Manuscripts, Chicago Historical Society, Chicago, Illinois
Manuscripts Collection, Minnesota State Historical Society Library, St. Paul, Minnesota
R. G. Dun and Company, Collection, Baker Library, Harvard Business School
Illinois, Volume 33, 35, 37
New York, Volume 179, 247, 329, 395, 409, 426
Philadelphia, Volume 1
Spencer Research Library, University of Kansas, Lawrence, Kansas
Kansas Collection, Spencer Research Library, University of Kansas, Lawrence, Kansas

Virginia Historical Society, Richmond, Virginia
Bernard Family Papers, 1821–1903
Bruce Family Papers 1836–1906
Garnett Family Papers, 1764–1944
Persinger Family Papers, 1865–1932
Washington County Historical Society, Fort Calhoun, Nebraska
Winterthur Museum and Country Estate
The Winterthur Library, Joseph Downs Collection of Manuscripts and Printed Ephemera
The Winterthur Library, Mobley Collection
The Winterthur Library, Printed Book and Periodical Collection

City Directories, Newspapers, Periodicals, and Trade Catalogs

City Directories, Chicago

Bailey and Edwards' Chicago Directory 1868. Chicago: Edwards and Co. Publishers, 1868.
Halpin's and Bailey's Chicago City Directory. Chicago: Halpin and Bailey, Publishers, 1862.
Halpin's Eighth Annual Edition Chicago City Directory, 1865–1866. Chicago: T. M. Halpin, 1865.

City Directories, Philadelphia

Boyd's Philadelphia City Business Directory. Wm. H. Boyd, compiler. Philadelphia: Joseph Monier, 1859.
Gopsill's Philadelphia City Directory for 1871. Philadelphia: James Gopsill, 1871.
Gopsill's Philadelphia City Directory for 1875. Philadelphia: James Gopsill, 1875.
Gopsill's Philadelphia City Directory for 1877. Philadelphia: James Gopsill, 1877.
Gopsill's Philadelphia City Directory for 1881. Philadelphia: James Gopsill, 1881.
Gopsill's Philadelphia City Directory for 1900. Philadelphia: James Gopsill, 1900.
Gopsill's Philadelphia City Directory for 1901. Philadelphia: James Gopsill, 1901.
McElroy's Philadelphia Directory, For 1855. Philadelphia: Edward C. and John Biddle, 1855.
McElroy's Philadelphia City Directory for 1861. Philadelphia: Edward C. & John Biddle and Company, 1861.

City Directories, Other

The Syracuse Directory. Syracuse, N.Y.: William H. Boyd, 1857.

Newspapers

Charleston City Gazette and Advertiser
Charleston Evening Gazette
Columbian Centinel (Boston)
Daily Gazette and Comet (Baton Rouge, Louisiana)
Federal Gazette (Philadelphia)
Fitchburg Sentinel (Massachusetts)
Gazette of the United States
General Advertiser (Philadelphia, Pennsylvania)
Maryland Gazette (Baltimore General Advertiser)
Maryland Journal (Baltimore)
New York Daily Tribune
New-York Times
Norfolk Herald
Pennsylvania Packet
Pennsylvania Packet (Dunlac's American Daily Advertiser)
Republican Daily Journal (Lawrence, Kansas)
Royal South Carolina Gazette (Charleston)
South Carolina and American General Gazette
South Carolina Gazette
Woods Newark Gazette and New-Jersey Advertiser

Periodicals

American Jeweler
The Delineator
Demorest's Magazine
Ehrich's Fashion Quarterly
Godey's Lady's Magazine and Book
Jewelers' Circular and Horological Review
Jewelers' Mercantile Agency Limited Directory for the Jobbing Trade Only
Le Bon Ton
Manufacturing Jeweller
Peterson's Magazine
The Watchmaker and Jeweler: Devoted to the Interests of Watchmakers, Jewelers, Silversmiths, etc.

Trade Catalogs

The A.C.B. Jewelers' Wholesale Price List for 1898. Chicago: A. C. Becken Company, 1898.

A. C. Becken Company. *Fourteenth Annual Illustrated Catalogue and Price List.* Chicago: A. C. Becken, 1905.

"Album of Hair Designs for Hair Jewelry." no author, no date [circa 1800].

Bloomingdale's Illustrated 1886 Catalog (Fashions, Dry Goods, and Housewares). New York: Dover Publications in association with the Henry Ford Museum and Greenfield Village, 1988.

Busiest House in America. *Illustrated Catalogue; Jeweler's Wholesale Supply Depot.* Chicago: 1883.

Busiest House in America. *Illustrated Catalogue; Jeweler's Wholesale Supply Depot.* Chicago: 1884.

Busiest House in America. *Illustrated Catalogue; Jeweler's Wholesale Supply Depot.* Chicago: 1888.

Clapp and Company. *Catalogue.* New York: Clapp and Company, 1888.

C. R. Hetter Jewelry Company. *Trade Price List (1907–1908).* St. Louis, 1901.

E. Burnham. *The Coiffure Catalog No. 37 (Illustrated).* Chicago: 1908.

G. M. Hansen. *Novelties, Notions, and Jewelry Catalogue,* no date [circa 1870s].

Graf Brothers. *Illustrated Catalogue and Price List.* New York, no date.

Henry Bristow, Price List. *Trade Catalogue: Ornaments, Novelties, Paper Flowers.* Washington, D.C.: Henry Bristow, 1886.

H. & G. Soule & Co. *Fine Jewelry and Ornamental Hair Work.* New York: Soule, 187-.

J. H. Purdy and Company. *Twentieth Century Catalogue of Supplies for Watchmakers, Jewelers and Kindred Trades.* Chicago: J. H. Purdy and Company, 1899.

Ladies' Art Company. *Illustrated Catalogue and Price List.* St. Louis, Mo.: Ladies' AA Company, 1897.

Madame Fried. *The Coiffure Beautiful.* New York: no date.

Montgomery Ward and Company. *Fall and Winter 1894–95 Catalogue and Buyers Guide No. 56.* Reprint, ed. Joseph T. Schroeder Jr. Northfield, Ill.: Gun Digest Books, 1970.

National Artistic Hair Work Company. *Catalogue of Designs for Artistic Hair Scenery and Ornaments Executed by National Artistic Hair Works of Chicago.* Chicago: National Artistic Hair Work Company, 1886.

Otto Young and Company. *53rd Annual Illustrated Price List of Jewelers' Merchandise.* Chicago: Otto Young and Company, 1924.

Our Salesman: Illustrated Price List and Jewelers' Reference Magazine. Chicago: F. M. Sproehnle & Co., 1891.

Sears, Roebuck and Company. *Catalogue No. 111.* Reprint edition. Introduction by Cleveland Amory. New York: Crown Publishers, 1969.

———. *Catalogue No. 117.* Reprint Edition. Joseph J. Schroeder, ed. Chicago: Follett Publishing, 1969.

The Restless and the Sleepless Standard Annual Price List. Chicago: B. F. Norn's Alister and Co., 1899.

S. F. Myers Company. *Catalogue No. 192.* New York: S. F. Myers Company, 1901.

S. H. Clement Company. *Wholesale Jewelers' Pamphlet.* Chicago: S. H. Clement, 1889.

Stellers' Jewelry. "Stellers Hair Jewelry." Pamphlet. Milwaukee, Wis.: Stellers, circa 1970s.

Waterman and Hunt. *Price List for Tools and Materials for Wax Flowers and Fruit-making*. Boston: circa 1885.

W[endell] & Company. *Book of Designs*. New York: 1920–1921.

Books and Pamphlets

Alcott, Louisa May. *Little Women*. 1868. New York: Puffin Books, 1952.

———. *Rose in Bloom*. Boston: Roberts Bros., 1876. Reprint, New York: Virago Press, 1990.

Arthur, Timothy Shay. "Taking Boarders." *Godey's Lady's Magazine* 42 (January 1851): 13–20; 42 (February 1851): 81–87; and 42 (March 1851): 160–167.

Bishop, J. Leander. *A History of American Manufactures from 1820–1868 . . . Comprising Annals of the Industry of the United States in Machinery, Manufacture, and Useful Arts*. Philadelphia: Edward Young and Company, 1866.

Blakelee, George E. *Blakelee's Industrial Cyclopedia: A Ready Reference and a Reservoir of Useful Information. A Simple, Practical Home Guide for Men, Women, and Children*. New York: Useful Information Exchange, 1887.

"The Blond Hair." *The Ladies' Magazine of Literature, Fashion and Fine Arts* (April 1844): 173–178.

Bradley, Mrs. "The Hair Ring." *Home Magazine* 5, no. 3 (March 1855): 71.

Britts, Mrs. Mattie D. "My Treasures." *Peterson's Magazine* 42 (October 1862): 290.

Campbell, Mark. Circular, "Ladies' Guide to M. Campbell's Self-Instructor. Art of Hair Work." Chicago: Mark Campbell, 1867.

———. *Hair Manual, or Self-Instructor in the Art of Dyeing Hair All Shades and Colors, Bleaching Hair White, Blonde, &c.* New York: Mark Campbell, 1879.

———. *Self-Instructor in the Art of Hair Work, Dressing Hair, Making Curls, Switches, Braids, and Hair Jewelry of Every Description/Compiled from Original Designs and the Latest Parisian Patterns by Mark Campbell*. New York: Mark Campbell, 1867.

———. *Self-Instructor in the Art of Hair Work, Dressing Hair, Making Curls, Switches, Braids, and Hair Jewelry of Every Description*. New ed. New York: Mark Campbell, 1875.

Carey, Alice. *Clovernook; or, Recollections of Our Neighborhood in the West*. 2nd ser. New York: Redfield, 1854.

Cassell, Peter. *Cassell's Household Guide: Being a Complete Encyclopedia of Domestic and Social Economy, and Forming a Guide to Every Department of Practical Life*. London: Peter Cassell and Galpin, 1869–71(?).

Catalogue of the Third Annual Exposition of the New England Manufacturers' and Mechanics' Institute (Boston, Massachusetts). Boston: Tolman and White, 1883.

Catalogue of the Thirteenth Exhibition of American Manufactures, held in Philadelphia, 1842. Philadelphia: William S. Young, 1842.

"A Chapter on Human Hair." *Peterson's Ladies National Magazine* 24 (1853): 33–34.

Coles, George S. *A Complete Dictionary of Dry Goods*. Chicago: J. B. Herring Publishing Company, 1894.

Cowles, Julia Darrow. *Artistic Home Furnishings for People of Moderate Means*. New York: F. M. Lupton Publishers, 1898.

Creer, Edwin. *Board-Work; or the Art of Wig-Making*. London: R. Hovendon and Sons, 1887.

Crofut, E. E. *The Art of Hair Chain Braiding*. Malta, Mont.: E. E. Crofut, 1911.

Cuyler, Theodore L., ed. *Golden Thoughts on Mother, Home and Heaven*. New York: E. B. Treat, 1882.

"The Daughter's Bedroom." *Demorest's Family Magazine* 28, no. 8 (June 1892): 497–499.

"Feather-Work." *Peterson's Magazine* 52 (July 1867): 76.

"A Few Objections to the Use of False Hair." *Manufacturer and Builder* 5, no. 7 (July 1873): 163–164.

"The Framing and Hanging of Pictures." *Ladies' Floral Cabinet*, November 1884, 363.

Francis, Mrs. Harriet E. "A Mother's Trial." *Godey's Book and Magazine* 65 (October 1862): 276.

Freeman, Mary E. Wilkins. "A Souvenir." *Harper's New Monthly Magazine* 70, no. 418 (March 1885): 590–596.

Frost, Annie S. *The Ladies' Guide to Needlework, Embroidery, etc.: Being a Complete Guide to All Kinds of Ladies' Fancy Work*. New York: Henry T. Williams, 1877.

Geniaux, Charles. "The Human Hair Harvest in Brittany." *Wide World Magazine* 4 (January 1900): 430–436.

Goodman, (Mrs.) D. Ellen. "The Two Shreds of Hair." *Peterson's Magazine* 13 (June 1848): 209–210.

Guyer, Isaac. *History of Chicago*. Chicago: Goodman and Cushing, 1862.

"The Hair." *The International Magazine of Literature, Art, and Science* 1, no. 4 (July 22, 1850): 103–104.

"Hair-Device Workers." *Cornhill Magazine* 52, no. S5 (July 1885): 62–65.

"Hair, Ornamental." *The New York, Boston, Philadelphia and Baltimore Business Directory for General Business Reference*. New York: Commercial Publishing Company, 1900.

Knight, Charles, editor. *The English Cyclopedia*. London: Bradbury and Evans, 1860.

Langford, Laura Carter Holloway. *The Hearthstone; or, Life at Home*. Beloit, Wis.: Inter-State Publishing House, 1883.

Lee, Jennette. "A Hair-Cut." *Living Age* 12, no. 230 (September 7, 1901): 659–661. From *A Pillar of Salt*. New York: Houghton Mifflin and Company, 1901.

Likins, Mrs. J. W. *Six Years' Experience as a Book Agent in California*. San Francisco: Women's Union and Job Printing Office, 1874.

Madam Worth's Kensington and Fancy Work Manual. Wallingford, Conn.: R. L. Spencer, 1886.

Mason, Amelia Gere. "Is Sentiment Declining?" *Century Illustrated Magazine* 61, no. 4 (February 1901): 626–634.

Neal, Alice B. "Gift-Making." *Godey's Book and Magazine* 55 (November 1857): 421–427.

Official Catalogue of the New York Exhibition of the Industry of All Nations. New York: G. P. Putnam, 1853.

Packard, Mrs. Clarissa. *Recollections of a Housekeeper.* New York: Harper and Brothers, 1834.

Palmer, John S. Patent Record No. 31,735. March 19, 1861.

Peltz, George A., ed. *The Housewife's Library.* Englewood, N.J.: Englewood Publishing Company, 1885.

Penny, Virginia. *How Women Can Make Money.* Springfield, Mass.: D. E. Fisk and Company, 1870. Reprint, New York: Arno and the New York Times, 1971.

Pullan, Mrs. Matilda Marian. *The Lady's Manual of Fancy-Work: A Complete Instructor in Every Variety of Ornamental Needle-Work.* New York: Dick & Fitzgerald, 1859.

A Record of the First Exhibition of the Metropolitan Mechanics' Institute. Washington, D.C.: H. Polkinhorn, 1853.

"Red Hair." *Bentley's Miscellany* 29 (1851): 532–537.

Reip, Mrs. Alfred H. "The Hair Neck-Lace." *The Ladies' Companion and Literary Expositor: A Monthly Magazine Embracing Every Department of Literature* (October 1843): 284–291.

"Remember Me." *The Souvenir.* (Philadelphia) July 18, 1827.

Report on the Twenty-Fourth Exhibition of American Manufactures. Philadelphia: Barnard and Jones, 1855.

Report of the Twenty-Seventh Exhibition of American Manufactures. Philadelphia: Barnard and Jones, 1874.

Reports of the First Exhibition of the Middlesex Mechanic Association. Lowell, Mass.: S. J. Varney, 1852.

Sargent, Charles E. *Our Home, or Influences Emanating from the Hearthstone.* Springfield, Mass.: King-Richardson Company, 1900.

Sauter, Lorenzo. Patent Record No. 56,618. July 24, 1866.

Scammell, Henry Bucklin. *Scammell's Universal Treasure-House of Useful Knowledge: An Encyclopaedia of Valuable Receipts in the Principal Arts of Life.* Philadelphia: Scammell and Company, 1885.

"Scrap-Books." *Harper's Bazaar* 9, no. 27 (July 1, 1876): 1.

Shaw, Louise F. Patent Application No. 96,275. October 26, 1869.

Sigourney, (Mrs.) Lydia H. "The Lock of Hair." *The Lady's Almanac for 1860.* Boston: Shepard, Clark, and Brown, 1860.

Smith, Pauline C[oggleshall]. "A Flower for Her Hair." In *Alfred Hitchcock: The Best of Mystery.* New York: Galahad Books, 1987: 28–34. Original version from *Alfred Hitchcock's Mystery Magazine* (July 1968).

"Specimens of Hair Work." In "Report on the New York Crystal Palace Exhibition." *Gleason's Pictorial Drawing-Room Companion*, August 13, 1853: 233.

Terhune, Mary Virginia (Hawes). *From My Youth Up.* New York: G. W. Carleton and Company, 1874.

———. *House and Home; a Complete Housewife's Guide by Marion Harland* [pseudonym]. New York: Union Publishing House, circa 1889.

"The Trade in Locks." *Every Saturday* 8, no. 184 (July 10, 1869): 40–44.

"The Trade in Locks." *London Society* 15 (May 1869): 547–552.

United States Centennial Commission. *Reports and Awards: International Exhibition, 1876, vol. v, Groups VIII–XIV.* Francis A. Walker, ed. Washington, D.C.: Government Printing Office, 1880.

Urbino, Madame Levina B., Henry Day, et al. *Art Recreations: Being a Complete Guide to Pencil Drawing, Oil Painting . . . Wax Work, Shell Work.* Boston: J. E. Tilton and Company, 1869.

Weld, H. Hastings. "The Mourning Ring." *Godey's Lady's Magazine* 26 (June 1843): 277–285.

Williams, Henry T., and "Daisy Eyebright." *The Ladies' Complete Manual of Home Duties.* New York: World Manufacturing Company, 1885.

Williams, Henry T., and Mrs. C. S. Jones. *Ladies' Fancy Work: Hints and Helps to Home Taste and Recreations.* New York: Henry T. Williams Publisher, 1876.

Wise, Reverend Daniel. *The Young Lady's Counsellor; or, Outlines and Illustrations of the Sphere, the Duties, and the Dangers of Young Women.* New York: Carlton and Phillips, 1852.

Wright, Julia McNair. *The Complete Home: An Encyclopaedia of Domestic Life and Affairs.* Philadelphia: J. C. McCurdy and Company, 1879.

The Young Lady's Companion: or, Sketches of Life, Manners, and Morals at the Present Day. Edited by a Lady. Philadelphia: H. C. Peck and Theodore Bliss, 1851.

Secondary Sources

Aarim-Heriot, Najia. *Chinese Immigrants, African Americans, and Racial Anxiety in the United States, 1848–82.* Urbana: University of Illinois Press, 2003.

Aiken, Carol. "The Emergence of the Portrait Miniature in New England." In *Painting and Portrait Making in the American Northeast.* Edited by Peter Benes. Dublin Seminar for New England Folklife Annual Proceedings 1994. Boston: Boston University, 1995: 30–45.

Abby Aldrich Rockefeller Folk Art Center. *American Folk Portraits: Paintings and Drawings from the Abby Aldrich Rockefeller Folk Art Center.* New York: Graphic Society, 1981.

Ambler, Cathy J. *The Look of the Fair: Kansas County Fairscapes, 1854–1994.* Ph.D. diss., University of Kansas, 1996.

Ames, Blanche Butler. *Adelbert Ames, 1835–1933; General, Senator, Governor; the Story of his Life and Times.* New York: Argosy-Antiquarian Press, 1964.

———, editor. *Chronicles from the Nineteenth Century: Family Letters of Blanche Butler Ames and Adelbert Ames.* Clinton, Mass.: Colonial Press, 1957.

Atherton, Lewis. *The Pioneer Merchant in Mid-America.* New York: Da Capo Press, 1969.

Baker, Jean H. *Mary Todd Lincoln: A Biography.* New York, W. W. Norton, 1987.

Ballaster, Ros Margaret, Elizabeth Frazer, and Sandra Hebron. *Women's Worlds: Ideology, Femininity, and the Woman's Magazine.* New York: Macmillan, 1991.

Balleisen, Edward J. *Navigating Failure: Bankruptcy and Commercial Society in Antebellum America.* Chapel Hill: University of North Carolina Press, 2001.

Banta, Martha. *Taylored Lives: Narrative Productions in the Age of Taylor, Veblen, and Ford.* Chicago: University of Chicago Press, 1993.

Bassin, Donna, Margaret Honey, and Meryle Mahrer Kaplan, eds. *Representations of Motherhood.* New Haven, Conn.: Yale University Press, 1994.

Benson, Susan Porter. *Counter Cultures: Saleswomen, Managers, and Customers in American Department Stores, 1890–1940.* Urbana: University of Illinois Press, 1988.

Bercaw, Nancy. "Solid Objects/Mutable Meanings: Fancywork and the Construction of Bourgeois Culture, 1840–1880." *Winterthur Portfolio* 26, no. 4 (Winter 1991): 231–247.

Bertolini, Vincent J. "Fireside Chastity: The Erotics of Sentimental Bachelorhood in the 1850s." *American Literature* 68, no. 4 (December 1996): 707–738.

Bertuca, David J., chief comp. *The World's Columbian Exposition: A Centennial Bibliographic Guide.* Westport, Conn.: Greenwood Press, 1996.

Bloch, Ruth H. "American Feminine Ideals in Transition: The Rise of the Moral Mother, 1785–1815." *Feminist Studies* 4, no. 21 (June 1978): 100–126.

Bolton-Smith, Robin. *Portrait Miniatures in the National Museum of American Art.* Chicago: University of Chicago Press, 1984.

Bonfield, Lynn A., and Mary C. Morrison. *Roxana's Children: The Biography of a Nineteenth-Century Vermont Family.* Amherst: University of Massachusetts Press, 1995.

Bowles, Ella Shannon. *Homespun Handicrafts.* Philadelphia: J. B. Lippincott Company, 1931.

Boydston, Jeanne. *Home and Work: Housework, Wages, and the Ideology of Labor in the Early Republic.* New York: Oxford University Press, 1990.

Breen, T. H. "'Baubles of Britain': The American and Consumer Revolutions of the Eighteenth Century." *Past and Present* 199 (1988): 73–104.

———. "'The Meaning of Likeness': Portrait-Painting in an Eighteenth-Century Consumer Society." In *The Portrait in Eighteenth-Century America.* Edited by Ellen G. Miles. Newark: University of Delaware, 1993: 37–60.

———. "Narrative of Commercial Life: Consumption, Ideology, and Community on the Eve of the American Revolution." *William and Mary Quarterly,* 3rd ser., 50, no. 3 (July 1993): 471–501.

Brown, Gillian. *Domestic Individualism: Imagining Self in Nineteenth-Century America.* Berkeley: University of California Press, 1990.

Bruchey, Stuart W., ed. *Small Business in American Life.* New York: Columbia University Press, 1980.

Brucken, Carolyn. "Victorian Privacy: An Analysis of Bedrooms in American Middle Class Homes from 1850–1880." Master's thesis, University of Delaware, 1991.

Buck, Solon J., ed. *William Watts Folwell: The Autobiography and Letters of a Pioneer of Culture.* Minneapolis: University of Minnesota Press, 1933.

Buckler, Patricia P., and C. Kay Leeper. "An Antebellum Woman's Scrapbook as

Autobiographical Composition." *Journal of American Culture* 14, no. 1 (Spring 1991): 1–8.

Bundles, A'Lelia. *On Her Own Ground: The Life and Times of Madam C. J. Walker.* New York: Scribner, 2001.

Carlisle, Lilian Baker. "Hair Today, Shorn Tomorrow (sorry!)." *Yankee* 38, no. 1 (January 1974), 95.

———. "Hair Work Flowers." *Antiques Journal* 26, no. 9 (September 1971): 35.

Carnes, Mark C. *Secret Ritual and Manhood in Victorian America.* New Haven, Conn.: Yale University Press, 1989.

Carrier, James G. "Alienating Objects: The Emergence of Alienation in Retail Trade." *Man: The Journal of the Royal Anthropological Institute* 29, no. 2 (June 1994): 359–380.

———. *Gifts and Commodities: Exchange and Western Capitalism Since 1700.* London: Routledge Press, 1995.

———. "The Symbolism of Possession in Commodity Advertising." *Man: The Journal of the Royal Anthropological Institute* 25, no. 4 (December 1990): 693–706.

Carson, Cary, Ronald Hoffman, and Peter J. Albert, eds. *Of Consuming Interests: The Style of Life in the Eighteenth Century.* Charlottesville: U.S. Capitol Historical Society by University Press of Virginia, 1994.

Caulfield, Sophia Frances Anne, and Blanche C. Saward. *Encyclopedia of Victorian Needlework [Dictionary of Needlework].* 2 vols. London: A. W. Cowan, 1887. Reprint, Mineola, N.Y.: Dover Publications, 1972.

Congram, Marjorie. *Horsehair: A Textile Resource.* Martinsville, N.J.: Dockwra Press, 1987.

Cooper, Wendy. *Hair: Sex Society Symbolism.* New York: Stein and Day, 1971.

Corson, Richard. *Fashions in Hair: The First Five Thousand Years.* New York: Hastings House, 1965.

Cott, Nancy F. *The Bonds of Womanhood: "Woman's Sphere" in New England, 1780–1835.* New Haven, Conn.: Yale University Press, 1977.

Cox, J. Stevens. *An Illustrated Dictionary of Hairdressing and Wigmaking.* Philadelphia: George S. MacManus Company, 1966.

Croly, Mrs. (Jenny June), ed. *Needlework: A Manual of Stitches and Studies in Embroidery and Drawn Work.* New York: A. L. Burt, 1885.

Curl, James Stevens. *A Celebration of Death: An Introduction to Some of the Buildings, Monuments, and Settings of Funerary Architecture in the West European Tradition.* New York: Scribner, 1980.

Davidoff, Leonore, and Catherine Hall. *Family Fortunes: Men and Women of the English Middle Class, 1780–1850.* Chicago: University of Chicago Press, 1987.

Day, Charles William. *The Art of Miniature Painting.* London: Winsor and Newton, 1905.

de Dillmont, Therese. *The Complete Encyclopedia of Needlework.* Philadelphia: Running Press, 1978.

de Grazia, Victoria, with Ellen Furlough, eds., *The Sex of Things: Gender and Consumption in Historical Perspective.* Berkeley: University of California Press, 1996.

Deutsch, Davida Tenenbaum. "Collector's Notes." *Antiques* 130 (September 1985).

———. "Jewelry for Mourning, Love, and Fancy, 1770–1830." *Antiques* 155 (April 1999): 566–575.

———. "Samuel Folwell of Philadelphia: An Artist for the Needlework." *Antiques* 119 (February 1981): 420–423.

Douglas, Ann. *The Feminization of American Culture.* New York: Anchor Books, 1977.

Duval, Cynthia. *Infinite Riches: Jewelry Through the Centuries.* Exhibition catalogue, Museum of Fine Arts, St. Petersburg, Florida, February 19–April 30, 1989.

Edmonds, Mary Jaene. *Samplers and Samplermakers: An American Schoolgirl Art, 1700–1850.* New York: Rizzoli for the Los Angeles County Museum of Art, 1991.

Farrell, James J. *Inventing the American Way of Death, 1830–1920.* Philadelphia: Temple University Press, 1980.

Felleman, Hazel. *The Best Loved Poems of the American People.* New York: Doubleday and Company, 1936.

Fitch, Josephine H. "Some Victorian Oddities." *Antiques* 6, no. 6 (December 1924): 316–318.

Foucault, Michel. *Discipline and Punish: The Birth of the Prison.* Translated by Alan Sheridan. New York: Vintage Books, 1977.

Foy, Jessica H., and Karal Ann Marling, eds. *The Arts and the American Home, 1890–1930.* Knoxville: University of Tennessee Press, 1994.

Frank, Robin Jaffee. *Love and Loss: American Portrait and Mourning Miniatures.* New Haven, Conn.: Yale University Press and Yale University Art Gallery, 2000.

Gamber, Wendy. *The Female Economy: The Millinery and Dressmaking Trades, 1860–1930.* Urbana: University of Illinois Press, 1997.

———. "Gendered Concerns: Thoughts on the History of Business and the History of Women." *Business and Economic History* 23 (1994): 129–140.

Gernes, Todd Steven. "Recasting the Culture of Ephemera: Young Women's Literary Culture in Nineteenth-Century America." Ph.D. diss., Brown University, 1987.

Gordon, Beverly. "Victorian Fancywork in the American Home: Fantasy and Accommodation." In *Making the American Home: Middle-Class Women and Domestic Material Culture, 1840–1940.* Edited by Marilyn Ferris Motz and Pat Browne. Bowling Green, Ohio: Bowling Green State University Popular Press, 1988: 48–56.

Green, Doris. "Hair Jewelry." *Antiques Journal* 18, no. 6 (June 1963): 16–17.

Green, Harvey. *The Light of the Home: An Intimate View of the Lives of Women in Victorian America.* New York: Pantheon Books, 1983.

Grier, Katherine C. *Culture and Comfort: Parlor Making and Middle-Class Identity, 1850–1930.* Rev. 2nd ed. Washington, D.C.: Smithsonian Institution Press, 1997.

———. *Culture and Comfort: People, Parlors, and Upholstery, 1850–1930.* Rochester, NY: Strong Museum, 1989.

Griffin, Clifford S. *The University of Kansas: A History*. Lawrence: University Press of Kansas, 1974.

Gutman, Herbert G. *The Black Family in Slavery and Freedom, 1750–1925*. New York: Pantheon Books, 1976.

Halttunen, Karen. *Confidence Men and Painted Women: A Study of Middle-Class Culture in America, 1830–1870*. New Haven, Conn.: Yale University Press, 1982.

Hamilton, Edith. *Mythology: Timeless Tales of Gods and Heroes*. 48th printing. New York: New American Library, 1969.

Hammond, Jennifer J. "The William Dunkling [sic] Mourning Pendant: Reflection of Early 19th-Century America." October 10, 1995. Winterthur Museum and Country Estate, Winterthur, Delaware. Unpublished paper.

Hemphill, C. Dallett. *Bowing to Necessities: A History of Manners in America, 1620–1860*. New York: Oxford University Press, 1999.

Herr, Patricia T. *The Ornamental Branches: Needlework and Arts from the Lititz Moravian Girls School Between 1800 and 1865*. Heritage Center Museum of Lancaster County, Pennsylvania, 1996.

Herzog, Don. "The Trouble with Hairdressers." *Representations* 53 (Winter 1996): 21–43.

Higham, John. *Strangers in the Land: Patterns of American Nativism, 1860–1925*. 2nd ed. New Brunswick, N.J.: Rutgers University Press, 1988.

Hoke, Donald R. *Ingenious Yankees: The Rise of the American System of Manufactures in the Private Sector*. New York: Columbia University Press, 1990.

Huber, Leonard V. *Clasped Hands: Symbolism in New Orleans Cemeteries*. Lafayette: University of Southwestern Louisiana, 1982.

Hulbert, Anne. *Victorian Crafts Revived*. New York: Hastings House, 1978.

Hunter, Margaret. "Mourning Jewellery: A Collector's Account." *Costume* 27 (1993): 9–22.

Illouz, Eva. *Consuming the Romantic Utopia: Love and the Cultural Contradictions of Capitalism*. Berkeley: University of California Press, 1997.

Jabour, Anya. "Albums of Affection: Female Friendship and Coming of Age in Antebellum Virginia." *Virginia Magazine of History and Biography* 107, no. 2 (Spring 1999): 125–158.

———. *Marriage in the Early Republic: Elizabeth and William Wirt and the Companionate Ideal*. Baltimore: Johns Hopkins University Press, 1998.

Jackson, Charles O., ed. *Passing: The Vision of Death in America*. Westport, Conn.: Greenwood Press, 1977.

Jaffee, David. "The Age of Democratic Portraiture: Artisan-Entrepreneurs and the Rise of Consumer Goods." In *Meet Your Neighbors: New England Portraits, Painters, and Society, 1790–1850*. Sturbridge: Old Sturbridge Village and University of Massachusetts Press, 1992: 35–46.

Jensen, Joan. *Loosening the Bonds: Mid-Atlantic Farm Women, 1750–1850*. New Haven, Conn.: Yale University Press, 1986.

Johnson, Dale T. *American Portrait Miniatures in the Manney Collection*. New York: Metropolitan Museum of Art, 1991.

Jones, William. *Finger-Ring Lore, Historical, Legendary and Anecdotal*. London: Chatto and Windus, 1898.

Kasson, John F. *Rudeness and Civility: Manners in Nineteenth-Century Urban America.* New York: Hill and Wang, 1990.

Kelley, Mary, ed. *The Power of Her Sympathy: The Autobiography and Journal of Catharine Maria Sedgwick.* Boston: Massachusetts Historical Society, 1993.

Kelly, Catherine E. " 'The Consummation of Rural Prosperity and Happiness': New England Agricultural Fairs and the Constructions of Class and Gender, 1810–1860." *American Quarterly* 49, no. 3 (September 1997): 574–602.

Kete, Mary Louise. "Sentimental Literature." In *Oxford Encyclopedia of American Literature,* vol. 3. Edited by Jay Parini. New York: Oxford University Press, 2004, 545.

Kerber, Linda. *Women of the Republic: Intellect and Ideology in Revolutionary America.* Chapel Hill: University of North Carolina Press, 1980.

Knobel, Dale T. *"America for the Americans": The Nativist Movement in the United States.* New York: Twayne Publishers, 1996.

Kwolek-Folland, Angel. "The Elegant Dugout: Domesticity and Moveable Culture in the United States, 1870–1900." *American Studies* 25 (Fall 1984): 21–37.

———. *Engendering Business: Men and Women in the Corporate Office, 1870–1930.* Baltimore: Johns Hopkins University Press, 1994.

———. *Incorporating Women: A History of Women and Business in the United States.* New York: Twayne Publishers, 1998.

———. "The Useful What-Not and the Ideal of 'Domestic Decoration.' " *Helicon Nine* 8 (1983): 72–83.

Kunz, George Frederick. *Rings for the Finger, from the Earliest Known Times to the Present.* Philadelphia: J. B. Lippincott Company, 1917.

Kyvig, David E., and Myron A. Marty. *Nearby History: Exploring the Past Around You.* 2nd ed. New York: Rowman and Littlefield, 2000.

Laurie, Bruce. *Artisans into Workers: Labor in Nineteenth-Century America.* New York: Hill and Wang, 1989.

———. " 'Spavined Ministers, Lying Toothpullers, and Buggering Priests': Third-Partyism and the Search for Security in the Antebellum North." In *American Artisans: Crafting Social Identity, 1750–1850.* Edited by Howard B. Rock, Paul A. Gilje, and Robert Asker. Baltimore: Johns Hopkins University Press, 1995: 98–123.

———. *Working People of Philadelphia, 1800–1850.* Philadelphia: Temple University Press, 1980.

Lears, T. J. Jackson. *No Place of Grace: Antimodernism and the Transformation of American Culture, 1880–1920.* 3rd ed. Chicago: University of Chicago Press, 1994.

Lehuu, Isabelle. *Carnival on the Page: Popular Print Media in Antebellum America.* Chapel Hill: University of North Carolina Press, 2000.

———. "Sentimental Figures: Reading *Godey's Lady's Book* in Antebellum America." In *The Culture of Sentiment: Race, Gender, and Sentimentality in Nineteenth-Century America.* Edited by Shirley Samuels. New York: Oxford University Press, 1992: 73–91.

Lemagny, Jean-Claude, and André Rouillé. *A History of Photography: Social and Cultural Perspectives.* Cambridge: Cambridge University Press, 1987.

Lewis, Jan. "Mother's Love: The Construction of an Emotion in Nineteenth-Century America." In *Social History and Issues in Human Consciousness: Some Interdisciplinary Connections.* Edited by Andrew E. Barnes and Peter N. Stearns. New York: New York University Press, 1989: 209–229.

Lewis, Susan Ingalls. "Female Entrepreneurs in Albany 1840–1885." *Business and Economic History.* 2nd Series. 21 (1992): 65–73.

Loomis, Mabel Todd, ed. *Letters of Emily Dickinson, vol. 1.* Boston: Roberts Brothers, 1894.

Lovell, Margaretta M. "Reading Eighteenth-Century American Family Portraits." *Winterthur Portfolio* 22, no. 4 (Winter 1987): 244–264.

Lystra, Karen. *Searching the Heart: Women, Men, and Romantic Love in Nineteenth-Century America.* New York: Oxford University Press, 1989.

Madison, James H. "The Evolution of Commercial Credit Reporting Agencies in Nineteenth-Century America." *Business History Review* 48, no. 2 (Summer 1974): 164–178.

Martinez, Katherine, and Kenneth L. Ames, eds. *The Material Culture of Gender / The Gender of Material Culture.* Hanover, N.H.: University Press of New England, 1997.

Marx, Leo. *The Machine in the Garden: Technology and the Pastoral Ideal in America.* New York: Oxford University Press, 1964.

Mayne, Arthur. *British Profile Miniaturists.* Boston: Boston Book and Art, 1970.

Mayo, Edith, ed. *American Material Culture: The Shape of Things Around Us.* Bowling Green, Ohio: Bowling Green State University Popular Press, 1984.

———. *Women in Mourning.* Exhibition catalogue of the Museum of the Confederacy, Richmond, Virginia, November 14, 1984–January 6, 1986.

McCracken, Grant. *Culture and Consumption: New Approaches to the Symbolic Character of Consumer Goods and Activities.* Bloomington: Indiana University Press, 1990.

McDannell, Colleen. *The Christian Home in Victorian America, 1840–1900.* Bloomington: Indiana University Press, 1986.

McKendrick, Neil, John Brewer, and J. H. Plumb. *The Birth of a Consumer Society: The Commercialization of Eighteenth-Century England.* Bloomington: Indiana University Press, 1982.

McKenney, Dorothy D. "Victorian Mourning Jewelry." *Spinning Wheel* June 1978: 8–11.

McMurry, Sally. *Families and Farmhouses in Nineteenth-Century America: Vernacular Design and Social Change.* New York: Oxford University Press, 1988.

Merish, Lori. "'The Hand of Refined Taste' in the Frontier Landscape: Caroline Kirkland's *A New Home, Who'll Follow Me?* and the Feminization of American Consumerism." *American Quarterly* 45, no. 4 (December 1993): 485–523.

Michaels, Walter Benn. *The Gold Standard and the Logic of Naturalism.* Berkeley: University of California Press, 1987.

Milham, Willis I. *Time and Timekeepers, Including the History, Construction, Care and Accuracy of Clocks and Watches.* New York: Macmillan, 1923.

Miller, Daniel, ed. *Unwrapping Christmas.* Oxford: Clarendon Press, 1993.

Mills, Betty J. *Calico Chronicle: Texas Women and Their Fashions, 1830–1910.* Lubbock: Texas Tech Press, 1985.

Mitford, Jessica. *The American Way of Death Revisited.* Rev. ed. New York: Alfred A. Knopf, 1998.

Mohr, James C., ed. *The Cormany Diaries: A Northern Family in the Civil War.* Pittsburgh: University of Pittsburgh Press, 1982.

Monfredo, Rachel Jean. "American Finger Rings: Representing Bonds of Relationships." Master's thesis, University of Delaware, 1990.

Morgan, John Hill. "Memento Mori: Mourning Rings, Memorial Miniatures, and Hair Devices." *Antiques* 17, no. 3 (March 1930): 226–230.

Morley, John. *Death, Heaven and the Victorians.* Philadelphia: Temple University Press, 1980.

Motz, Marilyn Ferris, and Pat Browne, eds. *Making the American Home: Middle-Class Women and Domestic Material Culture, 1840–1940.* Bowling Green, Ohio: Bowling Green State University Popular Press, 1988.

Nelson, Elizabeth White. *Market Sentiments: Middle-Class Market Culture in Nineteenth-Century America.* Washington, D.C.: Smithsonian Books, 2004.

Newhall, Beaumont. *The History of Photography: From 1839 to the Present.* 2nd ed. New York: Museum of Modern Art, distributed by New York Graphic Society Books, Little, Brown and Company, 1982.

Norgate, Edward. *Miniatura or the Art of Limning.* Edited, introduced, and annotated by Jeffrey M. Muller and Jim Murrell. New Haven, Conn.: Yale University Press, 1997.

Norris, James D. *R. G. Dun and Company, 1841–1900: The Development of Credit-Reporting in the Nineteenth Century.* Westport, Conn.: Greenwood Press, 1978.

Nutty, Colleen. "Cemetery Symbolism of Prairie Pioneers: Gravestone Art and Social Change in Story County, Iowa." *Journal of the Iowa Archeological Society* 31 (1984): 1–135.

O'Malley, Michael. *Keeping Watch: A History of American Time.* Washington, D.C.: Smithsonian Institution Press, 1996.

Obst, Janis. "Hair Wreaths and Ornaments." *Gopher Historian*, Winter 1966–67: 8–9.

Olton, Charles. *Artisans for Independence: Philadelphia Mechanics and the American Revolution.* Syracuse, N.Y.: Syracuse University Press, 1975.

Orvell, Miles. *The Real Thing: Imitation and Authenticity in American Culture, 1880–1940.* Chapel Hill: University of North Carolina Press, 1989.

Otnes, Cele, and Richard F. Beltramini, eds. *Gift Giving: A Research Anthology.* Bowling Green, Ohio: Bowling Green State University Popular Press, 1992.

Peiss, Kathy. *Cheap Amusements: Working Women and Leisure in Turn-of-the-Century New York.* Philadelphia: Temple University Press, 1986.

Perrot, Philippe. *Fashioning the Bourgeoisie: A History of Clothing in the Nineteenth Century.* Translated by Richard Bienvenu. Princeton, N.J.: Princeton University Press, 1994.

Peterson, Harold L. *Americans at Home: From the Colonists to the Late Victorians; a Pictorial Source Book of American Domestic Interiors with an Appendix on Inns and Taverns.* New York: Scribner, 1971.

Pike, Martha V., and Janice Gray Armstrong. *A Time to Mourn: Expressions of Grief in Nineteenth-Century America.* Stony Brook, N.Y.: Museums at Stony Brook, 1980.

Pointon, Marcia. "Intriguing Jewellery: Royal Bodies and Luxurious Consumption." *Textual Practice* 11, no. 3 (1997): 493–516.

———. "Valuing the Visual and Visualizing the Valuable: Jewellery and Its Ambiguities." *Cultural Values* 3, no. 1 (1999): 1–27.

Porter, Glenn, and Harold C. Livesay. *Merchants and Manufacturers: Studies in the Changing Structure of Nineteenth-Century Marketing.* Baltimore: Johns Hopkins University Press, 1971.

Potter, Parker B., Jr., and Mark P. Leone, eds. *The Recovery of Meaning: Historical Archaeology in the Eastern United States.* Washington, D.C.: Smithsonian Institution Press, 1988.

Price, Julius M. *Dame Fashion: Paris-London (1786–1912).* New York: Scribner, 1913.

Priddy, Sumter Turner. *Fancy: Acceptance of an Attitude, Emergence of a Style.* Master's thesis, University of Delaware, 1981.

Proctor, Molly J. *Victorian Canvas Work: Berlin Wool Work.* London: B. T. Batsford, 1972.

Rahm, Virginia L. "Human Hair Ornaments." *Minnesota History* Summer 1974: 70–74.

Restad, Penne L. *Christmas in America: A History.* New York: Oxford University Press, 1995.

Revi, Albert Christian, ed. *The Spinning Wheel's Complete Book of Antiques.* New York: Grosset & Dunlap, 1972: 416–417.

Riley, James Whitcomb. *The Complete Poetical Works of James Whitcomb Riley.* Bloomington: Indiana University Press, 1993.

Ring, Betty. *Girlhood Embroidery: American Samplers and Pictorial Needlework, 1650–1850.* New York: Alfred A. Knopf, 1993.

———. *Let Virtue Be a Guide to Thee: Needlework in the Education of Rhode Island Women, 1730–1830.* Providence: Rhode Island Historical Society, 1983.

———. "Needlework Pictures from Abby Wright's School in South Hadley, Massachusetts." *Antiques* 131 (September 1986): 482–493.

Rorabaugh, W. J. *The Craft Apprentice: From Franklin to the Machine Age in America.* New York: Oxford University Press, 1986.

Rose, Anne C. *Voices of the Marketplace: American Thought and Culture, 1830–1860.* New York: Twayne Publishers, 1995.

Rosenblum, Naomi. *A World of Photography.* 2nd ed. Rev. New York: Abbeville Press, 1989.

Rosswurm, Steven. *Arms, Country, and Class: The Philadelphia Militia and "Lower Sort" during the American Revolution, 1775–1783.* New Brunswick, N.J.: Rutgers University Press, 1987.

Rothman, Ellen K. *Hands and Hearts: A History of Courtship in America.* New York: Basic Books, 1984.

Rotundo, E. Anthony. *American Manhood: Transformations in Masculinity from the Revolution to the Modern Era.* New York: Basic Books, 1993.

R. W. Norton Art Gallery, *Portrait Miniatures in Early American History, 1750–1840.* April 18–June 13, 1976, exhibition, Shreveport, La.

Ryan, Mary P. *Cradle of the Middle Class: The Family in Oneida County, New York, 1790–1865.* Cambridge: Cambridge University Press, 1981.

———. *Women in Public: Between Banners and Ballots, 1825–1880.* Baltimore: Johns Hopkins University Press, 1990: 24–37.

Samuels, Shirley, ed. *The Culture of Sentiment: Race, Gender, and Sentimentality in Nineteenth-Century America.* New York: Oxford University Press, 1992.

Saum, Lewis O. *The Popular Mood of Pre-Civil War America.* Westport, Conn.: Greenwood Press, 1980.

Schorman, Robert. *Selling Style: Clothing and Social Change at the Turn of the Century.* Philadelphia: University of Pennsylvania Press, 2003.

Schorsch, Anita. "A Key to the Kingdom: The Iconography of a Mourning Picture." *Winterthur Portfolio* 14, no. 1 (Spring 1979): 41–71.

———. *Mourning Becomes America: Mourning Art in the New Nation.* Philadelphia, Pa.: Main Street Press, 1976.

Schultz, Ronald. "The Small-Producer Tradition and the Moral Origins of Artisan Radicalism in Philadelphia, 1720–1810." *Past and Present* 127 (May 1990) 84–116.

Scott, Alison. "Sensibility." In *Encyclopedia of the Romantic Era, 1760–1850,* vol. 2. Edited by Christopher John Murray. New York: Fitzroy Dearborn, 2004: 1039–1040.

Scranton, Philip. "Diversity in Diversity: Flexible Production and American Industrialization, 1880–1930." *Business History Review* 65 (Spring 1991): 27–90.

———. *Endless Novelty: Specialty Production and American Industrialization, 1865–1925.* Princeton, N.J.: Princeton University Press, 1997.

———. "Manufacturing Diversity: Production Systems, Markets, and an American Consumer Society, 1870–1930." *Technology and Culture* 35, no. 3 (July 1994): 476–505.

———. "The Politics of Production: Technology, Markets, and the Two Cultures of American Industry." *Science in Context* 8, no. 2 (1995): 369–395.

Seale, William. *The Tasteful Interlude: American Interiors through the Camera's Eye, 1860–1917.* Rev. 2nd ed. Nashville, Tenn.: American Association of State and Local History, 1981.

Severa, Joan L. *Dressed for the Photographer: Ordinary Americans and Fashion, 1840–1900.* Kent, Ohio: Kent State University Press, 1995.

———. *My Likeness Taken: Daguerrian Portraits in America.* Kent, Ohio: Kent State University Press, 2006.

Shawe-Taylor, Desmond. *The Georgians: Eighteenth-Century Portraiture and Society.* London: Barrie and Jenkins, 1990.

Sherman, Stuart. *Telling Time: Clocks, Diaries, and English Diurnal Form, 1660–1785.* Chicago: University of Chicago Press, 1996.

Shi, David. *The Simple Life: Plain Living and High Thinking in American Culture.* New York: Oxford University Press, 1985.

Smith, Billy G. *The "Lower Sort": Philadelphia Laboring People, 1750–1800.* Ithaca, N.Y.: Cornell University Press, 1990.

Smith, Gaye. *Sentimental Souvenirs: Victorian Scrap Albums from the Sir Harry Page Collection.* Catalog of exhibition, Holden Gallery, Faculty of Art and Design, Manchester Polytechnic, April 10–May 12, 1987, Manchester, England.

Smith-Rosenberg, Carroll. *Disorderly Conduct: Visions of Gender in Victorian America.* New York: Oxford University Press, 1985.

Sobieszek, Robert A., and Oddette M. Appel. *The Spirit of Fact: The Daguerreotypes of Southworth and Hawes, 1843–1862.* Boston: David R. Godine and the International Museum of Photography, 1976.

Spears, Timothy B. *100 Years on the Road: The Traveling Salesman in American Culture.* New Haven, Conn.: Yale University Press, 1995.

Stearns, Bertha. "Philadelphia Magazines for Ladies: 1830–1860." *Pennsylvania Magazine of History and Biography* 69 (July 1945): 207–219.

Stearns, Peter N. *Battleground of Desire: The Struggle for Self-Control in Modern America.* New York: New York University Press, 1999.

Steele, Valerie. *Fashion and Eroticism: Ideals of Feminine Beauty from the Victorian Era to the Jazz Age.* New York: Oxford University Press, 1985.

Stewart, Susan. *On Longing: Narratives of the Miniature, the Gigantic, the Souvenir, the Collection.* Baltimore: Johns Hopkins University Press, 1984.

Strickler, Susan. *American Portrait Miniatures: The Worcester Art Museum Collection.* Worcester, Mass.: Worcester Art Museum, 1989.

Swan, Susan Burrows. *Plain and Fancy: American Women and Their Needlework, 1700–1850.* New York: Holt, Rinehart and Winston, 1977.

Taylor, Lou. *Mourning Dress: A Costume and Social History.* London: Allen and Unwin, 1983.

Tebbutt, Melanie. *Making Ends Meet: Pawnbroking and Working-Class Credit.* New York: St. Martin's Press, 1983.

Theriot, Nancy M. *Mothers and Daughters in Nineteenth-Century America: The Biosocial Construction of Femininity.* Lexington: University Press of Kentucky, 1996.

Thompson, E. P. "Time, Work-Discipline, and Industrial Capitalism." *Past and Present* 38 (December 1967): 56–97.

Thornton, Tamara Plakins. *Handwriting in America: A Cultural History.* New Haven, Conn.: Yale University Press, 1996.

Todd, Janet. *Sensibility: An Introduction.* London: Methuen, 1986.

Tolman, Ruel Pardee. "A Document on Hair Painting." *Antiques* 17, no. 3 (March 1930): 231.

———. "Human Hair as a Pigment." *Antiques* 8, no. 6 (1925): 353.

Tomes, Nancy. *The Gospel of Germs: Men, Women, and the Microbe in American Life.* Cambridge, Mass.: Harvard University Press, 1998.

Ulrich, Laurel Thatcher. *The Age of Homespun: Objects and Stories in the Creation of an American Myth.* New York: Vintage Books, 2001.

———. *Good Wives: Image and Reality in the Lives of Women in Northern New England, 1650–1750.* New York: Vintage Books, 1982.

———. *A Midwife's Tale: The Life of Martha Ballard, Based on Her Diary, 1785–1812.* New York: Alfred A. Knopf, 1990.

Vincent, Margaret. *The Ladies' Work Table: Domestic Needlework in Nineteenth-*

Century America. Exhibition catalogue, Allentown Art Museum, Allentown, Pennsylvania. Allentown, Pa.: Allentown Art Museum. 1988.

Waits, William. *The Modern Christmas in America: A Cultural History of Gift Giving.* New York: New York University Press, 1993.

Walker, Juliet E. K. *The History of Black Business in America: Capitalism, Race, Entrepreneurship.* New York: Macmillan Library Reference Series (Twayne's Evolution of Modern Business Series), 1998.

Walton, Whitney. *France at the Crystal Palace: Bourgeois Taste and Artisan Manufacture in the Nineteenth Century.* Berkeley: University of California Press, 1992.

Watson, Samuel. "Flexible Gender Roles During the Market Revolution: Family, Friendship, Marriage, and Masculinity Among U.S. Army Officers, 1815–1846." *Journal of Social History* 29, no. 1 (1995): 81–107.

Welter, Barbara. *Dimity Convictions: The American Woman in the Nineteenth Century.* Athens, Ohio University Press, 1976.

Wharton, Anne Hollingsworth. *Heirlooms in Miniature.* Philadelphia: J. B. Lippincott Company, 1898.

White, Cynthia L. *Women's Magazines, 1693–1968.* London: Michael Joseph, 1970.

White, Elizabeth Alice. "Sentimental Enterprise: Sentiment and Profit in American Market Culture, 1830–1880." Ph.D. diss., Yale University Press, 1995.

Wilentz, Sean. *Chants Democratic: New York City and the Rise of the American Working Class, 1788–1850.* New York: Oxford University Press, 1984.

Williams, Raymond. *Keywords: A Vocabulary of Culture and Society.* London: Fontana/Croom Helm, 1976.

Winkler, Gail Caskey. "Influence of Godey's *Lady's Book* on the American Woman and Her Home: Contributions to a National Culture (1830–1877)." Ph.D. diss., University of Wisconsin—Madison, 1988.

Wright, Ila A. "Hair Watch Chains and Flowers." Interview in *Western Folklore* 18 (1959): 114–117.

Wurst, Louise Ann. "'A Rope of Sand': Second Great Awakening Symbolism on Gravestones of the Rural Elite in Broome County, New York." Master's thesis, Temple University, 1986.

Yarwood, Doreen. *English Costume from the Second Century B.C. to 1950.* New York: Crown Publishers, 1952.

Young, Alfred F. "Revolutionary Mechanics." In *Working for Democracy: American Workers from the Revolution to the Present.* Edited by Paul Buhle and Alan Dawley. Urbana: University of Illinois Press, 1985: 1–10.

Zakim, Michael. "Customizing the Industrial Revolution: The Reinvention of Tailoring in the Nineteenth Century." *Winterthur Portfolio* 33, no. 1 (Spring 1998): 41–58.

Index

Acknowledgments

I am grateful to have the opportunity to thank those who have aided me in this work. There are so many individuals whose insights, research skills, expertise, and scholarship have played a role in my efforts. I am conscious of how my own work reflects the contributions of so many.

First, I thank the staff at all the institutions listed in the bibliography. My love of the research process is due in part to the expertise of those who staff archives, museums, and libraries, from the desk clerks, paging clerks, photocopying interns, and security guards, to the curators, archivists, and directors.

In addition, I would like to thank the following individuals for their extraordinary efforts: at the Smithsonian Institution, National Museum of American History, Shelley Foote, former museum specialist of costume and textiles; Rodris Roth, now deceased and greatly missed former curator of the Domestic Life Division; Susan B. Strange of the Archives Center; and Fath Ruffin-Davis. The staff at the Winterthur Museum and Country Estate has been very supportive, with the most efficient photograph reproduction service around and an extraordinary collection of decorative arts. At Winterthur I especially thank Neville Thompson, who contributed a fearsome intelligence at an early stage of my research, and Gary Kulik, whose family invited me over for a holiday dinner when I was quite lonesome. At the University of Kansas, Cindy Pierard, then in the Reference section, and Deborah Dandridge of the Kansas Collection, Spencer Research Library, were each unfailingly helpful.

The research for this project was supported by the University of Kansas Summer Dissertation Research Grant; Winterthur Museum and Country Estate Pre-Doctorate Research Fellow Program; Smithsonian Institution Pre-Doctorate Research Fellow Program, and Minnesota State University–Moorhead Summer Faculty Research Fund. In addition, my parents and my brother Philip supported my travel and research costs over the years.

Most hairwork in this country is held by collectors, some of whom have been collecting since the 1950s. They have preserved an important part of our nineteenth-century cultural history. Leila Cohoon of Independence, Missouri, was exceptionally generous with her collection and private museum holdings. Jan Odegaard of the Wisconsin Historical Society let me examine her hairwork and letter; its contents have haunted me since.

I am pleased to thank the many scholars whose contributions of friendship, intellectual challenge, and enthusiasm infuse this work with their spirit. I thank Shirley Teresa Wajda, who has been an extraordinary resource. The careers of an entire generation of material culture scholars have been blessed by Shirley's willingness to provide feedback, encouragement, and collaboration. I also thank Beverly Gordon, Mark Hirsch, Charlie McGovern, Marcia Pointon, Laura Schiavo, Anne Schofield, and Robin Veder. My editor, Bob Lockhart, as well as Jean-Christophe Agnew, Valerie Steele, Susan Strasser, and the reviewers of the manuscript provided specific comments on the arguments in this volume.

Steven Mintz and Sarah Fishman at the University of Houston provided collegiality while I was teaching there. Laura Blunsom was an invaluable colleague at Minnesota State University–Moorhead; Mary Cayton and the Women's Writing Group at Miami University kept me going in the very last stages of writing this work.

I thank the following individuals and family groups whose friendship and scholarship have aided my own: Cathy Ambler, Beth Berninger, Dieter Berninger, Bradley Carter, Willy Dobak, Jon Earle, Tracey Floreani, Abigail Grotke, Dan Murtaugh, Todd Ormsbee, and Janet Rose. Natalie Dykstra, Leslie Tuttle, and I formed a dissertation writing group which sustained me through my graduate years. Every Sunday the three of us sat down and wrestled with arguments and literature and weighed the value of every word in each sentence. Angel Kwolek-Folland guided this work in its early phase, and is a mentor and friend.

Finally, I acknowledge the contributions of those whose lives I share. My parents, Rosemary Arendt Sheumaker and Richard Sheumaker, have endured years of discussion of this project and perhaps marveled at my persistence. My in-laws Katie Armitage and Kenneth Armitage have been wonderful friends, in part because their own exemplary careers as a scientist (Ken) and a local historian (Katie) have given them insight into this process. Kevin Armitage, my husband, has provided intellectual support, unending friendship, and constant and welcome companionship. My daughter Rita reminds me daily of the reasons why hairwork mattered so much to so many people in the nineteenth century. It was their children, their partners, their friends.